D0857344

Alzheimer Disease
SOURCEBOOK

Fourth Edition

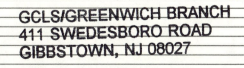

Health Reference Series

Fourth Edition

Alzheimer Disease SOURCEBOOK

Basic Consumer Health Information about Alzheimer Disease, Other Dementias, and Related Disorders, Including Multi-Infarct Dementia, Dementia with Lewy Bodies, Frontotemporal Dementia (Pick Disease), Wernicke-Korsakoff Syndrome (Alcohol-Related Dementia), AIDS Dementia Complex, Huntington Disease, Creutzfeldt-Jacob Disease, and Delirium

Along with Information about Coping with Memory Loss and Forgetfulness, Maintaining Skills, and Long-Term Planning for People with Dementia, and Suggestions Addressing Common Caregiver Concerns, Updated Information about Current Research Efforts, a Glossary of Related Terms, and Directories of Sources for Additional Help and Information

Edited by
Karen Bellenir

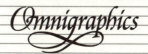

P.O. Box 31-1640, Detroit, MI 48231

Bibliographic Note

Because this page cannot legibly accommodate all the copyright notices, the Bibliographic Note portion of the Preface constitutes an extension of the copyright notice.

Edited by Karen Bellenir

Health Reference Series

Karen Bellenir, *Managing Editor*
David A. Cooke, M.D., *Medical Consultant*
Elizabeth Collins, *Research and Permissions Coordinator*
Cherry Stockdale, *Permissions Assistant*
EdIndex, Services for Publishers, *Indexers*

* * *

Omnigraphics, Inc.

Matthew P. Barbour, *Senior Vice President*
Kevin M. Hayes, *Operations Manager*

* * *

Peter E. Ruffner, *Publisher*
Copyright © 2008 Omnigraphics, Inc.
ISBN 978-0-7808-1001-3

Library of Congress Cataloging-in-Publication Data

Alzheimer disease sourcebook : basic consumer health information about Alzheimer disease, other dementias, and related disorders, including multi-infarct dementia, dementia with Lewy bodies, frontotemporal dementia (Pick disease), Wernicke-Korsakoff syndrome (alcohol-related dementia), AIDS dementia complex, Huntington disease, Creutzfeldt-Jacob disease, and delirium; along with information about coping with memory loss and forgetfulness, maintaining skills, and long-term planning for people with dementia, and suggestions addressing common caregiver concerns, updated information about current research efforts, a glossary of related terms, and directories of sources for additional help and information / edited by Karen Bellenir. -- 4th ed.

  p. cm. -- (Health reference series)
  Includes bibliographical references and index.
  Summary: "Provides basic consumer health information about Alzheimer disease and other dementias, with tips for coping with memory loss and related complications and advice for caregivers. Includes index, glossary of related terms and directory of resources"--Provided by publisher.
  ISBN 978-0-7808-1001-3 (hardcover : alk. paper) 1. Alzheimer's disease--Popular works. 2. Dementia--Popular works. I. Bellenir, Karen.
  RC523.2.A45 2008
  616.8'31--dc22

2007049332

Table of Contents

Visit www.healthreferenceseries.com to view *A Contents Guide to the Health Reference Series*, a listing of more than 13,000 topics and the volumes in which they are covered.

Part III: Coping with Alzheimer Disease and Other Dementias

Part IV: Caregiver Concerns

Part V: Alzheimer Disease and Dementia-Related Research

Part VI: Additional Help and Information

Preface

About This Book

According to recent statistics Alzheimer disease affects more than 5 million Americans. Medical researchers do not fully understand what causes it, and there is no cure. The risk for developing Alzheimer disease increases as a person ages. About five percent of men and women between the ages of 65 and 74 have Alzheimer disease, and nearly half of those 85 and older may have it. Because the U.S. population as a whole is aging, the estimated number of affected people is expected to grow dramatically. By the year 2050, as many as 14 million people may be victims—unless medical researchers can find a means of prevention or a cure.

Alzheimer Disease Sourcebook, Fourth Edition provides updated information about Alzheimer disease and other types of dementia, including multi-infarct dementia, frontotemporal dementia, Binswanger disease, Huntington disease, dementia with Lewy bodies, and Wernicke-Korsakoff syndrome. It explains recent advances made in understanding the causes of dementing disorders, improvements made in diagnostic procedures, and discoveries that have helped identify potential treatments. For people newly diagnosed with Alzheimer disease, it offers information about coping with mental changes and long-term planning. For caregivers, it offers suggestions about many practical aspects of daily life, including planning activities, managing behavior problems, and helping people with dementia maintain their skills. A glossary and directories of resources provide additional help and information.

How to Use This Book

This book is divided into parts and chapters. Parts focus on broad areas of interest. Chapters are devoted to single topics within a part.

Part I: What You Need to Know about Alzheimer Disease describes what is known about the causes and consequences of Alzheimer disease. It explains how thought, memory, and language functions are impaired, and it describes the stages that typically mark the progression of the disease. The part concludes with information from the National Institute on Aging discussing the hope that delaying the onset or advance of Alzheimer disease—or even preventing it entirely—might someday be possible.

Part II: Other Dementias and Related Disorders describes disorders other than Alzheimer disease characterized by brain dysfunction that impairs reasoning, problem solving abilities, memory, personality, behavior, social relationships, emotional control, and other mental processes. Individual chapters describe the symptoms and treatments of such dementing disorders as multi-infarct dementia, Lewy body dementia, and frontotemporal dementia and disorders for which dementia may be a component, including Huntington disease and Parkinson disease.

Part III: Coping with Alzheimer Disease and Other Dementias provides information for people who are concerned about cognitive and memory-related symptoms or who have recently been diagnosed with a dementing disorder. It explains the disease process, offers tips for coping with mental changes, and describes long-term strategies for making care-related decisions.

Part IV: Caregiver Concerns offers answers to people who find themselves giving care to a person with dementia. It discusses common questions about changing levels of ability and provides suggestions for dealing with difficult behavior or coping with other daily challenges. It also describes special concerns related to hiring in-home help, handling hospitalizations, and making decisions surrounding the end of life.

Part V: Alzheimer Disease and Dementia-Related Research summarizes the results of recent research regarding dementing disorders. It explains advances that have been made in identifying possible causes, pinpointing early warning signs, and refining diagnostic tools. It also describes the development of new medications and other treatment interventions that may alter the course of disease progression.

Part VI: Additional Help and Information offers a glossary of terms related to Alzheimer disease and other dementias, a directory of Alzheimer Disease Centers, a directory of additional resources, and suggestions for further reading.

Bibliographic Note

This volume contains documents and excerpts from publications issued by the following U.S. government agencies: Administration on Aging; Center for Medicare and Medicaid Services; Centers for Disease Control and Prevention; National Institute of Alcohol Abuse and Alcoholism; National Institute of Mental Health; National Institute of Neurological Disorders and Stroke; National Institute on Aging; National Institutes of Health; and the National Women's Health Information Center.

In addition, this volume contains copyrighted documents from the following organizations: Alzheimer Society of Canada; Alzheimer's Association; Alzheimer's Drug Discovery Foundation; American Academy of Family Physicians; American Federation for Aging Research; American Geriatrics Society Foundation for Health in Aging; Cleveland Clinic Foundation; Cognitive Neurology and Alzheimer's Disease Center, Northwestern University Feinberg School of Medicine; Consortium to Establish a Registry for Alzheimer's Disease, Duke University Medical Center; Family Caregiver Alliance; Fisher Center for Alzheimer's Research Foundation; HelpGuide.org (Center for Healthy Aging); Institute for the Study of Aging; Lewy Body Dementia Association, Inc.; National Association of Insurance Commissioners; National Down Syndrome Society; National Sleep Foundation; North Carolina Division of Aging and Adult Services; and Project Inform.

Acknowledgements

In addition to the organizations who have contributed to this *Sourcebook*, special thanks go to editorial assistant Nicole Salerno, research and permissions coordinator Liz Collins, permissions assistant Cherry Stockdale, and Bruce Bellenir (without whose help, nothing would ever get done).

About the Health Reference Series

The *Health Reference Series* is designed to provide basic medical information for patients, families, caregivers, and the general public. Each volume takes a particular topic and provides comprehensive coverage. This is especially important for people who may be dealing with a newly diagnosed disease or a chronic disorder in themselves or in a family member. People looking for preventive guidance, information about disease warning signs, medical statistics, and risk factors for health problems will also find answers to their questions in the *Health Reference Series*. The *Series*, however, is not intended to serve as a tool for diagnosing illness, in prescribing treatments, or as a substitute for the physician/patient relationship. All people concerned about medical symptoms or the possibility of disease are encouraged to seek professional care from an appropriate health care provider.

A Note about Spelling and Style

Health Reference Series editors use *Stedman's Medical Dictionary* as an authority for questions related to the spelling of medical terms and the *Chicago Manual of Style* for questions related to grammatical structures, punctuation, and other editorial concerns. Consistent adherence is not always possible, however, because the individual volumes within the *Series* include many documents from a wide variety of different producers and copyright holders, and the editor's primary goal is to present material from each source as accurately as is possible following the terms specified by each document's producer. This sometimes means that information in different chapters or sections may follow other guidelines and alternate spelling authorities. For example, occasionally a copyright holder may require that eponymous terms be shown in possessive forms (Crohn's disease *vs.* Crohn disease) or that British spelling norms be retained (leukaemia *vs.* leukemia).

Locating Information within the Health Reference Series

The *Health Reference Series* contains a wealth of information about a wide variety of medical topics. Ensuring easy access to all the fact sheets, research reports, in-depth discussions, and other material contained within the individual books of the *Series* remains one of our highest priorities. As the *Series* continues to grow in size and scope, however, locating the precise information needed by a reader may become more challenging.

A Contents Guide to the Health Reference Series was developed to direct readers to the specific volumes that address their concerns. It presents an extensive list of diseases, treatments, and other topics of general interest compiled from the Tables of Contents and major index headings. To access *A Contents Guide to the Health Reference Series*, visit www.healthreferenceseries.com.

Medical Consultant

Medical consultation services are provided to the *Health Reference Series* editors by David A. Cooke, M.D. Dr. Cooke is a graduate of Brandeis University, and he received his M.D. degree from the University of Michigan. He completed residency training at the University of Wisconsin Hospital and Clinics. He is board-certified in Internal Medicine. Dr. Cooke currently works as part of the University of Michigan Health System and practices in Brighton, MI. In his free time, he enjoys writing, science fiction, and spending time with his family.

Our Advisory Board

We would like to thank the following board members for providing guidance to the development of this *Series*:

- Dr. Lynda Baker, Associate Professor of Library and Information Science, Wayne State University, Detroit, MI
- Nancy Bulgarelli, William Beaumont Hospital Library, Royal Oak, MI
- Karen Imarisio, Bloomfield Township Public Library, Bloomfield Township, MI
- Karen Morgan, Mardigian Library, University of Michigan-Dearborn, Dearborn, MI
- Rosemary Orlando, St. Clair Shores Public Library, St. Clair Shores, MI

Health Reference Series *Update Policy*

The inaugural book in the *Health Reference Series* was the first edition of *Cancer Sourcebook* published in 1989. Since then, the *Series* has been enthusiastically received by librarians and in the medical community. In order to maintain the standard of providing high-quality health information for the layperson the editorial staff at Omnigraphics felt it was necessary to implement a policy of updating volumes when warranted.

Medical researchers have been making tremendous strides, and it is the purpose of the *Health Reference Series* to stay current with the most recent advances. Each decision to update a volume is made on an individual basis. Some of the considerations include how much new information is available and the feedback we receive from people who use the books. If there is a topic you would like to see added to the update list, or an area of medical concern you feel has not been adequately addressed, please write to:

Editor
Health Reference Series
Omnigraphics, Inc.
P.O. Box 31-1640
Detroit, MI 48231-1640
E-mail: editorial@omnigraphics.com

Part One

What You Need to Know about Alzheimer Disease

Chapter 1

Questions and Answers about Alzheimer Disease

Dementia is a brain disorder that seriously affects a person's ability to carry out daily activities. The most common form of dementia among older people is Alzheimer disease (AD), which initially involves the parts of the brain that control thought, memory, and language. Although scientists are learning more every day, right now they still do not know what causes AD, and there is no cure.

Scientists think that as many as 4.5 million Americans suffer from AD. The disease usually begins after age 60, and risk goes up with age. While younger people also may get AD, it is much less common. About five percent of men and women ages 65 to 74 have AD, and nearly half of those age 85 and older may have the disease. It is important to note, however, that AD is not a normal part of aging.

AD is named after Dr. Alois Alzheimer, a German doctor. In 1906, Dr. Alzheimer noticed changes in the brain tissue of a woman who had died of an unusual mental illness. He found abnormal clumps (now called amyloid plaques) and tangled bundles of fibers (now called neurofibrillary tangles). Today, these plaques and tangles in the brain are considered signs of AD.

Scientists also have found other brain changes in people with AD. Nerve cells die in areas of the brain that are vital to memory and other mental abilities, and connections between nerve cells are disrupted. There also are lower levels of some of the chemicals in the brain that

---

"Alzheimer Disease Fact Sheet," National Institute on Aging (http://www .nia.nih.gov), August 2006.

carry messages back and forth between nerve cells. AD may impair thinking and memory by disrupting these messages.

What causes AD?

Scientists do not yet fully understand what causes AD. There probably is not one single cause, but several factors that affect each person differently. Age is the most important known risk factor for AD. The number of people with the disease doubles every five years beyond age 65.

Family history is another risk factor. Scientists believe that genetics may play a role in many AD cases. For example, early-onset familial AD, a rare form of AD that usually occurs between the ages of 30 and 60, is inherited. The more common form of AD is known as late-onset. It occurs later in life, and no obvious inheritance pattern is seen in most families. However, several risk factor genes may interact with each other and with non-genetic factors to cause the disease. The only risk factor gene identified so far for late-onset AD is a gene that makes one form of a protein called apolipoprotein E (ApoE). Everyone has ApoE, which helps carry cholesterol in the blood. Only about 15 percent of people have the form that increases the risk of AD. It is likely that other genes also may increase the risk of AD or protect against AD, but they remain to be discovered.

Scientists still need to learn a lot more about what causes AD. In addition to genetics and ApoE, they are studying education, diet, and environment to learn what role they might play in the development of this disease. Scientists are finding increasing evidence that some of the risk factors for heart disease and stroke, such as high blood pressure, high cholesterol, and low levels of the vitamin folate, may also increase the risk of AD. Evidence for physical, mental, and social activities as protective factors against AD is also increasing.

What are the symptoms of AD?

AD begins slowly. At first, the only symptom may be mild forgetfulness, which can be confused with age-related memory change. Most people with mild forgetfulness do not have AD. In the early stage of AD, people may have trouble remembering recent events, activities, or the names of familiar people or things. They may not be able to solve simple math problems. Such difficulties may be a bother, but usually they are not serious enough to cause alarm.

However, as the disease goes on, symptoms are more easily noticed and become serious enough to cause people with AD or their family members to seek medical help. Forgetfulness begins to interfere with daily activities. People in the middle stages of AD may forget how to do simple tasks like brushing their teeth or combing their hair. They can no longer think clearly. They can fail to recognize familiar people and places. They begin to have problems speaking, understanding, reading, or writing. Later on, people with AD may become anxious or aggressive, or wander away from home. Eventually, patients need total care.

How is AD diagnosed?

An early, accurate diagnosis of AD helps patients and their families plan for the future. It gives them time to discuss care while the patient can still take part in making decisions. Early diagnosis will also offer the best chance to treat the symptoms of the disease.

Today, the only definite way to diagnose AD is to find out whether there are plaques and tangles in brain tissue. To look at brain tissue, however, doctors usually must wait until they do an autopsy, which is an examination of the body done after a person dies. Therefore, doctors can only make a diagnosis of "possible" or "probable" AD while the person is still alive.

At specialized centers, doctors can diagnose AD correctly up to 90 percent of the time. Doctors use several tools to diagnose "probable" AD, including the following:

- Questions about the person's general health, past medical problems, and ability to carry out daily activities
- Tests of memory, problem solving, attention, counting, and language
- Medical tests—such as tests of blood, urine, or spinal fluid
- Brain scans

Sometimes these test results help the doctor find other possible causes of the person's symptoms. For example, thyroid problems, drug reactions, depression, brain tumors, and blood vessel disease in the brain can cause AD-like symptoms. Some of these other conditions can be treated successfully.

How is AD treated?

AD is a slow disease, starting with mild memory problems and ending with severe brain damage. The course the disease takes and how fast changes occur vary from person to person. On average, AD patients live from eight to ten years after they are diagnosed, though some people may live with AD for as many as 20 years.

No treatment can stop AD. However, for some people in the early and middle stages of the disease, the drugs tacrine (Cognex, which is still available but no longer actively marketed by the manufacturer), donepezil (Aricept), rivastigmine (Exelon), or galantamine (Razadyne, previously known as Reminyl) may help prevent some symptoms from becoming worse for a limited time. Another drug, memantine (Namenda), has been approved to treat moderate to severe AD, although it also is limited in its effects. Also, some medicines may help control behavioral symptoms of AD such as sleeplessness, agitation, wandering, anxiety, and depression. Treating these symptoms often makes patients more comfortable and makes their care easier for caregivers.

What research is underway?

The National Institute on Aging (NIA), part of the National Institutes of Health (NIH), is the lead Federal agency for AD research. NIA-supported scientists are testing a number of drugs to see if they prevent AD, slow the disease, or help reduce symptoms. Researchers undertake clinical trials to learn whether treatments that appear promising in observational and animal studies actually are safe and effective in people. Some ideas that seem promising turn out to have little or no benefit when they are carefully studied in a clinical trial.

Neuroimaging: Scientists are finding that damage to parts of the brain involved in memory, such as the hippocampus, can sometimes be seen on brain scans before symptoms of the disease occur. An NIA public-private partnership—the AD Neuroimaging Initiative (ADNI)—is a large study that will determine whether magnetic resonance imaging (MRI) and positron emission tomography (PET) scans, or other imaging or biological markers, can see early AD changes or measure disease progression. The project is designed to help speed clinical trials and find new ways to determine the effectiveness of treatments. For more information on ADNI, call the NIA's Alzheimer's Disease Education and Referral (ADEAR) Center at 800-438-4380, or visit http://www.alzheimers.nia.nih.gov.

AD genetics: The NIA is sponsoring the AD Genetics Study to learn more about risk factor genes for late onset AD. To participate in this study, families with two or more living siblings diagnosed with

AD should contact the National Cell Repository for AD toll-free at 800-526-2839. Information may also be requested through the study's website: http://ncrad.iu.edu.

Mild cognitive impairment: During the past several years, scientists have focused on a type of memory change called mild cognitive impairment (MCI), which is different from both AD and normal age-related memory change. People with MCI have ongoing memory problems, but they do not have other losses such as confusion, attention problems, and difficulty with language. The NIA-funded Memory Impairment Study compared donepezil, vitamin E, or placebo in participants with MCI to see whether the drugs might delay or prevent progression to AD. The study found that the group with MCI taking donepezil were at reduced risk of progressing to AD for the first 18 months of a 3-year study, when compared with their counterparts on placebo. The reduced risk of progressing from MCI to a diagnosis of AD among participants on donepezil disappeared after 18 months, and by the end of the study, the probability of progressing to AD was the same in the two groups. Vitamin E had no effect at any time point in the study when compared with placebo.

Inflammation: There is evidence that inflammation in the brain may contribute to AD damage. Some studies have suggested that drugs such as nonsteroidal anti-inflammatory drugs (NSAIDs) might help slow the progression of AD, but clinical trials thus far have not demonstrated a benefit from these drugs. A clinical trial studying two of these drugs, rofecoxib (Vioxx) and naproxen (Aleve) showed that they did not delay the progression of AD in people who already have the disease. Another trial, testing whether the NSAIDs celecoxib (Celebrex) and naproxen could prevent AD in healthy older people at risk of the disease was suspended due to concerns over possible cardiovascular risk. Researchers are continuing to look for ways to test how other anti-inflammatory drugs might affect the development or progression of AD.

Antioxidants: Several years ago, a clinical trial showed that vitamin E slowed the progress of some consequences of AD by about seven months. Additional studies are investigating whether antioxidants—vitamins E and C—can slow AD. Another clinical trial is examining whether vitamin E or selenium supplements can prevent AD or cognitive decline, and additional studies on other antioxidants are ongoing or being planned, including a study of the antioxidant treatments—

vitamins E, C, alpha-lipoic acid, and coenzyme Q—in patients with mild to moderate AD.

Ginkgo biloba: Early studies suggested that extracts from the leaves of the ginkgo biloba tree may be of some help in treating AD symptoms. There is no evidence yet that ginkgo biloba will cure or prevent AD, but scientists now are trying to find out in a clinical trial whether ginkgo biloba can delay cognitive decline or prevent dementia in older people.

Estrogen: Some studies have suggested that estrogen used by women to treat the symptoms of menopause also protects the brain. Experts also wondered whether using estrogen could reduce the risk of AD or slow the disease. Clinical trials to test estrogen, however, have not shown that estrogen can slow the progression of already diagnosed AD. And one study found that women over the age of 65 who used estrogen with a progestin were at greater risk of dementia, including AD, and that older women using only estrogen could also increase their chance of developing dementia.

Scientists believe that more research is needed to find out if estrogen may play some role in AD. They would like to know whether starting estrogen therapy around the time of menopause, rather than at age 65 or older, will protect memory or prevent AD.

Advancing Our Understanding

Alzheimer Disease Prevention Initiative: Scientists have come a long way in their understanding of AD. Findings from years of research have begun to clarify differences between normal age-related memory changes, MCI, and AD. Scientists also have made great progress in defining the changes that take place in the AD brain, which allows them to pinpoint possible targets for treatment.

These advances are the foundation for the NIH Alzheimer Disease Prevention Initiative, which is designed to:

- understand why AD occurs and who is at greatest risk of developing it;
- improve the accuracy of diagnosis and the ability to identify those at risk;
- discover, develop, and test new treatments; and
- discover treatments for behavioral problems in patients with AD.

How can I participate in a clinical trial?

People with AD, those with MCI, or those with a family history of AD, who want to help scientists test possible treatments may be able to take part in clinical trials. Healthy people also can help scientists learn more about the brain and AD. The NIA maintains the AD Clinical Trials Database, which lists AD clinical trials sponsored by the Federal government and private companies. To find out more about these studies, contact the NIA's ADEAR Center at 800-438-4380 or visit the ADEAR Center website at www.nia.nih.gov/Alzheimers/ ResearchInformation/ClinicalTrials. You also can sign up for e-mail alerts on new clinical trials as they are added to the database. Additional clinical trials information is available at www.clinicaltrials.gov.

Many of these studies are being done at NIA-supported Alzheimer's Disease Centers located throughout the United States. These centers carry out a wide range of research, including studies of the causes, diagnosis, treatment, and management of AD. A list of these centers is included in the end section of this book.

Help for Caregivers

Most often, spouses and other family members provide the day-to-day care for people with AD. As the disease gets worse, people often need more and more care. This can be hard for caregivers and can affect their physical and mental health, family life, job, and finances.

The Alzheimer's Association has chapters nationwide that provide educational programs and support groups for caregivers and family members of people with AD. Contact information for the Alzheimer's Association is listed in the resources directory at the end of this book.

Chapter 2

Alzheimer Disease Facts and Figures

Prevalence

The Current Prevalence of Alzheimer Disease

An estimated 5.1 million Americans have Alzheimer disease in 2007. This number includes 4.9 million people age 65 and older. It also includes at least 200,000 individuals younger than 65 with early-onset Alzheimer disease. The Alzheimer's Association estimates there are approximately 500,000 Americans younger than 65 with Alzheimer disease or another dementia. At a conservative estimate, at least 40 to 50 percent of them are likely to have Alzheimer disease.

By age group, the proportion and number of the 4.9 million Americans age 65 and over with Alzheimer disease breaks down as follows:

- Age 65–74: 2 percent; 300,000 people
- Age 75–84: 19 percent; 2,400,000 people
- Age 85+: 42 percent; 2,200,000 people
- 13 percent, or one in eight, persons age 65 and over have Alzheimer disease.

Excerpted from "Every 72 Seconds Someone in America Develops Alzheimer's: Alzheimer's Disease Facts and Figures," © 2007 Alzheimer's Association. All rights reserved. Reprinted with permission. For additional information, call the Alzheimer's Association toll-free helpline, 800-272-3900, or visit their website at www.alz.org.

- Nearly half of persons over age 85 have Alzheimer disease.

- Every 72 seconds, someone in America develops Alzheimer disease; by mid-century, someone will develop Alzheimer disease every 33 seconds.

These figures reflect the total number of Americans estimated to have Alzheimer disease, whether or not they have ever been diagnosed with the disease. Many people with Alzheimer disease and other dementias have not been diagnosed, and even if they have, their diagnosis may not be noted in their medical record. In one recent study of patients age 65 and older in seven urban, racially diverse primary care practices in Indianapolis, less than one fifth of those with Alzheimer disease or another dementia had a diagnosis of the condition in their medical record.

Looking to the Future

The number of Americans surviving into their 80s and 90s is expected to grow because of national demographics as well as advances in medicine, medical technology and other social and environmental improvements. Since the incidence and prevalence of Alzheimer disease increase with advancing age, the number of persons with the disease is expected to grow as a proportion of this larger older population.

- In 2000, there were an estimated 411,000 new cases of Alzheimer disease. That number is expected to increase to 454,000 new cases a year by 2010, 615,000 new cases a year by 2030 and 959,000 new cases a year by 2050.

- The number of people age 65 and over with Alzheimer disease is estimated to be 7.7 million in 2030, a greater than 50 percent increase over the number currently affected.

- According to the U.S. Census Bureau, as of July 1, 2005, there were an estimated 78.2 million American baby boomers (those born between 1946 and 1964). In 2006, baby boomers began turning 60 at a rate of about 330 every hour. In 2011, baby boomers begin turning 65, reaching the age of greatest risk for Alzheimer disease.

- By 2050, the number of individuals age 65 and over with Alzheimer disease could range from 11 million to 16 million unless science finds a way to prevent or effectively treat the disease.

By that date, more than 60 percent of people with Alzheimer disease will be age 85+.

State-by-State Prevalence

The proportion of older adults in the age groups 65–74, 75–84 and 85+ varies by state. Because the incidence and prevalence of Alzheimer disease increase with age, states with a higher proportion of people in the older age groups are also likely to have a higher proportion of people with the disease.

Table 2.1 shows the estimated number of people age 65 and over with Alzheimer disease for each state in 2000 and 2010, and the percent change expected over this decade. The figures are based on state estimates for 2000, population projections from the U.S. Census Bureau and state-specific adjustments for gender, race, education, and mortality.

Table 2.1. Number and Percent Change in People Age 65+ With Alzheimer Disease Between 2000 and 2010 by State **(continued on next page)**

State	2000	2010	% change 2000–2010
Alabama	84,000	91,000	8
Alaska	3,400	5,000	47
Arizona	78,000	97,000	24
Arkansas	56,000	60,000	7
California	440,000	480,000	9
Colorado	49,000	72,000	47
Connecticut	68,000	70,000	3
Delaware	12,000	14,000	17
District of Columbia	10,000	9,100	-9
Florida	360,000	450,000	25
Georgia	110,000	120,000	9
Hawaii	23,000	27,000	17
Idaho	19,000	26,000	37
Illinois	210,000	210,000	0
Indiana	100,000	120,000	20
Iowa	65,000	69,000	6
Kansas	50,000	53,000	6
Kentucky	74,000	80,000	8
Louisiana	73,000	83,000	14

Table 2.1. (continued) Number and Percent Change in People Age 65+ With Alzheimer Disease Between 2000 and 2010 by State

State	2000	2010	% change 2000–2010
Maine	25,000	25,000	0
Maryland	78,000	86,000	10
Massachusetts	120,000	120,000	0
Michigan	170,000	180,000	6
Minnesota	88,000	94,000	7
Mississippi	51,000	53,000	4
Missouri	110,000	110,000	0
Montana	16,000	21,000	31
Nebraska	33,000	37,000	12
Nevada	21,000	29,000	38
New Hampshire	19,000	22,000	16
New Jersey	150,000	150,000	0
New Mexico	27,000	31,000	15
New York	330,000	320,000	-3
North Carolina	130,000	170,000	31
North Dakota	16,000	18,000	13
Ohio	200,000	230,000	15
Oklahoma	62,000	74,000	19
Oregon	57,000	76,000	33
Pennsylvania	280,000	280,000	0
Rhode Island	24,000	24,000	0
South Carolina	67,000	80,000	19
South Dakota	17,000	19,000	12
Tennessee	100,000	120,000	20
Texas	270,000	340,000	26
Utah	22,000	32,000	45
Vermont	10,000	11,000	10
Virginia	100,000	130,000	30
Washington	83,000	110,000	33
West Virginia	40,000	44,000	10
Wisconsin	100,000	110,000	10
Wyoming	7,000	10,000	43

Source: Hebert LE, Scherr PA, Bienias JL, Bennett DA, and Evans DA. "State-specific Projections Through 2025 of Alzheimer Disease Prevalence," *Neurology* 2004.

Mortality

Reporting Alzheimer Disease Deaths

The U.S. Standard Certificate of Death mandated by the Department of Health and Human Services provides for qualified medical personnel or coroners to record a single "underlying cause of death." This is commonly defined as the disease or injury initiating the train of events leading directly to death. Each certificate may list up to 20 additional diseases and conditions as "contributing causes" of death.

According to the Centers for Disease Control and Prevention (CDC), Alzheimer disease was listed as the "underlying cause of death" for 65,829 Americans in 2004. It was the seventh leading cause of death for people of all ages and the fifth leading cause of death in people age 65 and older.

The total number of deaths attributed to Alzheimer disease has increased over the last 15 years. In 1991, only 14,112 death certificates recorded Alzheimer disease as the underlying cause. From 2000 to 2004, deaths from Alzheimer disease increased by 32.8 percent, while the number one cause of death, heart disease, decreased by 8.0 percent.

Even though deaths attributed to Alzheimer disease are increasing, the number may fail to reflect the disease's real public health impact. Numerous studies have suggested that death certificates substantially underreport Alzheimer disease as a cause of death for people living in the community. Because most individuals with Alzheimer disease are age 65 and older, they also tend to have other serious co-existing medical conditions associated with aging, such as heart disease or stroke. Physicians may tend to attribute death primarily to one of these other conditions even when Alzheimer disease is present. In the large percentage of cases where the medical record fails to reflect an Alzheimer diagnosis, the certifying physician may not be aware the individual had Alzheimer disease.

In cases where Alzheimer disease is not listed as the underlying cause of death, it may not even be listed as a contributing factor. Nevertheless, people with Alzheimer disease in all age groups generally have decreased survival compared with survival in the general U.S. population. One 2004 study by Larson and colleagues noted that people newly diagnosed with Alzheimer disease survived about half as long as those of similar age who did not have the disease. In this study, average survival time was four to six years after diagnosis, but survival can be as long as 20 years from first symptoms.

The mechanisms by which dementia lead to death may create ambiguity about the underlying cause. Severe dementia frequently causes such complications as immobility, swallowing disorders, or malnutrition. These complications can significantly increase the risk of developing pneumonia, which has been found in several studies to be the most common identified cause of death among elderly persons with Alzheimer disease and other dementias. One researcher described the situation as a "blurred distinction between death with dementia and death from dementia."

Coexisting Medical Conditions

Other serious health conditions can develop or coexist in people with Alzheimer disease and other dementias, leading to major medical consequences and contributing to the higher likelihood of death for those with dementia. For example, 60 percent of Medicare beneficiaries age 65+ with Alzheimer disease and other dementias also suffer from hypertension, and 30 percent have coronary artery disease.

As a result of these coexisting conditions, people with Alzheimer disease and other dementias often face frequent hospitalizations for treatment of one or more of the conditions. These conditions also increase likelihood of entering a nursing home and dying there.

- The most common causes of hospitalization for nursing home residents with Alzheimer disease and other dementias are pneumonia and other infections.

- Cardiopulmonary resuscitation is three times less likely to be successful in a person with dementia.

State-by-State Deaths from Alzheimer Disease

The highest death rate attributed to Alzheimer disease in 2003 was in North Dakota, where the rate was 53 per 100,000 (336 deaths); the lowest rate was 8.6 per 100,000 in Alaska, or 56 deaths. Differences across states in death rates attributed to Alzheimer disease reflect state demographics, differences in reporting practices, and other factors.

Costs of Alzheimer Disease

Alzheimer disease and other dementias not only cause enormous suffering to the persons affected by the conditions and emotional and financial burden to their caregivers, they also rob the nation of vast resources. The drain on federal and state budgets and losses to American business rise each year as the number of persons with Alzheimer disease and other dementias grows with the aging of the population.

Costs to Federal and State Government and Business

Direct and indirect costs of Alzheimer disease and other dementias, including Medicare and Medicaid costs and the indirect cost to business

Table 2.2. Percent Change in Selected Leading Causes of Death from 2000 to 2004

Cause	2000	2004	% change
Heart disease	710,760	654,092	-8.0
Breast cancer	41,200	40,110	-2.6
Prostate cancer	31,900	29,900	-6.3
Stroke	167,661	150,147	-10.4
Alzheimer disease	49,558	65,829	+32.8

Source: Centers for Disease Control and Prevention, National Vital Statistics Reports, and Reports of the American Cancer Society.

Table 2.3. Percent of Medicare Beneficiaries Age 65+ with Alzheimer Disease and Other Dementias Who Had Specified Coexisting Medical Conditions (1999)

Coexisting Condition	% with the Condition
Hypertension	60
Coronary artery disease	30
Congestive heart failure	28
Osteoarthritis	26
Diabetes	21
Chronic obstructive pulmonary disease	17
Peripheral vascular disease	19
Stroke—late effects	10
Thyroid disease	16

Source: Bynum JPW, Rabins PV, Weller W, et al. *Journal of the American Geriatrics Society* 2004.

Table 2.4. Number of Deaths Due to Alzheimer Disease and Rate per 100,000 Population by State, 2003

State	Number of Deaths	Rate per 100,000
Alabama	1,268	28.2
Alaska	56	8.6
Arizona	1,703	30.5
Arkansas	552	20.3
California	6,585	18.6
Colorado	899	19.8
Connecticut	612	17.6
Delaware	147	18.0
District of Columbia	95	16.8
Florida	4,316	25.4
Georgia	1,630	18.8
Hawaii	161	12.8
Idaho	355	26.0
Illinois	2,626	20.8
Indiana	1,515	24.5
Iowa	887	30.1
Kansas	781	28.7
Kentucky	1,072	26.0
Louisiana	1,184	26.3
Maine	467	35.8
Maryland	865	15.7
Massachusetts	1,609	25.0
Michigan	2,133	21.2
Minnesota	1,243	24.6
Mississippi	583	20.2
Missouri	1,293	22.7
Montana	235	25.6
Nebraska	461	26.5
Nevada	309	13.8
New Hampshire	286	22.2
New Jersey	1,636	18.9
New Mexico	360	19.2
New York	1,866	9.7
North Carolina	2,145	25.5
North Dakota	336	53.0

Table 2.4. (continued) Number of Deaths Due to Alzheimer Disease and Rate per 100,000 Population by State, 2003

State	Number of Deaths	Rate per 100,000
Ohio	2,902	25.4
Oklahoma	794	22.6
Oregon	1,157	32.5
Pennsylvania	2,952	23.9
Rhode Island	303	28.2
South Carolina	1,051	25.3
South Dakota	174	22.8
Tennessee	1,466	25.1
Texas	4,015	18.2
Utah	332	14.1
Vermont	171	27.6
Virginia	1,466	19.8
Washington	2,380	38.8
West Virginia	470	21.6
Wisconsin	1,411	25.8
Wyoming	142	28.3
United States	63,457	21.8

Source: Centers for Disease Control and Prevention, National Center for Health Statistics, *National Vital Statistics Report* 2006: 54 (13). Number of deaths and the rate per 100,000 population are reported by the Centers for Disease Control and Prevention through the National Vital Statistics Reports. The most recent report by state is from Vol. 54, No. 13, published April 19, 2006.

of employees who are caregivers of persons with Alzheimer disease, amount to more than $148 billion annually.

- In 2005, Medicare spent $91 billion on beneficiaries with Alzheimer disease and other dementias, projected to increase to $160 billion by 2010 and $189 billion by 2015.

- State and federal Medicaid spending for nursing home care for people with Alzheimer disease and other dementias was estimated at $21 billion in 2005. It is projected to increase to $24 billion in 2010 and $27 billion in 2015.

- Costs to business for employees who are caregivers of people with Alzheimer disease and other dementias amount to $36.5

billion. These costs result from lost productivity, missed work, and costs to replace workers who leave their jobs to meet the demands of caregiving.

Costs to Individuals and Their Families

Although Medicare and Medicaid cover some health care costs for older beneficiaries, many expenses of caring for a person with Alzheimer disease or another dementia must be paid for by the person or family. According to an American Association of Retired Persons (AARP) analysis, Medicare beneficiaries age 65 and older spent an average of $3,455 (22 percent) of their income on health care in 2003. About 45 percent of those expenses were for Medicare Part B premiums, private Medicare plans (such as HMOs), and private supplemental insurance. Medicare beneficiaries age 65+ paid 37 percent of the cost of nursing home care out of pocket in 2002, the most recent year for which expenditure figures are available by type of medical service.

Out-of-pocket expenditures for health and long-term care are higher, on average, for older people with Alzheimer disease and other dementias than for other older people. One analysis based on a large, nationally representative sample from the Health and Retirement Study found that in 1995, average out-of-pocket expenditures for hospitalization, nursing home care stays, outpatient treatment, home care, and prescription medications were $1,350 for people with no dementia and $2,150 for people with mild or moderate dementia, an increase of $800. For people with severe dementia, average out-of-pocket expenditures were $3,010 in 1995, an increase of $1,660 over the average for people with no dementia.

The study found that the $1,660 increase in out-of-pocket expenses for people with severe dementia was greater than the increase in expenditures for people with any of the other conditions included in the analysis. The increases for those other conditions were: heart disease, $670; stroke, $820; diabetes, $760; hypertension, $630; cancer, $670; lung disease, $460; psychiatric problems, $630; and arthritis, $270. The $800 increase in out-of-pocket expenditures for people with mild-to-moderate dementia was greater than the increase for people with any of those other conditions except stroke.

No matter what the funding source, costs are high for care at home or in an adult day center, assisted living facility or nursing home.

• The average hourly rate for home health aides in 2006 was $19, or $152 for an eight-hour day. For homemaker or companion services, costs ran about $17 an hour.

- Adult day services cost an average of $56 per day, but can range from $25 to more than $100 per day, depending on the services offered and geographic region.

- The average monthly cost for a private, one-bedroom unit in an assisted living facility was $2,968, or $35,616 a year in 2006. (Assisted living facilities that provide specialized dementia care often charge additional fees ranging from $750 to $2,200 monthly for that care.)

- The average daily cost for a private room in a nursing home was $206 in 2006, or $75,190 a year.

Use of Services

Seventy percent of people with Alzheimer disease and other dementias live at home, where they are cared for by family and friends. Even when care is provided in the home, most families must also seek other sources of help, particularly as the disease progresses. People with Alzheimer disease and other dementias are high users of health care, residential care, and home and community services.

Care Settings

The estimated 13 percent of people age 65 and older in the United States with Alzheimer disease include 25 percent or more of all elderly users of hospital, nursing home, assisted living, home care, and adult day services. Many of these elders have never received a formal diagnosis of the disease.

- About 25 percent of all elderly hospital patients have Alzheimer disease or other dementias.

- An estimated 70 percent of all nursing home residents have some degree of cognitive impairment. About 47 percent of nursing home residents have a diagnosis of Alzheimer disease or another dementia in their medical record.

- Nursing home Alzheimer Special Care Units had about 91,000 beds in December 2006. Although the number of these units has grown since the 1980s, less than 13 percent of all residents with dementia had access to them in 2006.

- Half or more of all elderly residents of assisted living facilities have Alzheimer disease or another dementia.

- Twenty-four percent of people of all ages who received Medicare- or Medicaid-funded home health care have moderate to severe cognitive impairment.

- At least half of the elderly participants in adult day services have Alzheimer disease or another dementia.

Long-Term Care

The likelihood of needing long-term care services increases if an older person who cannot perform such daily activities as dressing, bathing, shopping, and managing money also has cognitive impairment. One 2002 study of community-living older adults who could not perform at least one customary daily activity found that:

- More than nine out of ten of those with cognitive impairment received assistance from family, friends, or paid workers, compared with slightly less than half of those who had no cognitive impairment.

- Nearly one-third of those with cognitive impairment who received any assistance used paid services, usually in combination with unpaid assistance; in contrast, only 12 percent of those who had no cognitive impairment used paid services.

- Those with cognitive impairment who used paid services used almost twice as many hours monthly of that assistance, on average, as those without cognitive impairment (200 hours compared to 108 hours for those without cognitive impairment).

- About 26 percent of these older community-living adults with severe disabilities (defined as those unable to perform three or more daily activities) were also cognitively impaired.

End-of-Life Care

Hospice can provide palliative or comfort care that can be helpful for people with Alzheimer disease and other dementias who are terminally ill. Medicare will cover hospice care if a physician certifies that a beneficiary is likely to die within six months. In general, the Medicare hospice benefit, and hospice care in general, is underutilized. A 2005 study estimated that only 43 percent of patients eligible for hospice ever receive services.

- A recent study investigated hospice referral in people age 65 and older with advanced dementia who died within one year of admission to either a nursing home in Michigan or the state's publicly funded home care and community-based services. The results showed that only 5.7 percent of nursing home residents and 10.7 percent home care clients dying with advanced dementia were referred to hospice.

- One study reported that when persons with Alzheimer disease were hospitalized for pneumonia or hip fracture, half died within six months compared to cognitively intact patients, who were less likely to die after receiving the same treatments.

- The study also indicated that hospital patients with Alzheimer disease often had untreated or under-treated pain.

- The number of hospice admissions for persons with dementia increased from 6.8 percent of all hospice admissions in 2001 to 9.8 percent of all hospice admissions in 2005.

Special Report: Caregiving

Caregivers of People with Alzheimer Disease and Other Dementias

Almost 10 million Americans are caring for a person with Alzheimer disease or another dementia. This figure constitutes about 29 percent of all caregivers of people aged 60 and older. These caregivers are often providing help for a person who has not only Alzheimer disease or another dementia, but also one or more other serious medical conditions, such as heart disease or stroke.

These unpaid caregivers provided the nation with an economic asset worth almost $83 billion in 2005, based on their hours of care. This figure is not reflected in any formal estimates of national health care costs.

The Challenges of Caregiving

Caring for a person with Alzheimer disease poses special challenges. Although memory loss is the most widely known symptom, as the disease progresses it also causes confusion, loss of orientation and, frequently, changes in personality, and behavior. Individuals require increasing levels of care, supervision, and provision for their safety. Because the disease gets worse slowly, caregivers tend to spend a long time in the caregiving role. A 2003 National Alliance for Caregiving/ AARP survey found that:

23

- Nearly one in four of the caregivers of people with Alzheimer disease and other dementias provide 40 hours a week or more of care. Seventy-one percent sustain this commitment for more than a year, and 32 percent do so for five years or more.

- Sixty-five percent of Alzheimer caregivers perform physically demanding kinds of personal care—for example, bathing, feeding, helping the person to the toilet, and dealing with loss of bladder or bowel control. These tasks are made more difficult by the confused and disoriented state of the person with dementia, who may be unable to help with the tasks or may resist assistance from the caregiver.

- Caregivers of people with Alzheimer disease and other dementias are much more likely than other caregivers to help with loss of bladder or bowel control (32 percent of Alzheimer/dementia caregivers, compared with 13 percent of other caregivers) and bathing (35 percent v. 25 percent).

Stress Associated with Caregiving

These challenges often affect the health and income of caregivers of people with Alzheimer disease and other dementias. Over 40 percent of these caregivers report high levels of emotional stress. Many of them are working full- or part-time, but their work responsibilities can be seriously affected by the demands of caregiving.

- Almost one-quarter of caregivers of people with Alzheimer disease and other dementias report that caring for their family member is very stressful, compared to 15 percent of other caregivers who reported that high a level of stress.

- Two-thirds of working caregivers of people with Alzheimer disease and other dementias report that they missed work because of caregiving responsibilities, compared with 57 percent of other caregivers.

- Eight percent of working caregivers of people with Alzheimer disease and other dementia turned down a promotion (4 percent of other caregivers), and 7 percent lost job benefits (3 percent for other caregivers).

- Almost a third of caregivers of people with Alzheimer disease and other dementias got less exercise than they did before they began their caregiving, compared with about a quarter of other caregivers.

A recent study found that among elderly people, hospitalization of a spouse for dementia was associated with an increased risk of death for the non-hospitalized partner. Among men, 8.6 percent died within a year after a spouse's hospitalization for dementia compared to 6.4 percent that died after a spouse's hospitalization for colon cancer and 6.9 percent after a spouse's hospitalization for stroke. Among women, the rate was 5 percent in the year after a spouse's hospitalization for dementia compared to 3 percent that died after a spouse's hospitalization for colon cancer and 3.7 percent after a spouse's hospitalization for stroke.

Another study assessed the type and intensity of care provided by family caregivers of persons with dementia during the year before the care recipient's death. End-of-life care for people with dementia was "extremely demanding of family caregivers," the study found, particularly during a "protracted and stressful" period preceding death. The stress was so great, many of the caregivers said, that they experienced relief when death finally occurred.

The Economic Value of Caregiving

Caregivers of people with Alzheimer disease and other dementias make significant personal investments of time and energy in caring for their loved ones. Their unpaid care also contributes billions in value to the nation. A total of approximately 9.8 million caregivers of people with Alzheimer disease and other dementias nationwide provided care worth almost $83 billion in 2005. A million of these caregivers in California, for example, provided an estimated $8.5 billion of care that year. Even Rhode Island, the smallest state, had almost 37,000 caregivers of people with Alzheimer disease and other dementias, and those caregivers provided 32 million hours of care worth $310.7 million.

Chapter 3

The Brain and Alzheimer Disease: New Insights

Structure and Function of the Brain

The brain is essential to our survival. With the help of motor and sensory nerves throughout the body, it integrates, regulates, initiates, and helps control the body's functions. The brain governs thinking, personality, moods, the senses, and physical action. We can speak, move, remember, and feel emotions and physical sensations because of the complex interplay of chemical and electrical processes that takes place in our brains. The brain and the rest of the nervous system also regulate body functions that happen automatically, such as breathing and digesting food.

The healthy human brain is made up of billions of neurons that share information with one another through a diverse array of biological and chemical signals. A typical neuron has a cell body, an axon, and many dendrites, all surrounded by a cell membrane. The nucleus, which is found inside the cell body and contains genes composed of deoxyribonucleic acid (DNA), helps to regulate the cell's activities in response to signals from outside and inside the cell. The axon, which extends from the cell body, transmits messages to other neurons, sometimes

Excerpted from "Progress Report on Alzheimer's Disease: New Discoveries, New Insights," National Institute on Aging (NIA), 2004-2005, NIH Pub. No. 05-5724, 2005. The section titled "New Developments in Tau Research," was excerpted from "Progress Report on Alzheimer's Disease: Journey to Discovery, 2005-2006," NIH Pub. No. 06-6047, 2007.

over very long distances. Dendrites, which also branch out from the cell body, receive messages from axons of other nerve cells or from specialized sense organs. Axons and dendrites collectively are called neurites. Neurons are surrounded by glial cells, which support and nourish them.

Neurons generally communicate with each other and with sense organs by producing and releasing special chemicals called neurotransmitters. As a neuron receives messages from the dendrites of surrounding cells, an electrical charge (nerve impulse) builds up within the cell. This charge travels down the axon until it reaches the end. Here, it triggers the release of the neurotransmitters that move from the axon across a gap, called a synapse, between it and the dendrites or cell bodies of other neurons. Scientists estimate that a typical neuron has up to 15,000 synapses. Neurotransmitters bind to specific receptor sites on cell bodies and the receiving end of dendrites of adjacent nerve cells. In this way, signals travel between neurons in a fraction of a second. Millions of signals continuously flash through the brain.

Groups of neurons in the brain have specific jobs. For example, some neurons are involved in thinking, learning, remembering, and planning. Others are responsible for vision or hearing, regulating the body's biological clock, or managing the many other tasks that keep the human body functioning.

The survival of neurons in the brain depends on the healthy functioning of several processes all working in harmony. These processes are communication, metabolism, and repair. The first process, communication between neurons, depends on the integrity of the neuron and its synapses, as well as the production of neurotransmitters.

The second process is metabolism, or all the chemical reactions that take place in the cell. Some of these reactions break down substances, which releases energy. Other reactions involve building complex substances that the cell needs to function out of simple "building block" molecules. Efficient metabolism requires adequate blood circulation to supply the cells with oxygen and glucose (a sugar), the brain's major fuel.

The third process is repair. Unlike most other body cells, most neurons are already formed at birth. Neurons are programmed to live a long time—even more than 100 years. In an adult, when neurons die because of disease or injury, they are usually not replaced, although we now know that new neurons can be generated in several areas of the brain. To prevent their own death, living neurons must constantly maintain, repair, and remodel themselves.

Alzheimer Disease Damages the Brain

Research shows that the damage seen in AD involves changes in all three of these neuronal processes: communication, metabolism, and repair.

In healthy aging, nerve cells (neurons) in the brain are not lost in large numbers. In Alzheimer disease (AD), however, many nerve cells stop functioning, lose connections with other nerve cells, and die. At first, AD destroys neurons in parts of the brain that control memory,

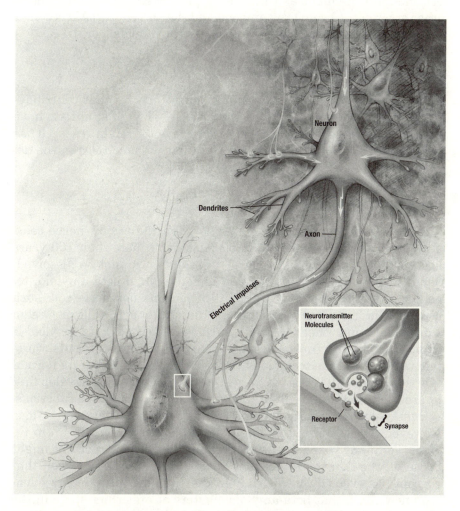

Figure 3.1. Normal neuronal functioning (Source: NIA).

including the entorhinal cortex and the hippocampus (structures in the brain that help form and store short-term memories) and related structures. As nerve cells in these structures stop working properly, short-term memory fails, and a person's ability to do easy and familiar tasks can begin to decline. AD later attacks the cerebral cortex (the outer layer of neurons in the brain), particularly the areas responsible for language and reasoning. At this point, AD begins to take away language skills and changes a person's ability to make judgments. Personality changes also may occur. Emotional outbursts and disturbing behaviors, such as wandering, begin to happen and can become more frequent as the disease progresses. Eventually, many other areas of the brain are damaged and the person with AD becomes bedridden, helpless, and unresponsive to the outside world.

Main Characteristics of the Brain in AD

The brain in AD has three major characteristics that contribute to the pathology, or damage, of the disease. Though scientists have known about these characteristics for many years, recent research has revealed much about their nature and their possible roles in the development of AD.

Amyloid Plaques

Plaques are found in the spaces between the brain's nerve cells. They were first discovered by Alois Alzheimer more than 100 years ago, in 1906. They consist of largely insoluble (cannot be dissolved) deposits of a protein peptide, or fragment, called beta-amyloid, together with other proteins, remnants of neurons, non-nerve cells such as microglia (cells that surround and digest damaged cells or foreign substances), and other glial cells, such as astrocytes. Beta-amyloid is snipped, or cleaved, from a larger protein called amyloid precursor protein (APP). APP is associated with the cell membrane, but its normal function in the cell is not yet fully known. In AD, plaques develop first in areas of the brain used for memory and other cognitive functions.

Most people develop some plaques in their brain tissue as they age. However, the AD brain has many more plaques in certain brain regions. For many years, scientists thought that these structures might cause all the damage to neurons that is seen in AD. However, that concept has evolved considerably in the past few years. Many scientists now think that beta-amyloid clusters at an earlier stage in the plaque development process—called Aβ-derived diffusible ligands, or

ADDLs (also known as soluble oligomers)—may be a major culprit. Many also think that plaques are a late-stage attempt by the brain to get harmful beta-amyloid away from neurons.

Neurofibrillary Tangles

The second hallmark of AD pathology, also found by Alois Alzheimer, consists of abnormal collections of twisted protein threads found inside nerve cells. The chief component of these structures, called neurofibrillary tangles (NFTs), is a protein called tau. Healthy neurons are internally supported in part by structures called microtubules, which help transport nutrients and other cellular components from the body of the cell down to the ends of the axon and back. Tau, which normally has a certain number of phosphate molecules attached to it, binds to microtubules and stabilizes them. In AD, an abnormally high number of additional phosphate molecules attach to tau. As a result of this "phosphorylation" process, tau disengages from the microtubules and begins to aggregate with other threads of tau. Ultimately, these tau threads become enmeshed with one another, forming tangles. When this happens, the microtubules disintegrate and the neuron's transport system collapses. This may result first in malfunctions in communication between neurons and later in the death of the cells.

Loss of Connections Between Cells and Cell Death

The third major pathological feature of AD, described only in the past 30 years, is the gradual loss of connections between neurons. This process damages neurons to the point that they cannot function properly. Eventually, they die. As the death of neurons spreads through the brain, affected regions begin to shrink in a process called brain atrophy. By the final stage of AD, damage is widespread, and brain tissue has shrunk significantly.

Causes of AD

In a very few families, about half of the children of a parent with AD develop the disease in their 30s, 40s, and 50s. These people have inherited mutations in one of three genes. So, in these "early-onset" cases, we know exactly what causes AD. However, the vast majority of AD cases—more than 90 percent—develop in people older than 65. This form of AD is called "late-onset" AD. We don't yet completely understand the causes of late-onset AD, but they probably include a mix of genetic, environmental, and lifestyle factors. The importance of these factors in increasing or decreasing the risk of developing the disease may differ from person to person.

Although many questions about the players and steps involved in the causes and development of AD have been answered, our knowledge still has some surprising gaps. For example, we don't yet fully understand the normal function of several key players, such as APP. Certainly a better knowledge of normal function would give us clues about the causes of AD.

Perhaps the greatest mystery is why AD largely strikes the elderly. Why does it take 30 to 50 years for people to develop signs of the disease, even those individuals who are born with disease-causing mutations? One possibility is that the environment of the aging brain is subtly different from that of the young brain. We may need to understand more about how the brain changes normally as we age before we can fully understand AD.

Scientists supported by the NIH are working in laboratories and research institutions all across the U.S. and in other countries to assemble the many bits of new knowledge that, combined with our existing understanding, will some day explain this complex biological puzzle.

Brain Transformation from Healthy Aging to AD

As people age, changes occur in all parts of the body, including the brain:

- Some neurons shrink, especially large ones in areas important to learning, memory, planning, and other complex mental activities. This translates into some shrinkage of brain volume over the course of years, even in healthy older people (Resnick et al., 2003).

- Tangles develop inside neurons and plaques develop in the spaces between neurons.

- Damage by free radicals increases (free radicals, also called reactive oxygen species, are a kind of molecule that reacts easily with other molecules).

The impact of these changes differs among people as they age. Some older people may notice only a modest reduction in their ability to learn new things, retrieve information from memory, and plan and make decisions. Their performance on complex tasks of attention, learning, and memory may decline. However, if given enough time, they may ultimately score as well on the task as a younger person. Other people, however, experience much greater declines in these cognitive abilities as they grow older. Understanding the differences between healthy aging and a neurodegenerative process is an important key to unlocking the secrets of AD.

Long ago, before we knew much about AD, many people thought that "senile dementia" was just a part of aging. Now, of course, we know that AD is a distinct disease that affects the brain. Several recent studies and reviews of the scientific literature have provided some evidence that cognitive decline with age and AD are, in some respects, separate entities that follow different pathways as they evolve. For example, an investigator from Washington University in St. Louis recently published a review of a vast array of data on memory and executive function (the cognitive abilities involved in planning, organizing, and decision-making) in aging and AD (Buckner, 2004). The review suggested that factors that influence executive function more commonly falter with normal aging. In contrast, factors that influence long-term memory function are more impaired in AD. Some of the changes that can take place in normal aging may not necessarily be the cause of AD. In a more direct assessment of this idea, this investigator and colleagues at Washington University used MRI to measure volumes of the hippocampal region and the white matter region between the two hemispheres of the brain in 150 people aged 18 to 93 years (Head et al., 2005). They found that early-stage AD did not make age-associated reductions in the white matter region worse. They also found that early-stage AD was characterized by significant reductions in hippocampal volume, whereas age alone was associated with only mild reductions in hippocampal volume. These results suggest that AD manifests itself early and significantly in the area of the brain encompassing the hippocampus, whereas normal aging affects the white matter connecting the front regions of the brain. These frontal white matter reductions may underlie the executive function difficulties that are common in normal aging.

Columbia University scientists funded by the National Center for Research Resources (NCRR) and NIA, in collaboration with researchers at the California National Primate Research Center, conducted neuroimaging studies in older monkeys and rats to distinguish the effects of healthy aging and AD on the structure of the brain (Small et al., 2004). The selection of the animals for this study was important because neither monkeys nor rats naturally develop AD. They found that the brain region known as the dentate gyrus (a region within the hippocampus) was changed by aging in both species. However, AD predominantly affected a different region of the hippocampus, thus indicating that some processes affecting normal aging and AD may be distinct.

New Thinking about Cognitive Reserve

Two questions have fascinated investigators for years:

- Why do some people remain cognitively healthy all their lives while others develop dementia?

- Why do some people remain cognitively healthy even though examination of their brain tissue after death shows significant deposits of plaques and tangles?

One possible explanation revolves around the concept of "cognitive reserve." Reserve refers to the brain's ability to operate effectively even when function is disrupted and to the amount of damage that the brain can sustain before the damage is clinically apparent. Individual variability in reserve may reflect genetic differences or differences in life experiences, such as education, occupational experience, or leisure activities.

Lifelong engagement in activities that help to build and maintain cognitive reserve is generally beneficial to health and may even help keep people cognitively healthy as they age. A number of research teams are looking intensively at these activities. For example, new information from the Religious Orders Study, a long-term study of aging among members of 40 religious communities, has revealed that years of formal education may modify the relationship between level of cognitive functioning and AD pathology (Bennett et al., 2003). After comparing participants' brain tissue after their deaths and the results of earlier cognitive function tests, study investigators at the Rush University Medical Center ADC in Chicago, found that the density of plaques in the brain tissue was linked to cognitive function. This relationship was modified by the number of years of education the person had received, such that a person with a higher level of education retained a higher level of cognitive function even in the presence of AD damage to the brain.

In another study, scientists from Columbia University periodically tested the memory performance of 136 cognitively healthy older people over the course of 5 years (Manly et al., 2003). The scientists accounted for the participants' age at the beginning of the study and their years of education. They found that participants with low levels of literacy (a proxy for quality of education) had a steeper decline in their ability to remember a word list immediately after seeing it, as well as after a delay, as compared to those with a higher literacy level. These findings suggest that literacy may be an important measure of cognitive reserve, or even that literacy itself builds cognitive reserve, protecting against memory decline in older people without dementia.

Rush ADC investigators from the Chicago Health and Aging Project (CHAP), an epidemiologic study of AD risk factors in a racially diverse urban population, looked at the issue of cognitive reserve from a slightly different angle (Barnes et al., 2004). They wondered whether an important life experience, such as the level of engagement in social networks of family and friends, could be related to changes in cognitive function. The 6,102 African-Americans and whites in the study participated in up to three interviews over the course of about 5 years. The researchers found that more social networks and a higher level of social engagement were associated with a higher initial level of cognitive function. These factors also were related to a reduced rate of cognitive decline over time. Additional research is clearly necessary to sort out cause and effect. Does increased involvement with social networks increase cognitive reserve, or are people who later develop dementia less involved because they are already in the early stages of AD, before symptoms are evident?

Findings from recent studies suggest that the brain has an inherent ability to cope with age- and disease-associated changes. It may attempt to compensate for these changes through various mechanisms, such as the use of alternate brain networks to bypass those that are not functioning or the use of new cognitive strategies (Buckner, 2004). A number of scientists are exploring these compensatory mechanisms. For example, researchers at Columbia University examined whether engaging in various intellectual, social, and physical activities, such as gardening, reading, traveling, and going to the movies, might enhance cognitive reserve (Scarmeas et al., 2003). Cognitively healthy older people and people with early AD were scanned for blood flow in the brain using PET. The researchers found that study participants with AD who had a higher leisure activity score also had prominent deficits in cerebral blood flow, despite being at the same level of clinical disease. Those participants who had engaged in more lifestyle activities before disease onset were able to sustain more pathology, as shown by greater cerebral blood flow deficits.

Understanding that AD is a process that develops over many years and is the result of many factors creates opportunities for early interventions that may prevent or delay the onset of the disease. It may be that because of the physical properties of a person's brain and his or her genetic makeup and life experiences, the person is able to tolerate and adapt to a certain amount of change and damage that occurs to the brain during aging. This tolerance level differs from person to person depending on cognitive reserve and other factors. At some point in the life of some people, the balance may tip in favor of a disease process. For others, the balance may remain in favor of healthy aging. Learning about the earliest developments in the disease process will help researchers understand this complex, lifelong balancing act.

The Journey from Healthy Aging to AD: Damage in the Brain

Since the earliest days of AD research, investigators have focused on the basic disease process in the brain—on trying to understand exactly what happens in neurons to damage and ultimately kill them. In the last several years, scientists have made enormous progress in characterizing the individual players in this process, describing their activities, and determining the exact steps in the disease process. These advances mean that scientists are increasingly able to move away from studies of these players in isolation and focus on their complex relationships and how their effects on each other affect the development of AD.

New Discoveries about Beta-Amyloid and Plaque Formation

Recent studies have dramatically improved scientists' understanding of how beta-amyloid plaques are formed. These discoveries have fundamentally changed how scientists think about this critical component of AD pathology.

APP, the starting point for beta-amyloid plaques, is one of many proteins associated with cell membranes, the lipid barrier that encloses the cell. As it is being made inside the cell, APP becomes embedded in the neuron's membrane, 4/5 on the outside and 1/5 on the inside, like a toothpick stuck in an orange. While APP is embedded in the cell membrane, certain enzymes (proteins that cause or speed up a chemical reaction) cleave it into discrete fragments. Several years ago, scientists identified the enzymes responsible for cleaving APP into these peptides. These enzymes are called alpha-secretase, beta-secretase, and gamma-secretase. In a major breakthrough, scientists then discovered that, depending on which enzyme does the cleaving and the segment of APP within which the cleaving occurs, APP processing can follow one of two pathways that have very different consequences.

In one pathway, alpha-secretase cleaves the APP molecule within the portion that has the potential to become beta-amyloid. Cleaving at this site results in the release from the neuron of a fragment called sAPPα. This fragment has beneficial properties, such as promoting neuronal growth and survival. The remaining APP fragment, still tethered in the neuron's membrane, is then cleaved by gamma-secretase at the end of the beta-amyloid segment. The smaller of the resulting fragments also is released into the space outside the neuron, while the larger fragment remains within the neuron and interacts with factors in the nucleus.

In the second pathway, beta-secretase cleaves the APP molecule at one end of the beta-amyloid peptide, releasing a fragment called sAPPβ from the cell. Gamma-secretase then cleaves the resulting fragment at the other end of the beta-amyloid peptide. Following its cleavage at both ends, the beta-amyloid peptide is released into the space outside the neuron and begins to stick to other peptides of beta-amyloid. These small, soluble clumps of two, three, four, or even up to a dozen beta-amyloid peptides are called ADDLs. The number of individual beta-amyloid peptides within ADDLs varies, but collectively, they are referred to as oligomers. It is likely that some oligomers may be cleared from the brain. Those that cannot be cleared clump together with more beta-amyloid peptides and other proteins and cellular material. As the process continues, these oligomers grow larger, becoming increasingly insoluble entities called protofibrils and fibrils. Eventually these entities coalesce into the well-known plaques that are characteristic of AD.

Until recently, scientists thought that fibrils and plaques were somehow responsible for all the neuronal damage and death in AD. Now, new evidence suggests that the formation of plaques may actually be a kind of clearance mechanism that the brain uses to get harmful beta-amyloid clumps away from neurons.

Researchers also are increasingly convinced that oligomers that are not cleared from the brain and that do not become part of a plaque may be one of the neuron-damaging culprits. A research team at Northwestern University has even suggested how oligomers damage neurons and cause the memory loss that features so prominently in AD (Cleary et al., 2005; Lacor et al., 2004). Working with cell cultures and tissue extracts taken from AD and rat brains, the scientists found that some oligomers attach themselves to the synapses located on

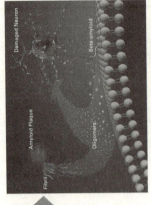

Single beta-amyloid peptides clump into soluble oligomers. Some oligomers attach to neurites, disrupting synapse function. Some oligomers clump together with other cellular material, forming increasingly insoluble fibrils. Eventually this clumping process leads to the insoluble plaques that are found in abundance in AD.

Pathway to Harm

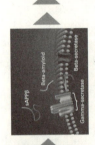

Beta-secretase cleaves APP at one end of the beta-amyloid peptide; sAPPβ is released into the space outside the neuron.

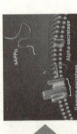

Gamma-secretase cleaves APP at the other end of the beta-amyloid peptide, releasing it into the space outside the neuron. The other fragment stays within the neuron.

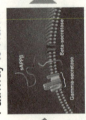

As it is being made, APP sticks through the neuron's membrane, partly inside and partly outside the cell.

Pathway to Healthy Aging

Alpha-secretase cleaves the APP molecule within the portion that would have formed beta-amyloid. sAPPα is released into the space outside the neuron.

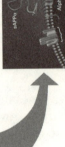

Gamma-secretase cleaves the remaining fragment. The smaller portion is released into the space outside the neuron; the larger stays within the neuron.

Figure 3.2. Two pathways, two outcomes (Source: NIA).

neurites (the structures that branch out from the cell body). When this happens, the synapses are not able to function properly and therefore cannot receive messages from other neurons. Unable to communicate, the neuron ultimately ceases to function and dies. As this destructive process accelerates, essential cognitive operations, such as memory formation and retrieval, are disrupted.

University of California at San Francisco investigators funded by the National Institute of Neurological Disorders and Stroke (NINDS), NIA, and other research institutions are contributing to this understanding through their studies of an enzyme called fyn kinase, which is thought to increase the susceptibility of neurons to beta-amyloid toxicity. In their studies with transgenic mice, the investigators found that fyn kinases were necessary for the toxic effects of beta-amyloid on neuronal synapses and contributed to premature death in the mice, but they were not involved in all elements of the pathologic process in neurons (Chin et al., 2004).

This expanding knowledge about the stages of plaque formation and the toxicity of molecules formed at each stage is giving scientists new therapeutic targets. For example, because toxic forms of beta-amyloid build up most rapidly when they are at high concentrations in the brain, one strategy is to investigate whether high levels of beta-amyloid in the brain might be partly due to how rapidly these molecules are removed from brain tissue into the blood stream through the blood-brain barrier. Several groups are trying to understand which receptors on the surface of cells at the blood-brain barrier are responsible for this transport and whether their ability to move beta-amyloid in and out of the brain might be related to AD pathology.

One research team based at the University of Rochester Medical Center is working on receptors that remove beta-amyloid from the brain (Deane et al., 2004). A receptor called low-density lipoprotein receptor-related protein (LRP) was previously found to be primarily responsible for this task. The new studies show that LRP binds to beta-amyloid at the blood-brain barrier. Interestingly, LRP's efficiency in clearing beta-amyloid from the brain into the blood was greatest for the most soluble form of normal beta-amyloid. In contrast, mutated forms (such as one found in a Dutch family where mutated beta-amyloid accumulated around blood vessels) and less soluble forms of normal beta-amyloid were cleared from the brain much less rapidly. However, at high concentrations, all forms of beta-amyloid directly caused an increased rate of LRP breakdown, reducing the ability of LRP to clear beta-amyloid from the brain. Together, these results indicate that preserving LRP activity at the blood-brain barrier may be an important component of strategies to remove beta-amyloid from the brain.

A receptor called p75[NTR] also is coming under scientific scrutiny. Among other actions, p75[NTR] makes many kinds of neurons more susceptible to beta-amyloid. In a recent study funded by NINDS and other organizations, a research team from the University of Rochester studied the effects of beta amyloid on p75[NTR] levels in cell cultures of human neurons. They expected that increasing p75[NTR] would make the neurons more susceptible to beta-amyloid. Instead, they found that exposure to beta-amyloid increased p75[NTR] activity in the neurons and that the increased activity actually protected the cells, even when cells were exposed to levels of beta-amyloid 2,500 times higher than those usually found in people with AD (Zhang et al., 2003). These findings open the door to future studies to examine the possibility that activating the p75[NTR] receptor may be a useful strategy for treating AD in humans.

Scientists funded by the National Institute of Environmental Health Sciences, NIA, and the Wisconsin Distinguished Rath Graduate Fellowship in Medicine have investigated another protein that may be protective because it binds beta-amyloid (Stein et al., 2004). This research team, from the University of Wisconsin at Madison, studied why transgenic mice that had defective genes from people with early-onset AD inserted into their DNA had high levels of beta-amyloid deposits but did not exhibit any neurodegenerative symptoms. Further investigations led the research team to discover that these mice were producing high levels of transthyretin, a carrier of the thyroid hormone thyroxine. When the mice were given antibodies that prevented transthyretin from interacting with the beta-amyloid protein, the mice showed an increased level of brain cell death. Cell culture studies of human brain cells treated with transthyretin and beta-amyloid showed minimal amounts of cell death while beta-amyloid alone caused significant cell death. These studies indicated that transthyretin can block the progression of AD in this mouse model by inhibiting the effects of beta-amyloid protein. Although we do not yet know whether transthyretin protects against beta-amyloid in humans, this discovery suggests that it may be possible to develop a drug that increases the production of transthyretin and thus protects people at risk of AD, possibly including those who are at higher genetic risk of developing the disease. The findings also may improve the detection of environmental agents that may play a role in the development of AD by allowing scientists to determine which of these agents upsets the balance between transthyretin and beta-amyloid proteins.

Avenues of beta-amyloid research involving new pathways are proving to be rich ground for discovery. The possibility that blocking the production of beta-amyloid in the brain might prevent the development of AD is one such avenue. Scientists funded by the National Institute of Mental Health and the National Institute on Aging at the Howard Hughes Medical Institute and the University of Pennsylvania built on previous research suggesting that an enzyme called glycogen synthase kinase-3alpha (GSK-3α) may be crucial to the development of AD because inhibiting the action of GSK-3α also inhibits the formation of beta-amyloid plaques and neurofibrillary tangles. In the new study, the investigators examined the potential of the mood-stabilizing medication lithium to inhibit GSK-3α and minimize the biological changes leading to AD (Phiel et al., 2003). The researchers first showed that lithium inhibited GSK-3α in cultured cells, reducing the production of beta-amyloid. Then, they demonstrated that administering therapeutic doses of lithium to transgenic mice markedly reduced the accumulation of beta-amyloid in the mouse brains. These results appear promising and are opening new lines of investigation about the association of lithium and AD.

For example, it may be useful to investigate whether patients who have taken lithium for bipolar disorder show a lower incidence of AD. However, even if lithium does prove to be useful as an AD intervention, its known side effects, such as nausea, fatigue, and hand tremor, particularly in older patients, may require the development of new agents that provide the therapeutic effects without the negative side effects.

New Developments in Tau Research

One of the hallmarks of AD is the formation of neurofibrillary tangles (NFTs), which consist largely of an abnormal form of tau. Long considered by many investigators to have a secondary role in AD, tau has, in recent years, come into its own as a leading player in AD research. Findings from the past several years clearly show why tau is generating new excitement.

NFTs are found in a variety of human diseases other than AD, including corticobasal degeneration, progressive supranuclear palsy, and frontotemporal dementia and Parkinsonism linked to chromosome 17 (FTDP-17). These diseases are called "tauopathies." Even though no mutations have been found in the tau gene in AD, inherited mutations do occur in other tauopathies that can change the structure of the protein from normal to abnormal. Previously, only transgenic mice that

41

had been bred to have mutated tau demonstrated NFTs. Now, a research group at the Albert Einstein College of Medicine in New York, has developed a new mouse model of human AD (Andorfer et al., 2005). These "hTau" mice have nonmutant human tau protein and accumulate an excessive amount of an abnormal form of tau. They also form clumps of tau filaments in a region-specific fashion that is similar to AD. This new mouse model will allow researchers to investigate the relationship between cell death, accumulation of altered tau, and the development of NFTs. This study also provides compelling evidence that neuronal death in AD may not result directly or primarily from NFT formation, but rather from disrupted axon transport (in other words, a loss of normal tau function). The scientists found that the presence of tau filaments did not directly correlate with death within individual cells. Instead, they found that it was associated with the appearance of cell-cycle molecules and the initiation of DNA synthesis, which suggests that cell death can occur independently of NFT formation. Possibly, the neurodegeneration occurring in the hTau mice may be at least partially due to abnormal, incomplete initiation of the cell-cycle process.

In a second tau advance, scientists at the University of Minnesota Medical School were able to partially rescue memory function in a transgenic mouse model that had a form of a mutant tau gene whose synthesis could be suppressed by a drug (SantaCruz et al., 2005). This meant that production of the mutant tau could be precisely regulated. As the mice aged, they produced more mutant tau and began to accumulate NFTs. Their neurons began to die, brain tissue shrank, and memory was lost. The researchers were able to stop the production of the mutant tau by giving the mice the drug that turned off the gene. Once the mutant gene was suppressed, the scientists found, much to their surprise, that not only did the memory loss stop, it actually was partially reversed. Even more striking, memory function improved even though NFTs formed from tau that had already been made continued to accumulate in the brains of the mice. The fact that memory function improved in mice carrying the mutant tau gene when the gene was turned off, despite continued NFT accumulation, implies that the processes that lead to memory loss and those that cause NFTs are separate. Perhaps NFTs do not invariably cause neuronal death, but an earlier, toxic form of abnormal tau does. Some investigators are suggesting that NFTs, like beta-amyloid plaques, may even be a protective response by the brain that is aimed at preventing abnormal tau from damaging the neuron (Tanzi, 2005).

Tau studies are one of the most active areas of AD research, and, as with other areas of AD research, new findings are emerging all the

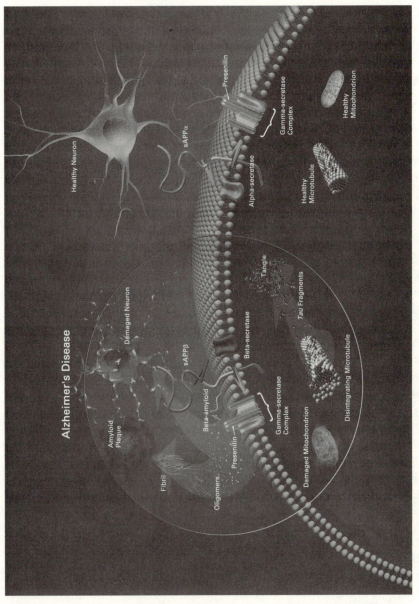

Figure 3.3. Players on the AD stage: Putting it all together (Source: NIA)

time. Current and future studies in animal models are examining whether it might, in fact, be possible to "turn on and off" the synthesis of abnormal, damaging tau and beta-amyloid and exploring whether the brain could even regain some cognitive function once the disease process has begun.

Exploring Commonalities in the Transformation from Healthy Aging to Neurodegenerative Disease

For some time, scientists have realized that a number of devastating diseases—such as AD, dementia with Lewy bodies, frontotemporal dementia, Parkinson disease, Huntington disease, and prion diseases—are characterized by aggregations of abnormally folded proteins. In AD, the abnormal proteins are beta-amyloid and tau; in PD, it's synuclein; and in frontotemporal dementia, it's tau. Scientists think, therefore, that the pathological process in these diseases must share some characteristics, though these overlaps are not fully understood.

For example, research on beta-amyloid aggregates has provided evidence that the actual structure of oligomers may help to explain the pathology seen in these diseases. In one series of experiments, scientists at the University of California at Irvine made an antibody in rabbits that specifically recognizes soluble beta-amyloid oligomers. The antibody failed to recognize soluble lower-molecular weight and fibrillar forms of this peptide (Kayed et al., 2003). This antibody also reacted with a variety of soluble protein oligomers that are involved in other neurodegenerative diseases, regardless of their specific amino acid sequence. Importantly, this particular antibody blocked the toxicity of these oligomers on cells in culture, including that of beta-amyloid oligomers. These results suggest that many types of soluble oligomers contain a common structural feature, independent of their amino acid sequence, and that the toxicity and pathogenesis of these oligomers may be mediated by a common mechanism.

Scientists also know that many neurodegenerative diseases have some clinical characteristics in common. For example, some people with AD have trouble moving, the most obvious symptom of PD. Many of those with PD also have dementia. Sleep-wake disorders, delusions, psychiatric disturbances, and memory loss occur in all of these diseases. Finally, it is clear that all of these diseases develop over many years and occur as a result of complex interactions of genes, lifestyle and environmental factors, and factors affecting all parts of the body (such as hormonal changes).

By investigating these diseases individually and together, scientists hope to shed light on their causes and, possibly, on future common treatment and prevention strategies.

References

Andorfer C, Acker CM, Kress Y, Hof PR, Duff K, Davies P. Cell-cycle reentry and cell death in transgenic mice expressing nonmutant human tau isoforms. *Journal of Neuroscience* 2005;25(22):5446-5454.

Barnes LL, Mendes de Leon CF, Wilson RS, Bienias JL, Evans DA. Social resources and cognitive decline in a population of older African Americans and whites. *Neurology* 2004;63(12):2322-2326.

Bennett DA, Wilson RS, Schneider JA, Evans DA, Mendes de Leon CF, Arnold SE, Barnes LL, Bienias JL. Education modifies the relation of AD pathology to level of cognitive function in older persons. *Neurology* 2003;60(12):1909-1915.

Buckner RL. Memory and executive function in aging and AD: multiple factors that cause decline and reserve factors that compensate. *Neuron* 2004;44(1):195-208.

Chin J, Palop JJ, Yu GQ, Kojima N, Masliah E, Mucke L. Fyn kinase modulates synaptotoxicity, but not aberrant sprouting, in human amyloid precursor protein transgenic mice. *Journal of Neuroscience* 2004;24(19):4692-4697.

Cleary JP, Walsh DM, Hofmeister JJ, Shankar GM, Kuskowski MA, Selkoe DJ, Ashe KH. Natural oligomers of the amyloid-beta protein specifically disrupt cognitive function. *Nature Neuroscience* 2005;8(1): 79-84.

Deane R, Wu Z, Sagare A, Davis J, Du Yan S, Hamm K, Xu F, Parisi M, LaRue B, Hu HW, Spijkers P, Guo H, Song X, Lenting PJ, Van Nostrand WE, Zlokovic BV. LRP/amyloid beta-peptide interaction mediates differential brain efflux of Abeta isoforms. *Neuron* 2004;43(3):333-344.

Head D, Snyder AZ, Girton LE, Morris JC, Buckner RL. Frontal-hippocampal double dissociation between normal aging and Alzheimer's disease. *Cerebral Cortex* 2005;15(6):732-739.

Kayed R, Head E, Thompson JL, McIntire TM, Milton SC, Cotman CW, Glabe CG. Common structure of soluble amyloid oligomers implies common mechanism of pathogenesis. *Science* 2003;300(5618):486-489.

Lacor PN, Buniel MC, Change L, Fernandez SJ, Gong Y, Viola KL, Lambert MP, Velasco PT, Bigio EH, Finch CE Krafft, GA, Klein WL.

Synaptic targeting by Alzheimer's–related amyloid beta oligomers. *Journal of Neuroscience* 2004;24(45):10191-10200.

Manly JJ, Touradji P, Tang MX, Stern Y. Literacy and memory decline among ethnically diverse elders. *Journal of Clinical and Experimental Neuropsychology* 2003;25(5):680-690.

Phiel CJ, Wilson CA, Lee VM, Klein PS. GSK-3alpha regulates production of Alzheimer's disease amyloid-beta peptides. *Nature* 2003;423 (6938):435-439.

Resnick SM, Pham DL, Kraut MA, Zonderman AB, Davatzikos C. Longitudinal magnetic resonance imaging studies of older adults: a shrinking brain. *Journal of Neuroscience* 2003;23(8):3295-3301.

SantaCruz K, Lewis J, Spires T, Paulson J, Kotilinek L, Ingelsson M, Guimaraes A, DeTure M, Ramsden M, McGowan E, Forster C, Yue M, Orne J, Janus C, Mariash A, Kuskowski M, Hyman B, Hutton M, Ashe KH. Tau suppression in a neurodegenerative mouse model improves memory function. *Science* 2005;309(5733):476-481.

Scarmeas N, Zarahn E, Anderson KE, Habeck CG, Hilton J, Flynn J, Marder KS, Bell KL, Sackeim HA, Van Heertum RL, Moeller JR, Stern Y. Association of life activities with cerebral blood flow in Alzheimer disease: implications for the cognitive reserve hypothesis. *Archives of Neurology* 2003;60(3):359-365.

Small SA, Chawla MK, Buonocore M, Rapp PR, Barnes CA. Imaging correlates of brain function in monkeys and rats isolates a hippocampal subregion differentially vulnerable to aging. *Proceedings of the National Academy of Sciences, USA* 2004;101(18):7181-7186.

Stein TD, Anders NJ, DeCarli C, Chan SL, Mattson MP, Johnson JA. Neutralization of transthyretin reverses the neuroprotective effects of secreted amyloid precursor protein (APP) in APPSW mice resulting in tau phosphorylation and loss of hippocampal neurons: support for the amyloid hypothesis. *Journal of Neuroscience* 2004;24(35):7707-7717.

Tanzi RE. Tangles and neurodegenerative disease—a surprising twist. *New England Journal of Medicine* 2005;353(17):1853-1855.

Zhang Y, Hong Y, Bounhar Y, Blacker M, Roucou X, Tounekti O, Vereker E, Bowers WJ, Federoff HJ, Goodyer CG, LeBlanc A. p75 neurotrophin receptor protects primary cultures of human neurons against extracellular amyloid beta peptide cytotoxicity. *Journal of Neuroscience* 2003;23(19):7385-7394.

Chapter 4

Understanding Alzheimer Disease Risk Factors

Can Certain Factors Protect Against or Increase Risk of AD?

We've known for some time that certain genetic and non-genetic factors can increase the risk of developing Alzheimer Disease (AD). Recent evidence has suggested that other factors may actually help to reduce AD risk. The combined weight of these advances is making scientists eager to understand how these risk and protective factors balance each other over the course of a lifetime. They also want to know more about the types of interventions that may be useful in changing this balance in the direction of healthy aging and the times in the life cycle at which these interventions might be most effective.

Ideas about what these risk and protective factors might be are derived from a variety of different types of studies, including genetics studies, studies of individual lifestyles and behavioral patterns, and studies of large groups or populations. Findings from these studies are important because they point the way to potential therapeutic approaches that might be worth investigating in controlled clinical trials. If confirmed in trials, they may suggest ways that people can change their lifestyles or environments to reduce risk. The genetics

Excerpted from "Progress Report on Alzheimer's Disease: New Discoveries, New Insights," National Institute on Aging (NIA), 2004-2005, NIH Pub. No. 05-5724, 2005. Text under the heading "Vascular Disease and AD" was excerpted from "Progress Report on Alzheimer's Disease: Journey to Discovery, 2005-2006," NIH Pub. No. 06-6047, 2007.

studies, in particular, will help identify pathways that affect the development or progression of AD. They also will help researchers develop new animal models to understand early events in the disease, as well as identify potential targets for treatment and prevention.

New Discoveries about AD Genetics

Genetic studies of complex neurodegenerative diseases such as AD have focused on two key issues—whether a gene might influence a person's overall risk of developing a disease and whether a gene might influence some particular aspect of a person's risk, such as the age at which the disease begins ("age at onset"). To date, only four of the approximately 30,000 genes in the human genetic map (the "genome") have been conclusively shown to affect AD development. Mutations in three genes—the APP gene found on chromosome 21, the PS1 gene on chromosome 14, or the PS2 gene on chromosome 1—are linked to the rare early-onset form of familial AD. The APP gene is responsible for making APP, the precursor to beta-amyloid. The presenilin genes code for proteins that are components of enzymes that play an important part in cleaving APP to form beta-amyloid. Presenilin gene mutations promote the breakdown of APP, leading to increased production of harmful beta-amyloid.

A fourth gene on chromosome 19 encodes a protein called apolipoprotein E (ApoE). ApoE carries lipids in the bloodstream and is important in clearing lipids from the blood. APOE, the gene that encodes ApoE, has three common forms, or alleles—ε2, ε3, and ε4. The ε4 allele is a risk factor gene for the common late-onset AD. The ε2 allele may provide some protection against AD and ε3 is thought to play a neutral role.

Scientists estimate that an additional four to seven risk factor genes exist for late-onset AD. A study from researchers at Massachusetts General Hospital, who are participating in the National Institute of Mental Health's (NIMH) Alzheimer Disease Genetics Initiative and who are also supported by the National Institute on Aging (NIA) funding, is shedding light on these genes. The researchers screened the entire genomes of a large number of families with AD using 382 genetic markers and complex statistical analysis to identify regions of the genome that were associated with AD and might contain additional susceptibility genes (Blacker et al., 2003). The study identified 12 additional chromosomal regions that might be linked to AD. Some of these regions will probably be found not to contribute to AD. However, other regions may well harbor genuine AD susceptibility genes, particularly the regions that yielded strong statistical evidence during the genome analysis. Even though it will be difficult to identify and characterize the genes in these chromosomal regions, the results will greatly facilitate the development of strategies for AD treatment, early intervention, and prevention.

Another team of researchers examined genetic associations with AD in a different population. This Boston University School of Medicine team worked with a population in Wadi Ara, an Arab community in northern Israel that has an unusually high prevalence of AD (Farrer et al., 2003). A genomic scan conducted on people from this community with and without AD revealed markers with significant AD allelic association on chromosomes 2, 9, 10, and 12. The researchers then analyzed the distribution of allele frequencies to narrow the potential regions on these chromosomes where the genes might be found. The unique characteristics of the Wadi Ara populations and the fact that findings from this analysis replicate those from other genome scans may help scientists more rapidly identify AD risk factor genes on these chromosomes.

Other studies have shown that a region on chromosome 10 is likely to harbor at least one AD risk factor gene and several research teams have made advances in this area. For example, scientists from the Karolinska Institute in Stockholm, Sweden, examined a stretch of genetic material on chromosome 10 that contains the insulin degrading enzyme (IDE) gene (Prince et al., 2003). This enzyme is of interest because it also degrades beta-amyloid. Genetically engineered mice that do not have the IDE gene develop high insulin levels, glucose intolerance, and increased brain levels of beta-amyloid. The scientists compared genetic material from people with and without AD to assess the IDE gene and two other close-by genes. They were interested in finding differences between individuals at a single point in the genetic code (these points are called SNPs) and in stretches of DNA that are inherited in common among groups of people (these stretches of DNA are called haplotypes). Results strongly indicated that this region contains alleles and haplotypes that confer AD risk. These findings provide substantial evidence that genetic variation within or extremely close to IDE affects both disease risk and traits related to the severity of the disease. The study also indicated that an analysis of this type can be an effective way to assess genetic variation in complex diseases like AD.

Other scientists have focused on chromosomes 12 and 19. In one study, conducted collaboratively by scientists from NIA and Celera Diagnostics of Alameda, California, the researchers examined regions of chromosomes 12 and 19 from three separate sample sets that included people with and without AD (Li et al., 2004). The researchers found that single nucleotide polymorphisms (SNP) in the glyceralde-hyde 3 phosphate dehydrogenase (GAPD) gene family were significantly associated with AD risk in all three sample sets. They also found that some GAPD SNPs on chromosome 12 were associated with an age of onset of 75 years and older, whereas some GAPD SNPs on chromosome 19 were associated with an age of onset of less than 75 years. Individually, the GAPD SNPs made different contributions to AD risk in each of the sample sets, and the investigators speculate that variants in functionally similar genes may account for this heterogeneity of AD risk.

In addition, knowledge gained from studying Down syndrome (DS) is revealing much about chromosome 21 and its possible role in AD. Most people have two copies of chromosome 21, but people with DS have three. Therefore, they have an extra copy of the APP gene. Every individual with DS who survives into his or her third decade develops the signature brain pathology of AD, although the location and distribution of these features are much more variable than in traditional AD.

Another genetics area of great interest to investigators is APOE-ε4, the risk factor gene found on chromosome 19. A number of recent studies have shed additional light on the role of this APOE allele in AD. For example, studies using positron emission tomography (PET) scans have found that people with AD have abnormally low rates of glucose metabolism in certain areas of the cerebral cortex (the outer layer of neurons in the brain that controls conscious thought, mental activity, and voluntary movement, and that processes sensory information from the outside world). Building on earlier PET studies that showed that cognitively healthy older carriers of the APOE-ε4 allele had abnormally low rates of glucose metabolism in those same brain regions, investigators at the Banner Good Samaritan Medical Center in Phoenix, Arizona, examined whether this was true for relatively young adults as well (Reiman et al., 2004). The investigators performed PET and magnetic resonance imaging (MRI) scans and conducted neuropsychological tests on 24 healthy participants, 12 of whom were APOE-ε4 carriers and 12 were not. The two groups did not differ significantly in gender, age, educational level, neuropsychological test scores, or other characteristics. Results of this study were consistent with previous studies in that the researchers found that APOE-ε4 carriers had abnormally low rates of glucose metabolism in the selected brain regions. This study is important because it documents the earliest brain changes yet seen in living persons at risk of AD. These results also provide evidence that AD-like changes in the brains of APOE-ε 4 carriers can occur in cognitively healthy young adults. Tracking brain and cognitive changes over time will be necessary to determine how this pattern of AD-like brain changes relates to the likelihood that APOE-ε4 carriers will develop AD at a later age. If these functional brain changes are eventually validated as an early predictor of AD, very early intervention and treatment will become a possibility.

Another study from the same group compared memory decline and new learning in APOE-ε4 carriers and noncarriers aged 48 to 77 over a two-year period. These investigators and colleagues from several other research sites in Arizona found that APOE-ε4 carriers aged 60 and older showed a decline in new learning as compared with noncarriers (Baxter et al., 2003). No difference in cognitive performance was seen in those younger than 60 years old. These findings suggest that repeat testing of new learning over time may be a sensitive measure for detecting early cognitive changes in older people who are at increased risk of AD.

A group of investigators from the Cache County Study has reported on recent genetic findings about whether AD is an inevitable consequence of aging (Khachaturian et al., 2004). The Cache County Study, a long-term study of 5,000 people in Cache County, Utah, provides a unique perspective on AD because the participating population is one of the longest lived in the United States. It includes about 700 individuals older than 85 and almost 250 who are 90 years old and older. This aspect of the study allowed the investigators to explore one AD puzzle: We know that the risk of AD increases with age, but we don't know much about the proportion of people who would be likely to get AD over an extended life-time, say 100 years, or about the effect of APOE-ε4 over that time period. Using several types of analytic models, these investigators set out to estimate the risk of developing AD as a function of age and number of APOE-ε4 alleles. The models estimated that 28 percent of individuals would not develop AD over any reasonable life expectancy. They confirmed that AD onset is accelerated in individuals with one, and especially two, APOE-ε4 alleles, but did not see any meaningful difference in lifetime risk of developing AD related to number of APOE-ε4 alleles. The authors concluded that this population contains individuals who are not susceptible to developing AD at an advanced age, regardless of which APOE allele they may carry. Discovering the genetic or environmental factors that are responsible for this resilience is clearly a high priority for future research.

Finally, scientists have used a genetics approach to examine late-life depression, a condition that is often associated with cognitive impairment and is a risk factor for the development of dementia and

AD. To determine whether the presence of APOE-ε4 could explain the linkage of this form of depression with dementia, University of Pittsburgh investigators funded by NIMH and NIA analyzed how frequently the different forms of APOE occurred in patients with depression compared to healthy older adults and people with AD (Butters et al., 2003). As expected, APOE-ε4 occurred more frequently in individuals with AD. However, the frequency of APOE-ε4 was not higher in those with depression compared to the healthy study participants. APOE-ε4 frequency also did not differ among depressed participants with and without accompanying cognitive impairment. Unexpectedly, the onset of depression occurred at a younger age for APOE-ε4 carriers compared to noncarriers. These results indicate that APOE-ε4 is associated with the age of onset of late-life depression, but not cognitive functioning in that condition. Further studies will be required to elucidate the avenues through which late-life depression may contribute to the onset of AD.

Lifestyle and Dietary Patterns

The possible impact of environmental and lifestyle factors, such as intellectually stimulating activities, physical activity, and diet, on AD risk is becoming an increased focus of research. A number of studies over the past few years have provided intriguing hints that these factors may be linked to a reduced risk of AD, and they are consistent with what we know about other benefits associated with health-promoting behaviors throughout life. It is important to note, however, that these factors have been identified in observational and animal studies, and at present, they are only associated with changes in AD risk. Only further research, including clinical trials, will reveal whether, in fact, these factors can help prevent AD.

Recent studies have looked at these environmental and lifestyle issues from various aspects. For example, researchers from the Rush Alzheimer Disease Center (ADC) found reduced AD risk among participants in a Chicago Health and Aging Project (CHAP) study who consumed fish frequently and whose diet was high in unsaturated, unhydrogenated fats (Morris et al., 2003a; Morris et al., 2003b). In this CHAP study, complete dietary intake and disease diagnosis data were available on 815 people, and the length of follow-up between dietary assessment and clinical evaluation was about 2.3 years. CHAP investigators found that participants who consumed one or more fish meals per week had a 60 percent reduced risk of AD compared to participants who seldom or never ate fish. People whose diets were higher in polyunsaturated and vegetable fats also had a reduced AD risk compared to those whose fat intake was predominantly saturated fats. Though these studies support other research showing health benefits related to fish and unsaturated fat consumption and provide some intriguing hints about AD, the authors caution that further studies are needed before dietary recommendations can be made based on a relationship to AD risk.

A considerable amount of research also has been devoted to examining the role of educational attainment on AD risk. One recent study, conducted by investigators at Harvard Medical School, used data from the long-term Nurses' Health Study of 16,596 older female registered nurses to assess the relationship of educational attainment, husband's education, household income, and childhood socioeconomic status to cognitive function and decline (Lee et al., 2003). The study participants had an initial cognitive assessment in the late 1990s and a second assessment about two years later. The investigators found that women with a graduate degree had substantially decreased odds of a low initial cognitive score and of cognitive decline over the two years compared to women with less education. The other measures of socioeconomic status considered in this study had little, if any, relation to cognitive function or decline in later life.

In the past few years, several research groups have attempted to link participation in leisure activities with a lower risk of dementia. However, the exact relationship remains unclear. Scientists do not know whether increased participation in leisure activities lowers the risk of dementia or whether people who later develop dementia participate less in leisure activities because they are already in the early phase of dementia, before symptoms are evident. Investigators from the Albert Einstein College of Medicine in New York City explored this issue in a group of 469 cognitively healthy people who were older than age 75 and still living in the community (Verghese et al., 2003). Over a period of about five years, 124 people developed dementia. Based on a statistical analysis, the investigators concluded that participation in leisure activities was associated with a reduced risk of dementia, even after adjusting for participants' initial cognitive status and after excluding participants with possible preclinical dementia. Controlled clinical trials are needed to explore this issue further and assess the protective effect of leisure activities on the risk of dementia.

In addition to these studies, which suggest an association between particular lifestyle factors and actual AD risk reduction, other research provides indirect indications that lifestyle factors may be related in some way to AD risk. For example, a recent collaborative study by investigators at the University of Toronto and the University of California at Irvine assessed whether long-term treatment with a combination of "behavioral enrichment" (extra attention and lots of training and stimulation) and a diet rich in antioxidants, including vitamins E and C, and fruit and vegetable extracts could reduce age-related cognitive decline in dogs (Milgram et al., 2004). Dogs are a good model for studying AD because they can perform sophisticated and complex cognitive behaviors, their brains accumulate beta-amyloid plaques with age, and the degree of beta-amyloid deposition is related to the severity of cognitive decline. This study included both old and young dogs. Some received the fortified food and the enriched environment, some received one or the other enrichment, and some received neither. At the end of a year, the researchers tested the dogs on two learning tasks. Not surprisingly, the researchers found that the old dogs performed less well than the young dogs. However, the performance of the old dogs was improved by the fortified food and behavioral enrichment. The effects of the treatments were most evident in the dogs who received both interventions.

Accumulating evidence also suggests that being physically active may benefit more than just our hearts and waistlines. Research in animals has shown that aspects of both brain function and cognitive function improve with physical exercise. Several studies in aging adults have shown similar results. One study, conducted by researchers at the University of Illinois at Urbana-Champaign, used a form of magnetic resonance imaging (MRI) to measure changes in brain activity in healthy adults aged 58 to 78 before and after a six-month program of brisk walking (Colcombe et al., 2004). The researchers found that the function of neurons in key parts of the brain increased along with improvements in the participants' cardiovascular fitness. Compared to a physically inactive group, the walkers were able to pay attention better and focus more clearly on goals while disregarding unimportant information. Scientists working in this area speculate that physical activity may be beneficial because it may improve blood flow to the brain. Another possibility under investigation is that physical activity triggers cellular mechanisms that protect the brain from damage and promote its repair.

Vascular Disease and AD

Even though the brain makes up only 2 percent of the body's mass, it receives 20 percent of the body's blood flow. The blood delivers oxygen and glucose to neurons. Maintaining a constant and adequate blood flow in the brain is essential for neuronal survival and brain function, and decreased blood flow in parts of the brain affected by AD is an early feature of the disease.

Recent research has focused on the many micro blood vessels that constitute a critical part of the brain's blood supply. Two aspects of these capillaries are important in AD:

- The brain's ability to grow new micro vessels is diminished in AD.

- The brain uses the micro vessels to get rid of toxic beta-amyloid peptides. It appears that clearance of beta-amyloid across the blood-brain barrier (BBB) into the circulation is impaired in AD. The BBB is a protective barrier formed by the blood vessels of the brain to prevent large molecules from entering the brain.

For some time now, the study of the brain's blood vessel system (vasculature) in the context of AD has been a productive line of inquiry. A scientific team at the University of Rochester Medical Center has proposed a "neurovascular hypothesis of AD," which pulls together a decade's worth of disparate research on the brain and its blood vessels (Zlokovic, 2005).

This hypothesis states that faulty clearance of beta-amyloid peptides across the BBB, abnormal development of new micro vessels, and accelerated or abnormal aging of the brain's blood vessel system could start a process that leads to BBB compromise, chemical imbalances in the neuronal environment, and synaptic and neuronal dysfunction.

If it is true that diminished or abnormal functioning of the neurovascular system contributes substantially to AD, then a recent study by the University of Rochester team may go some of the way toward explaining the role of vasculature cells in the damage done by AD (Wu et al., 2005). This study focused on lipoprotein receptor-related protein 1 (LRP), a protein located in the endothelial cells that line the inside of brain micro vessels. LRP is responsible for transporting beta-amyloid peptides out of the brain across the BBB into the body's circulation. The endothelial cells in the brains of people with AD produce less LRP compared to healthy older people. As a result, clearance of beta-amyloid is impaired and the toxic peptide accumulates in the brain. Until now, scientists have not been able to understand why LRP production falls.

The researchers approached this important question by comparing the pattern of expression of genes in endothelial cells isolated from brain tissue of people who had died of AD to the genetic expression pattern of endothelial cells isolated from brain tissue of cognitively healthy old and young people who had died of other causes. They found that the expression of a gene called MEOX2, which is known to be involved in the growth and development of brain micro vessels, was specifically reduced in AD. They also discovered that when the expression of this gene was stopped, a protein involved in endothelial cell death began to be produced. Using transgenic mice that express half the normal amount of MEOX2, the investigators discovered that when production of MEOX2 was reduced, the brain also was less able to grow new micro vessels in response to injury. When MEOX2 expression was reduced, the amount of LRP also was reduced, and the brain was not able to remove beta-amyloid efficiently across the BBB.

Clearly, much more work needs to be done to answer remaining questions about beta-amyloid, the cell-cycle process, tau, vascular dysfunction, and other factors that may promote or retard the AD process. However, these and other basic research studies are making an invaluable contribution to our understanding of AD, and they are opening promising new avenues in the search for AD therapeutic strategies.

Diabetes and AD

The possible association of diabetes, insulin, and AD also is garnering increasing attention. Type II diabetes mellitus is a serious public health problem in the U.S. The condition affects about one in five people over age 65 and has been associated with a variety of adverse health effects. Evidence from a number of epidemiologic studies suggests a possible link between diabetes and cognitive impairment, and this has spurred researchers to examine this link on many levels, from test tube investigations to population studies. The idea behind this area of research is to determine whether or not diabetes is a risk factor for cognitive decline, and if so, whether therapies for diabetes may help lower risk of cognitive decline or AD.

Researchers from the University of California at San Francisco investigated whether diabetes and impaired fasting glucose (IFG, an indicator of increased diabetes risk) were linked to cognitive function (Yaffe et al., 2004). The data for the study came from the Multiple Outcomes of Raloxifene Evaluation (MORE), a long-term osteoporosis study of more than 7,000 women between the ages of 31 and 80. The investigators found that the cognitive abilities of women with IFG were lower than those of women with normal blood glucose levels but higher than those with diabetes. They also found a higher risk of developing cognitive impairment among the women with IFG or diabetes than among the women with normal blood glucose levels.

Another University of California at San Francisco team of researchers examined the change in cognitive performance over a four-year period among older adults participating in a study called the Rancho Bernardo Study (Kanaya et al., 2004). Participants, who were divided into three groups—normal glucose tolerance, impaired glucose tolerance, and diabetic—were given three different cognitive tests at the beginning of the study and again four years later. The researchers found that scores on all three cognitive function tests did not differ across the groups at the beginning of the study, but that the women with diabetes had a more rapid decline in performance on the verbal fluency test over the study period compared with women in either of the other two groups.

Other researchers, such as one team from New York University School of Medicine, are studying diabetes and cognition through studies with animals and small numbers of individuals (Convit et al., 2003). We know that age is a risk factor for both impaired cognition and impaired glucose metabolism, and a relationship between these deficits is suspected. It is not clear, however, how poor glucose metabolism may exert its effect on memory function. One possibility is through the hippocampus, the brain structure that is important for learning and memory and is one of the earliest regions damaged by AD. Rodent studies have shown that during performance of a memory task, the hippocampus is activated, and hippocampal glucose levels drop in specific locations depending on the difficulty of the task. In older rodents, the drop in hippocampal glucose levels is more profound and lasts longer, perhaps forming a basis for impairments in memory performance seen in some older animals. Because of this vulnerability, subtle metabolic insults may lead to damage and volume loss. Using these findings as a starting point, the New York University investigators conducted memory tests with 30 nondiabetic middle-aged and older individuals who did not have dementia. Simultaneously, they administered a glucose tolerance test to measure the participants' ability to regulate glucose. The size of the hippocampus and other brain regions was measured with MRI. A decreased ability to regulate glucose was associated with decreased general cognitive performance, memory impairments, and atrophy of the hippocampus. This association was not related to the participants' ages. The investigators also found no association between the volume of other brain regions and glucose regulation. They concluded that a decreased ability to regulate glucose is associated with modest impairments of memory and that the impairments may be the result of a direct impact of poor glucose metabolism on brain structures important for memory. Based on these findings, the researchers suggest that memory deficits among older people with poorer glucose tolerance may be caused by an inability to compensate for the drops in hippocampal glucose levels that normally occur with activation of brain circuits during performance of a memory task. Perhaps better lifetime management of blood sugar may help maintain memory function in old age and perhaps even reduce the risk of hippocampal damage.

References

Baxter LC, Caselli RJ, Johnson SC, Reiman E, Osborne D. Apolipoprotein E epsilon 4 affects new learning in cognitively normal individuals at risk for Alzheimer's disease. *Neurobiology of Aging* 2003;24(7): 947-952.

Blacker D, Bertram L, Saunders AJ, Moscarillo TJ, Albert MS, Wiener H, Perry RT, Collins JS, Harrell LE, Go RC, Mahoney A, Beaty T, Fallin MD, Avramopoulos D, Chase GA, Folstein MF, McInnis MG, Bassett SS, Doheny KJ, Pugh EW, Tanzi RE, NIMH Genetics Initiative Alzheimer's Disease Study Group. Results of a high-resolution genome screen of 437 Alzheimer's disease families. *Human Molecular Genetics* 2003;12(1):23-32.

Butters MA, Sweet RA, Mulsant BH, Ilyas Kamboh M, Pollock BG, Begley AE, Reynolds CF, DeKosky ST. APOE is associated with age-of-onset, but not cognitive functioning, in late-life depression. *International Journal of Geriatric Psychiatry* 2003;18(12):1075-1081.

Colcombe SJ, Kramer AF, Erickson KI, Scalf P, McAuley E, Cohen NJ, Webb A, Jerome GJ, Marquez DX, Elavsky S. Cardiovascular fitness, cortical plasticity, and aging. *Proceedings of the National Academy of Sciences, USA* 2004;101(9):3316-3321.

Convit A, Wolf OT, Tarshish C, de Leon MJ. Reduced glucose tolerance is associated with poor memory performance and hippocampal atrophy among normal elderly. *Proceedings of the National Academy of Sciences, USA* 2003;100(4):2019-2022.

Farrer LA, Bowirrat A, Friedland RP, Waraska K, Korczyn AD, Baldwin CT. Identification of multiple loci for Alzheimer disease in a consanguineous Israeli-Arab community. *Human Molecular Genetics* 2003;12(4):415-422.

Kanaya AM, Barrett-Connor E, Gildengorin G, Yaffe K. Change in cognitive function by glucose tolerance status in older adults: a 4-year prospective study of the Rancho Bernardo study cohort. *Archives of Internal Medicine* 2004;164(12):1327-1333.

Khachaturian AS, Corcoran CD, Mayer LS, Zandi PP, Breitner JC, Cache County Study Investigators. Apolipoprotein E epsilon 4 count affects age at onset of Alzheimer disease, but not lifetime susceptibility: The Cache County Study. *Archives of General Psychiatry* 2004; 61(5):518-524.

Lee S, Kawachi I, Berkman LF, Grodstein F. Education, other socioeconomic indicators, and cognitive function. *American Journal of Epidemiology* 2003;157(8):712-720.

Li Y, Nowotny P, Holmans P, Smemo S, Kauwe JS, Hinrichs AL, Tacey K, Doil L, van Luchene R, Garcia V, Rowland C, Schrodi S, Leong D, Gogic G, Chan J, Cravchik A, Ross D, Lau K, Kwok S, Chang SY, Catanese J, Sninsky J, White TJ, Hardy J, Powell J, Lovestone S, Morris JC, Thal L, Owen M, Williams J, Goate A, Grupe A. Association of late-onset Alzheimer's disease with genetic variation in multiple members of the GAPD gene family. *Proceedings of the National Academy of Sciences, USA* 2004;101(44):15688-15693.

Milgram NW, Head E, Zicker SC, Ikeda-Douglas C, Murphey H, Muggenburg BA, Siwak CT, Tapp PD, Lowry SR, Cotman CW. Long-term treatment with antioxidants and a program of behavioral enrichment reduces age-dependent impairment in discrimination and reversal learning in beagle dogs. *Experimental Gerontology* 2004;39(5):753-765.

Morris MC, Evans DA, Bienias JL, Tangney CC, Bennett DA, Aggarwal N, Schneider J, Wilson RS. Dietary fats and risk of incident Alzheimer disease. *Archives of Neurology* 2003a;60(2):194-200.

Morris MC, Evans DA, Bienias JL, Tangney CC, Bennett DA, Wilson RS, Aggarwal N, Schneider J. Consumption of fish and n-3 fatty acids and risk of incident Alzheimer disease. *Archives of Neurology* 2003b; 60(7):940-946.

Prince JA, Feuk L, Gu HF, Johansson B, Gatz M, Blennow K, Brookes AJ. Genetic variation in a haplotype block spanning IDE influences Alzheimer disease. *Human Mutation* 2003;22(5):363-371.

Reiman EM, Chen K, Alexander GE, Caselli RJ, Bandy D, Osborne D, Saunders AM, Hardy J. Functional brain abnormalities in young adults at genetic risk for late-onset Alzheimer's dementia. *Proceedings of the National Academy of Sciences, USA* 2004;101(1):284-289.

Verghese J, Lipton RB, Katz MJ, Hall CB, Derby CA, Kuslansky G, Ambrose AF, Sliwinski M, Buschke H. Leisure activities and the risk of dementia in the elderly. *New England Journal of Medicine* 2003; 348(25):2508-2516.

Wu Z, Guo H, Chow N, Sallstrom J, Bell RD, Deane R, Brooks AI, Kanagala S, Rubio A, Sagare A, Liu D, Li F, Armstrong D, Gasiewicz T, Zidovetzki R, Song X, Hofman F, Zlokovic BV. Role of the MEOX2 homeobox gene in neurovascular dysfunction in Alzheimer disease. *Nature Medicine* 2005;11(9):959-965.

Yaffe K, Blackwell T, Kanaya AM, Davidowitz N, Barrett-Connor E, Krueger K. Diabetes, impaired fasting glucose, and development of cognitive impairment in older women. *Neurology* 2004;63(4):658-663.

Zlokovic BV. Neurovascular mechanisms of Alzheimer's neurodegeneration. *Trends in Neuroscience* 2005;28(4):202-208.

Chapter 5

Genetics and Alzheimer Disease

Scientists do not yet fully understand what causes Alzheimer disease (AD). However, the more they learn about AD, the more they become aware of the important function genes play in the development of this devastating disease.

Genes

All living things are made up of basic units called cells, which are so tiny that you can only see them through the lens of a strong microscope. Most of the billions of cells in the human body have one nucleus that acts as a control center, housing our 23 pairs of chromosomes. A chromosome is a thread-like structure found in the cell's nucleus, which can carry hundreds, sometimes thousands, of genes. In humans, one of each pair of 23 chromosomes is inherited from each parent. The genetic material on these chromosomes is collectively referred to as the human genome. Scientists now believe that there are about 30,000 genes in the human genome. Genes direct almost every aspect of the construction, operation, and repair of all living things. For example, genes contain information that determines eye and hair color and other traits inherited from our parents. In addition, genes ensure that we have two hands and can use them to do things, like play the piano.

"Alzheimer's Disease Genetics Fact Sheet," National Institute on Aging (http://www.nia.nih.gov), August 2006.

Genes alone are not all-powerful. Most genes can do little until spurred on by other substances. Although they are necessary in their own right, genes basically wait inside the cell's nucleus for other molecules to come along and read their messages. These messages provide the cell with instructions for building a specific protein.

Proteins are essential building blocks in all cells. Bones and teeth, muscles and blood, for example, are formed from different proteins. They help our bodies grow, work properly, and stay healthy. Amino acids are the building blocks of proteins. A gene provides the code, or blueprint, for the type and order of amino acids needed to build a specific protein. Sometimes a genetic mutation (or defect in a gene) can occur, leading to the production of a faulty protein. Faulty proteins can cause cell malfunction, disease, and death.

Scientists are studying genes to learn more about the proteins they make and what these proteins actually do in the body. They also hope to discover what illnesses are caused when proteins don't work right.

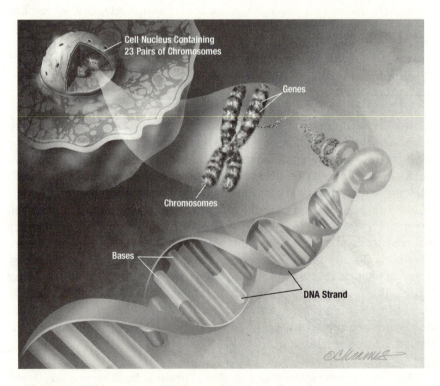

Figure 5.1. Chromosomes, housed in the cell nucleus, carry genes.

The Genetics of Alzheimer Disease

Diseases such as cystic fibrosis, muscular dystrophy, and Huntington disease are single-gene disorders. If a person inherits the gene that causes one of these disorders, he or she will usually get the disease. AD, on the other hand, is not caused by a single gene. More than one gene mutation can cause AD, and genes on multiple chromosomes are involved.

The two basic types of AD are familial and sporadic. Familial AD (FAD) is a rare form of AD, affecting less than 10 percent of AD patients. All FAD is early-onset, meaning the disease develops before age 65. It is caused by gene mutations on chromosomes 1, 14, and 21. Even if one of these mutated genes is inherited from a parent, the person will almost always develop early-onset AD. This inheritance pattern is referred to as autosomal dominant inheritance. In other words, all offspring in the same generation have a 50/50 chance of developing FAD if one of their parents had it.

Genes in Late-Onset Disease

The majority of AD cases are late-onset, usually developing after age 65. Late-onset AD has no known cause and shows no obvious inheritance pattern. However, in some families, clusters of cases are seen. Although a specific gene has not been identified as the cause of late-onset AD, genetic factors do appear to play a role in the development of this form of AD. Only one risk factor gene has been identified so far.

Researchers have identified an increased risk of developing late-onset AD related to the apolipoprotein E gene found on chromosome 19. This gene codes for a protein that helps carry cholesterol in the bloodstream. The APOE gene comes in several different forms, or alleles, but three occur most frequently: APOE ε2, APOE ε3, and APOE ε4.

People inherit one APOE allele from each parent. Having one or two copies of the ε4 allele increases a person's risk of getting AD. That is, having the ε4 allele is a risk factor for AD, but it does not mean that AD is certain. Some people with two copies of the ε4 allele (the highest risk group) do not develop clinical signs of Alzheimer disease, while others with no ε4s do. The ε3 allele is the most common form found in the general population and may play a neutral role in AD. The rarer ε2 allele appears to be associated with a lower risk of AD. The exact degree of risk of AD for any given person cannot be determined based on APOE status. Therefore, the APOE ε4 gene is called a risk factor gene for late-onset AD.

Scientists are looking for genetic risk factors for late-onset AD on other chromosomes as well. They think that additional risk factor genes may lie on regions of chromosomes 9, 10, and 12.

The National Institute on Aging (NIA) has launched a major study to discover remaining genetic risk factors for late-onset AD. Geneticists from the NIA's Alzheimer's Disease Centers are working to collect genetic samples from families affected by multiple cases of late-onset AD. Researchers are seeking large families with two or more living relatives with late-onset AD. Families interested in participating in this study can contact the National Cell Repository for Alzheimer's Disease at 800-526-2839. Information may also be requested through their website, http://ncrad.iu.edu.

ApoE Testing in Research or Diagnosis

A blood test is available that can identify which APOE alleles a person has. However, because the APOE ε4 gene is only a risk factor for AD, this blood test cannot tell whether a person will develop AD or not. Instead of a yes or no answer, the best information a person can get from this genetic test for APOE is maybe or maybe not. Although some people want to know whether they will get AD later in life, this type of prediction is not yet possible. In fact, some researchers believe that screening measures may never be able to predict AD with 100 percent accuracy.

In a research setting, APOE testing may be used to identify study volunteers who may be at a higher risk of getting AD. In this way, researchers can look for early brain changes in some patients. This test also helps researchers compare the effectiveness of treatments for patients with different APOE profiles. Most researchers believe that the APOE test is useful for studying AD risk in large groups of people but not for determining one person's individual risk. Predictive screening in otherwise healthy people will be useful if an accurate/reliable test is developed and effective ways to treat or prevent AD are available.

In diagnosing AD, APOE testing is not a common practice. The only definite way to diagnose AD is by viewing a sample of a person's brain tissue under a microscope to determine if there are plaques and tangles present. This is usually done after the person dies. However, through a complete medical evaluation (including a medical history, laboratory tests, neuropsychological tests, and brain scans), well-trained doctors can diagnose AD correctly up to 90 percent of the time. Doctors look to rule out other diseases and disorders that can cause the same symptoms of AD. If no other cause is identified, a person is said to have "probable" or "possible" AD. In some cases, APOE testing may be used in combination with these other medical tests to strengthen the diagnosis of a suspected case of AD. Currently, there is no medical test to establish if a person without the symptoms of AD is going to develop the disease. APOE testing as a patient screening (predictive) method is not recommended.

Concerns about Confidentiality

APOE testing, and indeed all genetic testing, raises ethical, legal, and social questions for which we have few answers. Generally, confidentiality laws protect APOE information gathered for research purposes. On the other hand, information obtained in APOE testing may not remain confidential if it becomes part of a person's medical records. Thereafter, employers, insurance companies, and other health care organizations could find out this information, and discrimination could result. For example, employment opportunities or insurance premiums could be affected.

Genetic Counseling

Depending on the study, research volunteers may occasionally have the opportunity to learn the results of their APOE testing. The meaning of these results is complex. Since the results of APOE testing can be hard to understand, and more importantly, devastating to those tested, the NIA and the Alzheimer's Association recommend that research volunteers and their families receive genetic counseling before and after testing, if they have the option of learning the results.

People who learn through testing that they have an increased risk of getting AD may experience emotional distress and depression about the future, because there is not yet an effective way to prevent or cure the disease. Through counseling, families can learn about the genetics of AD, the tests themselves, and possible meanings of the results. Due to privacy, emotional, and health care issues, the primary goal of genetic counseling is to help people explore and cope with the potential consequences of such knowledge.

The National Society for Genetic Counselors (NSGC) can provide a list of genetic counselors in your area, as well as information about creating a family history. Search their online database at www.nsgc .org/consumer. The NSGC does not provide information about specific genetic disorders.

Experts still do not know how limited information about AD risk can benefit people. Among the issues are privacy and confidentiality policies related to genetic information and AD, and the small number of genetic counselors now trained in neurodegenerative disorders. In addition, little is known about how stigma associated with an increased risk for AD may affect people's families and their lives.

Research Questions

Learning more about the role of APOE ε4 and other risk factor genes in the development of AD may help scientists identify who would benefit from prevention and treatment efforts. Age, still the most important known risk factor for AD, continues to be associated with the disease even when no known genetic factors are present. Research focusing on advancing age may help explain the role that other genes play in most AD cases. Many AD researchers are studying the genetics of AD. In addition, researchers, ethicists, and health care providers are developing policies about the appropriate use of genetic testing and counseling for AD.

Chapter 6

Can Alzheimer Disease Be Prevented?

These days, it seems that newspapers, magazines, and TV are full of stories about ways to stay healthy, eat right, and keep fit. Lots of people are concerned about staying healthy as they get older. They wonder whether they can do anything to prevent diseases that happen more often with age, such as Alzheimer disease (AD).

AD has no known cure, and the secrets to preventing it are not yet known. But research supported by the National Institute on Aging (NIA) and other public and private agencies offers tantalizing clues about the origins and development of AD. These findings are raising hopes that someday it might be possible to delay the onset of AD, slow its progress, or even prevent it altogether. Delaying by even five years the time when AD symptoms begin could greatly reduce the number of people who have the disease.

Preventing a Complex Disease Like AD Is a Challenge

Many diseases, such as diabetes, heart disease, and arthritis, are complex. They develop when genetic, environmental, and lifestyle factors work together to cause a disease process to start and then progress. The importance of these factors may differ for each person. AD is one of these complex diseases. It develops over many years, and it appears to be affected by a number of factors that may increase or decrease a

"Genes, Lifestyles, and Crossword Puzzles: Can Alzheimer's Disease Be Prevented?" National Institute on Aging, NIH Pub. No. 06-5503, June 2006.

person's risk of developing the disease. We don't have control over some of the risk factors for AD. We can do something about other possible AD risk factors, though. The effect on any particular person of risk factor changes will likely depend on his or her genetic makeup, environment, and lifestyle.

AD Risk Factors We Can't Control

Age is the most important known risk factor for AD. The risk of developing the disease doubles every five years over age 65. Several studies estimate that up to half the people older than 85 have AD. These facts are significant because of the growing number of people 65 and older. More than 34 million Americans are now 65 or older. Even more significant, the group with the highest risk of AD—those older than 85—is the fastest growing population group in the country.

Genetics is the other known AD risk factor that a person can't control. Scientists have found genetic links to the two forms of AD. Early-onset AD is a very rare form of the disease that can occur in people between the ages of 30 and 65. In the 1980s and early 1990s, researchers found that mutations (or changes) in certain genes on three chromosomes cause early-onset AD. If a parent has any of these genetic mutations, his or her child has a 50-50 chance of inheriting the mutant gene and developing early-onset AD.

Late-onset AD, the more common form, develops after age 65. In 1992, researchers found that certain forms of the apolipoprotein E (ApoE) gene can influence AD risk:

- ApoE ε2, a rarely occurring form, may provide some protection;

- ApoE ε3, the most common form, plays a neutral role; and

- ApoE ε4, which is found in about 40 percent of people with AD; ApoE ε4 lowers the age of onset and thus increases risk. (Having this gene form does not mean that a person will definitely develop AD; it only increases risk. Many people who develop AD do not have the ApoE ε4 form.)

Researchers are now intensively searching for other risk factor genes that may be linked to late-onset AD. Discovering these genes is essential for understanding the very early biological steps leading to AD and for pinpointing targets for drug development and other prevention or treatment strategies. It's also critical for developing better ways to identify people at risk and determining how AD risk factor genes may interact with other genes or with lifestyle or environmental factors to affect AD risk in any one individual.

In 2003, the National Institute of Aging (NIA) announced a major expansion of AD genetics research efforts. The AD Genetics Study is collecting genetic material from individuals in families with two or more living brothers or sisters who have late-onset AD. This valuable resource will allow geneticists to speed up the discovery of additional AD risk factor genes.

The Search for AD Prevention Strategies

Though we can't do much about our age or genetic profile, recent research suggests that maintaining good overall health habits may help lower the chances of developing several serious diseases, including ones affecting the brain. This chapter describes a number of health, lifestyle, and environmental factors that could make a difference in AD and that are being actively studied by scientists.

Many of these potential factors have been identified in observational and animal studies. At present, they are only associated with changes in AD risk. Only further research, including clinical trials, will reveal whether, in fact, these factors can help to prevent AD. It is important to understand that the degree to which a person might be helped by any of these factors may be very slight, especially if the person has inherited a bad form of a risk factor gene. That is why it is so important to also focus on other parts of the AD prevention research mission. At the same time that scientists are examining lifestyle factors, many others are developing drugs that can enhance protective biochemical pathways or block pathways that lead to cognitive decline and AD.

Investigating Heart Disease Risk

High levels of blood cholesterol are a known risk factor for heart disease. In recent years, basic research in laboratories as well as population and animal studies have suggested there may also be a connection between high levels of blood cholesterol and development of AD. These findings led scientists to wonder whether drugs that lower blood cholesterol might also lower the risk of developing AD or reduce its rate of progression. Recent population and animal studies have raised the possibility that statins, the most commonly prescribed cholesterol lowering drugs, may reduce the risk of dementia. Other studies, though, have found no association between statins and dementia risk. Thus, it is not clear at this time whether statins affect the onset or progression of AD. To help answer this question, the NIA is currently funding a clinical trial to determine whether one particular statin slows the progression of AD.

Other research has found that a high level of the amino acid homocysteine is associated with an increased risk of developing AD. High levels of homocysteine are known to increase heart disease risk, and NIA studies in mice have shown that high levels of this amino acid can make neurons stop working and die. The relationship between AD risk and homocysteine levels is particularly appealing because blood levels of homocysteine can be reduced by increasing intake of folic acid and vitamins B_6 and B_{12}. An NIA-funded clinical trial is currently studying whether reducing homocysteine levels with folic acid and vitamin B_6 and B_{12} supplements will slow the rate of cognitive decline in older adults with AD.

Examining High Blood Pressure

Scientists also have found associations among AD, high blood pressure that begins in midlife, and other risk factors of stroke, such as age, diabetes, and cardiovascular disease. It is known that even in relatively healthy older adults, high blood pressure and other stroke risk factors can damage blood vessels in the brain and reduce the brain's oxygen supply. This damage may disrupt nerve cell circuits that are thought to be important to decision-making, memory, and verbal skills. Scientists are studying the connections between AD and high blood pressure in hopes that knowledge gained will provide new insights into both conditions.

Learning about Diabetes and Insulin Resistance

Large-scale population studies suggest that diabetes is associated with several types of dementia, including AD and vascular dementia (a type of dementia associated with strokes, sometimes referred to as multi-infarct dementia). These studies have found that AD and type 2 diabetes share several characteristics, including increasing prevalence with age, genetic predisposition, and deposits of two different kinds of damaging amyloid protein (in the brain for AD and in the pancreas for type 2 diabetes). Abnormal glucose (a type of sugar) regulation, a key element of diabetes, also has been associated with development of AD. Scientists are working to learn more about this association.

Researchers also are becoming increasingly interested in the possible role of insulin resistance (a condition in which the body produces insulin but cells do not use it properly) in AD. Too much insulin in the blood (which happens as a result of insulin resistance) may encourage inflammation and oxidative stress, both of which contribute to the damage seen in AD.

Possible relationships between cognitive decline, AD, and diabetes are being explored in the Religious Orders Study, which involves a large group of older priests, nuns, and brothers who have been working with scientists funded by the NIA since 1993. This study has provided a wealth of information about many aspects of AD, including the possible link between diabetes and cognitive decline and AD. In one analysis involving more than 800 study participants, researchers examined tests of five "cognitive systems" involved with word and event memory, information processing speed, and the ability to recognize spatial patterns. They found that diabetes was associated with declines in some cognitive systems but not others. The researchers also found a link between those with diabetes and an increased risk of developing AD.

The NIA is funding several clinical trials to determine whether treating different aspects of diabetes might affect AD development or progression. For example, the NIA is supporting clinical trials to evaluate the effect of a drug called rosiglitazone on changes in cognitive abilities in people with mild cognitive impairment (MCI, a condition in which a person has memory problems but not other AD problems; this condition often progresses to AD). Rosiglitazone makes cells more sensitive to insulin. The NIA is also supporting a study that is evaluating cognitive and brain structure changes using magnetic resonance imaging (MRI). This study, called ACCORD-MIND (Memory in Diabetes) has been added to the ongoing National Heart, Lung, and Blood Institute ACCORD (Action to Control Cardiovascular Risk in Diabetes) clinical trial. ACCORD is evaluating a variety of approaches for managing glucose, blood pressure, and blood lipids.

Examining Social Engagement and Intellectually Stimulating Activities

Findings from studies of animals, nursing home residents, and older people living in the community have suggested a link between social engagement and cognitive abilities. Having lots of friends and acquaintances and participating in many social activities is associated with reduced cognitive decline and decreased risk of dementia in older adults. In the NIA-funded Chicago Health and Aging Project, a high level of social engagement was associated with a significant reduction in cognitive decline.

Studies also have shown that keeping the brain active is associated with reduced AD risk. In the Religious Orders Study, for example, investigators periodically asked more than 700 participants to describe the amount of time they spent in seven activities that involve significant information processing. These activities included listening to the radio, reading newspapers, playing puzzle games, and going to museums. After following the participants for 4 years, investigators found that the risk of developing AD was 47 percent lower, on average, for those who did the activities most frequently than for those who did them least frequently. Other studies have shown similar results. In addition, a growing body of research, including other findings from the Religious Orders Study, suggests that, even in the presence of AD plaques, the more formal education a person has, the better his or her memory and learning ability.

Another NIA-funded study also supports the value of lifelong learning and mentally stimulating activity. In this study of healthy older people and people with possible or probable AD, scientists found that during their early and middle adulthood, the healthy older people had engaged in more mentally stimulating activities and spent more hours doing them than did those who ultimately developed AD.

The reasons for these findings aren't entirely clear, but scientists have come up with four possibilities:

- These activities may protect the brain in some way, perhaps by establishing a "cognitive reserve."

- Perhaps these activities help the brain become more adaptable and flexible in some areas of mental function so that it can compensate for declines in other areas.

- Less engagement with other people or in intellectually stimulating activities could be the result of very early effects of the disease rather than its cause.

- Perhaps people who engage in these activities have other lifestyle features that may protect them against developing AD.

The only way to really evaluate some of these possibilities is by testing them in a controlled way in a clinical trial.

Several clinical trials have directly examined whether memory training and similar types of mental skills training can actually improve the cognitive abilities of healthy older adults and people with mild AD. In the Advanced Cognitive Training for Independent and Vital Elderly (ACTIVE) trial, certified trainers provided 10 sessions of memory training, reasoning training, or speed of processing training to healthy adults 65 years old and older. The sessions improved participants' mental skills in the area in which they were trained. Even better, these improvements persisted for at least two years after the training was completed. In another study, 25 participants with mild AD worked with researchers to learn how to improve their ability to carry out various tasks, such as how to put names and faces together, recall the names of objects, and pay bills correctly. Compared to another group with mild AD who received more generic mental stimulation activities, people in the "cognitive rehabilitation" group improved their abilities more, and their abilities were still improved three months later.

Investigating Physical Activity

Accumulating evidence suggests that being physically active may benefit more than just our hearts and waistlines. Research in older animals has shown that both physical and mental function improve with aerobic fitness. Two studies in aging adults have shown similar results. The first study used magnetic resonance imaging (MRI) to measure changes in brain activity in healthy adults aged 58–78 before and after a 6-month program of brisk walking. The researchers found that improvements in the participants' cardiovascular fitness were associated with increased functioning in certain regions of the brain. Compared to a physically inactive group, the walkers were able to pay attention better and focus more clearly on goals while disregarding unimportant information.

In a second study, investigators studied the relationship of physical activity and mental function in nearly 6,000 healthy women 65 years old and older over a period of up to eight years. The investigators found that the women who were more physically active were less likely to experience a decline in their mental function than were inactive women. The NIA is currently funding several clinical trials that are studying the effects of physical activity programs on the cognitive abilities and brain function of healthy older adults and older adults with MCI.

Scientists have speculated about why physical activity may help our brains as much as our bodies. It may be that physical activity improves blood flow to the brain so that it responds better to a task.

Or, it may activate cellular mechanisms that improve brain function. However, we still don't know whether physical activity can actually prevent cognitive decline or postpone the development of AD, especially in people with a high genetic risk.

Examining Nonsteroidal Anti-Inflammatory Drugs (NSAIDs)

Inflammation of tissues in the brain is a common feature of AD, but it is not clear whether it is a cause or effect of the disease. Some population studies suggest an association between a reduced risk of AD and commonly used NSAIDs, such as ibuprofen, naproxen, and indomethacin.

Clinical trials thus far have not demonstrated a benefit for AD from these drugs or from the newer cyclooxygenase-2 (COX-2) inhibitors, such as rofecoxib and celecoxib. A trial testing whether naproxen or celecoxib could prevent AD in healthy older people at risk of the disease has been halted, but investigators are continuing to conduct followup examinations with participants and to examine data about cognitive changes and possible cardiovascular risk. Scientists continue to look for ways to test how anti-inflammatory drugs targeting particular pathways might affect the development or progression of AD.

Learning about Antioxidants and Other Interventions

Another promising area of research focuses on highly active molecules called free radicals. Damage from these free radicals during aging can build up in nerve cells and result in a loss of cell function, which could contribute to AD. Some population and laboratory studies suggest that antioxidants from dietary supplements or food may provide some protection against this damage (called oxidative damage), but other studies show no effect. Clinical trials may provide some answers. Several trials are investigating whether two antioxidants—vitamins E and C—can slow cognitive decline and development of AD in healthy older individuals. The NIA is conducting a clinical trial that will examine whether taking vitamin E or selenium supplements over a period of 7 to 12 years can help prevent memory loss and dementia. This trial has been added on to a prostate cancer prevention clinical trial funded by the National Cancer Institute. The NIA is also conducting a clinical trial to determine whether antioxidant supplements can prevent cognitive decline in healthy older women or older women at increased risk of dementia.

Another just-completed study focused on the use of vitamin E supplements in people with MCI. This NIA study, the Memory Impairment Study, compared donepezil (Aricept), vitamin E supplements, or placebo (an inactive substance) in participants with MCI to see whether the drugs might delay or prevent progression to AD. The study found that taking the vitamin E had no effect on progression to AD at any time in the study when compared with placebo. It may be that this antioxidant may not help after memory declines have already started. Donepezil, however, did seem to delay progression to AD over the first year of treatment. Interestingly, there seemed to be an interaction between the genetic makeup of participants and their response to treatment: People carrying the risk factor ApoE ε4 allele delayed the risk of developing AD for the three years of the trial. Scientists caution, however, that people with MCI should not be tested to see whether they carry the ApoE ε4 allele because more research is still needed to understand how the drug works in the body and to answer other questions.

Expanding Knowledge about Estrogen

This hormone is produced by a woman's ovaries during her childbearing years. After this time, estrogen production declines dramatically. Over the past 25 years, some laboratory and animal research, as well as observational studies in women, have suggested that estrogen used by women to treat the symptoms of menopause also protects the brain. Experts have wondered whether using estrogen could reduce the risk of AD or slow disease progression.

A number of clinical trials have shown that estrogen does not slow the progression of already-diagnosed AD. Clinical trials testing whether estrogen might prevent AD in women who have already gone through menopause have also found that using estrogen to treat or prevent AD may not be effective, if treatment is begun in later life. A large trial found that women older than 65 who took estrogen (Premarin) alone or estrogen with a synthetic progestin were actually at increased risk of developing dementia, including AD. Some questions remain unanswered, however, such as whether some forms of estrogen might help if started somewhat earlier than the older ages tested in this trial. These questions are now being investigated.

Researchers also are trying other ways to work with estrogen's potentially positive effects for the brain. For example, scientists have developed estrogen-like molecules called SERMs (selective estrogen-receptor modulators) that protect against bone loss and other consequences of estrogen levels falling after menopause. These molecules may retain estrogen's neuron-protecting ability but may not have some of its other harmful effects on the body. A large clinical trial tested a SERM called raloxifene, which is used in the prevention and treatment of osteoporosis. The study showed that this SERM lowered the risk of MCI among a group of postmenopausal women with osteoporosis. A newly funded clinical trial is ongoing to test whether raloxifene can slow the rate of AD progression.

Investigating Ginkgo Biloba

This readily available natural product has been proposed as a potential treatment or preventive agent for AD. A 1997 study in the U.S. suggested that a ginkgo extract may be of some help in treating the symptoms of AD and multi-infarct dementia, but no evidence exists that ginkgo biloba will prevent AD. At the National Institute of Health (NIH), the National Center for Complementary and Alternative Medicine and the NIA are currently supporting a large clinical trial to explore whether ginkgo has any effect on preventing AD or delaying cognitive decline in older adults.

Exploring Immunization

Will a vaccine someday prevent AD? Early vaccine studies in mice were so successful in reducing deposits of beta-amyloid (the major component of the plaques that develop in the brains of people with AD) and improving brain performance on memory tests that investigators conducted preliminary clinical trials in humans with AD. These studies had to be stopped because of life-threatening inflammation that occurred in some participants. However, the pharmaceutical industry and NIH-funded scientists are continuing to refine this strategy in animal models of AD, hoping to find ways of maintaining the therapeutic effects while reducing the unwanted side effects. Several pharmaceutical companies have recently obtained permission from the Food and Drug Administration (FDA) to test several of these new strategies for safety in early stage clinical trials.

The Search for Other Clues That May Contribute to Prevention Strategies

Investigators are pursuing still other strategies that may eventually help to prevent or delay AD. For example, they are trying to discover whether changes in certain biological compounds in blood, urine, or cerebrospinal fluid could indicate early AD changes in the brain. Understanding more about these biological markers, how they work, and what causes their levels to change is important in helping scientists answer questions about what makes AD begin and develop. Learning more about these markers also may help scientists track whether certain medications are having their intended effects and may some day lead to new prevention strategies.

One major effort involves the use of imaging techniques, such as MRI and positron emission tomography (PET), to measure brain structure and function. An NIA public-private partnership—the AD Neuroimaging Initiative—is a large study that will determine whether MRI and PET scans or other imaging or biological markers can be used to identify early AD changes and disease progression. One day, these measurements may be able to identify those people who are at risk of AD before they develop symptoms. The measurements may also help physicians assess the response to treatment much more rapidly and less expensively than is possible today.

What Can You Do?

Our knowledge is growing rapidly as scientists expand their understanding of the many factors involved in the development of AD. Even though no treatments, drugs, or pills have yet been proven to prevent AD or even delay its development, people can take some actions that might reduce the effect of possible AD risk factors. These actions include:

- lowering cholesterol and homocysteine levels
- lowering high blood pressure levels
- controlling diabetes
- exercising regularly
- engaging in social and intellectually stimulating activities

All of these strategies are good to do anyway because they lower risk of other diseases and help maintain and improve overall health and well-being. However, it is important to remember that pursuing any of these strategies will not necessarily prevent or delay AD in any one individual. Even if the strategies were eventually proven to be effective, they might not offset a person's individual genetic and other risk factors enough to prevent AD from developing.

Another important action a person can take is to volunteer for the Genetics Study, the Neuroimaging Initiative, or an AD clinical trial. People who participate in these studies say that the biggest benefit is having regular contact with experts on AD who have lots of practical experience and a broad perspective on the disease. They also feel they are making a valuable contribution to future knowledge that will help scientists, people with AD, and their families. Families interested in participating in the Genetics Study can call the National Cell Repository for Alzheimer's Disease (NCRAD) toll-free at 800-526-2839. Information may also be requested through its website at http://ncrad .iu.edu. People who are interested in joining the Neuroimaging Initiative or an AD clinical trial should contact the ADEAR Center at www.alzheimers.nia.nih.gov, or call the ADEAR Center toll-free at 800-438-4380 for a referral to the nearest participating study site.

A Final Word of Caution

Because AD is such a devastating disease, caregivers and patients may be tempted by untried, unproven, and unscientific cures, supplements, or prevention strategies. Before trying pills or anything else that promises to prevent AD, people should check with their doctor first. These purchases might be unsafe or a waste of money. They might even interfere with other medical treatments that have been prescribed.

For More Information

Becoming well informed is another important thing that people can do to protect their health. Thousands of internet websites provide health-related information, including information on AD. Some of the information on these websites is reliable, but some is not. Health websites sponsored by the Federal Government are good sources of information, as are websites of large professional organizations and well-known medical schools.

Chapter 7

Stages of Alzheimer Disease

The Progression of Alzheimer Disease: Introduction

Alzheimer disease is a progressive, degenerative disease that destroys vital brain cells. As each area of the brain is affected, certain functions or abilities can be lost. The losses affect the individual's ability to think, to remember, to understand, and to make decisions. In addition to affecting a person's mental abilities, Alzheimer disease affects moods and emotions. Along with loss of abilities, changes in behavior occur. Gradually, independence disappears.

Duration of the Disease

The progression of Alzheimer disease varies from person to person and can span three to 20 years (the average length of the disease is between eight and 12 years[1]). The progression can be described as a series of stages, providing a guide to the pattern of the disease, which can help when making care decisions.

One staging system explains the disease in three stages: early, middle, and late. Another staging system, often used by medical professionals, is the Global Deterioration Scale (also called the Reisberg Scale[2]). This scale divides the disease into seven stages.

This chapter includes "The Progression of Alzheimer's Disease: Introduction," "The Progression of Alzheimer's Disease: The Three Stages," and "The Progression of Alzheimer's Disease: Global Deterioration Scale (GDS)," © 2005 Alzheimer Society of Canada (www.alzheimer.ca); reprinted with permission.

79

Whichever staging system is used, or if none is used, it's important to remember that the disease affects each person differently. The order in which the symptoms appear and the length of each stage will vary from person to person. There is no clear line when one stage ends and another begins. In many cases, stages will overlap. Some people experience many of the symptoms in each stage, while others experience only a few. There may be fluctuations from day to day with a person appearing more confused one day, for example, and less so another.

The Three Stages

Early Stage

A person in this stage will usually be aware of the diagnosis and will be able to participate in decisions affecting future care.

Symptoms can include mild forgetfulness and communication difficulties, such as finding the right word and following a conversation. Some people stay involved in activities while others become passive or withdrawn. The individual may also be frustrated by changing abilities and may become depressed or anxious. It is important to monitor the emotional well-being of the person.

Table 7.1. Early Stage Symptoms

Abilities Affected	Typical Symptoms
Mental Abilities	Mild forgetfulness; difficulty learning new things and following conversations; difficulty concentrating or limited attention span: problems with orientation, such as getting lost or not following directions; communication difficulties such as finding the right word
Moods and Emotions	mood shifts; depression
Behaviors	passiveness; withdrawal from usual activities; restlessness
Physical Abilities	mild coordination problems

Middle Stage

This stage brings a further decline in the person's mental and physical abilities. Memory will continue to deteriorate as the person forgets personal history and no longer recognizes family and friends. Increased confusion and disorientation to time and place will result in requiring assistance in many daily tasks, such as dressing, bathing, and using the toilet.

In this stage, some people become restless and pace or wander. Registering the person with the Safely Home™—Alzheimer Wandering Registry program will provide peace of mind should she become lost. You can register for this program through your local Alzheimer Society (visit http://www.alzheimer.ca for information).

In response to the loss of abilities, a person may react in a number of ways. For example, he or she may become less involved in activities or repeat the same action or word over and over again. It can be helpful to understand more about the disease and develop strategies to deal with these situations. Your local Alzheimer Society can provide education, resources, and support.

Table 7.2. Middle Stage Symptoms

Abilities Affected	Typical Symptoms
Mental Abilities	continued memory problems; forgetfulness about personal history; inability to recognize friends and family; disorientation about time and place
Moods and Emotions	personality change; confusion; anxiety/apprehension; suspiciousness; mood shifts; anger; sadness/depression; hostility
Behaviors	declining ability to concentrate; restlessness (pacing, wandering); repetition; delusions; aggression; uninhibited behavior; passiveness
Physical Abilities	assistance required for daily tasks (for example, dressing, bathing, using the toilet); disrupted sleep patterns; appetite fluctuations; language difficulties; visual spatial problems

Late Stage

In this last stage, the person becomes unable to remember, communicate, or look after herself. Care is required 24 hours a day. Eventually, the person will become bed-ridden, have difficulty eating or swallowing, and lose control of bodily functions. This stage eventually ends with the person's death, often from secondary complications such as pneumonia.

Table 7.3. Late Stage Symptoms

Abilities Affected	Typical Symptoms
Mental Abilities	loss of ability to remember, communicate, or function; inability to process information; severe speaking difficulties; severe disorientation about time, place, and people
Moods and Emotions	possible withdrawal
Behaviors	non-verbal methods of communicating (eye contact, crying, groaning)
Physical Abilities	sleeps longer and more often; becomes immobile (bed-ridden); loses ability to speak; loses control of bladder and bowels; has difficulty eating and/or swallowing; unable to dress or bathe; may lose weight

Global Deterioration Scale (GDS)

Some health-care professionals use the Global Deterioration Scale, also called the Reisberg Scale, to measure progression of Alzheimer disease. This scale divides Alzheimer disease into seven stages of decreasing ability.

Stage 1: No Cognitive Decline

- Experiences no problems in daily living.

Stage 2: Very Mild Cognitive Decline

- Forgets names and locations of objects.
- May have trouble finding words.

Stage 3: Mild Cognitive Decline

- Has difficulty traveling to new locations.
- Has difficulty handling problems at work.

Stage 4: Moderate Cognitive Decline

- Has difficulty with complex tasks (finances, shopping, planning dinner for guests).

Stage 5: Moderately Severe Cognitive Decline

- Needs help to choose clothing.

- Needs prompting to bathe.

Stage 6: Severe Cognitive Decline

- Needs help putting on clothing.
- Requires assistance bathing; may have a fear of bathing.
- Has decreased ability to use the toilet or is incontinent.

Stage 7: Very Severe Cognitive Decline

- Vocabulary becomes limited, eventually declining to single words.
- Loses ability to walk and sit.
- Becomes unable to smile.

Footnotes:

1. *The Canadian Journal of Neurological Sciences Supplement*; Canadian Consensus Conference on Dementia, Volume 28 (Supplement 1), February 2001, p. S22.

2. Reisberg, B., Ferris, S.H., de Leon, M.J., and Crook, T., *American Journal of Psychiatry*, 139:1136–1139, 1982.

Chapter 8

Can the Progression of Alzheimer Disease Be Slowed?

What Can be Done to Slow the Progression of Alzheimer Disease or Lessen its Effects?

Research advances have vastly increased our understanding of brain function, the transformation from healthy aging to Alzheimer disease (AD), and the factors that influence the development of AD. These findings have opened doors to a range of potential therapeutic approaches being investigated in various ways by the National Institute of Aging (NIA), other National Institute of Health (NIH) Institutes, other research institutions, and private industry. Studies are underway on dozens of compounds and strategies to help people with AD maintain cognitive function over the short-term; treat AD-associated behavioral and neuropsychiatric symptoms; slow the progression of the disease; and prevent AD.

AD research has progressed to a point where scientists are increasingly able to think about how they can intervene to treat AD or perhaps even to prevent it. They think about the importance of timing—when is it best to intervene and what interventions are most appropriate at what time? For example, a physician would certainly provide different treatments to a patient who is having a stroke than to a patient who

Excerpted from "Progress Report on Alzheimer's Disease: New Discoveries, New Insights," National Institute on Aging (NIA), 2005. Text under the heading "Lifestyle Modifications" was excerpted from "Progress Report on Alzheimer's Disease: Journey to Discovery," NIA, 2007.

is seemingly healthy but at higher risk of having a stroke at some point in the future. AD develops over the course of years or decades, and a person's brain is affected well before any symptoms are evident. It may be that one kind of intervention with a particular compound or approach may be most effective if it is applied well before any symptoms are evident. Other interventions may be most appropriate for use after AD is established.

Investigators are working to develop an array of options from which clinicians can choose. For example, developing new and better drugs and broadening the range of non-drug therapeutic approaches are critically important for those who already have AD because of the long-term nature of the disease and its high emotional and physical toll. Slowing the progress of the disease and alleviating psychiatric and behavioral problems could do much to delay or prevent institutionalization, maintain the dignity of people with AD, reduce physical and emotional stress on caregivers, and reduce the financial costs associated with the disease. Finding ways to prevent the disease altogether is an increasingly urgent priority because of the enormous impact of AD on our society. Scientists use clinical trials to pursue all of these goals.

Clinical Trials

Clinical trials, which compare a potential new treatment with a standard treatment or with a placebo, are the only way to determine whether a drug, other compound, or non-drug approach is effective. These complex and expensive studies involve hundreds or even thousands of people and are often conducted over a long period of time. Some clinical trials are focused on treatment strategies—helping people with AD preserve cognitive function for as long as possible, for example, or helping people with behavioral or psychiatric problems associated with AD. Other clinical trials are focused on prevention strategies—using specific compounds to help people reduce the risk of developing AD in the future. The sections that follow describe some of NIH's AD treatment and prevention clinical trials. Recruitment is ongoing for a number of these trials.

AD Treatment Clinical Trials

The NIH is currently supporting clinical trials of treatments for people who already have AD. Many of these are conducted as part of the Alzheimer's Disease Cooperative Study (ADCS), an NIA-supported national consortium of more than 50 research sites that conduct clinical trials for both cognitive and behavioral symptoms of AD. Here are highlights of just a few of these trials.

Divalproex sodium and agitation: An ADCS clinical trial of divalproex sodium (Valproate), conducted among 150 nursing home residents, was designed to see whether this medication could ease agitation in people with severe AD. A second trial that has recently begun will examine whether divalproex sodium can delay or prevent agitation and psychosis in individuals with mild to moderate AD. Researchers are also interested in seeing whether its possible neuroprotective properties have any effect on slowing the rate of cognitive decline.

Simvastatin and AD progression: This ADCS trial, which began in 2003, is testing whether simvastatin (Zocor), a commonly prescribed cholesterol-lowering drug, can safely and effectively slow the rate of disease progression in people with mild to moderate AD. Data from epidemiologic and animal studies indicate that high cholesterol levels increase the risk of AD and that statin drugs specifically may help reduce this risk. The trial, which is being conducted in about 40 sites nationwide, will enroll 400 participants. Some participants will receive 20 mg of simvastatin for six weeks and then 40 mg of the statin for the rest of the study period. Others will receive a placebo during the entire study. Clinical trial staff are tracking changes in participants' cognitive health by measuring a number of indicators, including mental status, functional ability, behavioral disturbances, and quality of life.

Huperzine A and cognitive function: This ADCS trial is evaluating whether huperzine A, a natural cholinesterase inhibitor derived from the Chinese herb, *Huperzia serrata*, can slow the progression of cognitive decline in people with mild to moderate AD. A number of small, randomized controlled trials in China have indicated that people with AD who were treated with huperzine performed better on memory tests than those on placebo. Investigators also are interested in huperzine because it has antioxidant and neuroprotective properties that suggest it may be useful in treating AD. Participants will be randomly assigned to three equal groups—two groups will receive varying amounts of huperzine A every day and the third group will receive a placebo. All participants will receive huperzine A during the last eight weeks of the 24-week trial.

Supplements to reduce homocysteine and slow the rate of cognitive decline: High homocysteine levels are associated with increased

AD risk. Levels of this amino acid can be reduced by high-dose supplements of folate and vitamins B_6 and B_{12}. This ADCS clinical trial is designed to determine whether reduction of homocysteine levels with high-dose supplements of folate, vitamin B_6, and vitamin B_{12} will slow the rate of cognitive decline in older adults with AD. Participants in this clinical trial were divided into two groups: 60 percent of participants will receive daily high-dose supplements (5 mg of folate, 25 mg of vitamin B_6, 1 mg of vitamin B_{12}) and 40 percent will receive a placebo.

AD Pilot Treatment Trials

Before beginning a full-scale clinical trial, NIH Institutes often conduct pilot clinical trials to collect initial data on the safety, effectiveness, and best dosage of a potential treatment. These data help the Institutes determine which interventions should go to the next step. Here are highlights of a few current pilot clinical trials in AD:

Combination vitamin supplement in the treatment of AD in Down syndrome: This high-potency supplement consists of two cellular antioxidants (vitamins E and C) and a mitochondrial antioxidant (alpha-lipoic acid). The aims of this 24-month intervention trial are to determine whether cognitive function improves with antioxidant supplementation and to determine its safety and tolerability.

Nicotine skin patch and amnestic MCI: Some of the 60 participants in this study will be given the nicotine patch and others a placebo patch. Research has suggested that one of the causes of memory disorders may be a reduction in the neurotransmitter acetylcholine. Acetylcholine is critically important in the process of forming memories, and nicotine imitates many of the actions of acetylcholine. Preliminary studies have suggested that short-term administration of nicotine appears to improve memory in patients with mild memory loss and early AD. Furthermore, nicotine administration appears to have significant neuroprotective effects, and it may have positive influences on APP processing. The primary goal of this pilot trial is to demonstrate whether the nicotine patch is safe to administer to the nonsmoking amnestic MCI participants over a 1-year period. Study investigators also hope to determine whether nicotine can improve memory loss symptoms over the longer term and whether it can help delay the progression of memory loss symptoms.

Rosiglitazone and amnestic mild cognitive impairment (MCI): This clinical trial will test whether rosiglitazone (Avandia), a drug that has anti-inflammatory properties and that improves sensitivity to insulin, can improve memory in people who have amnestic MCI. Epidemiologic studies indicate that people with insulin resistance are at increased risk for both MCI and AD. Insulin resistance also is associated with inflammation, which may increase AD risk through several mechanisms. These findings provide the rationale for this novel treatment strategy. Study participants will be divided into two groups—one group will receive the rosiglitazone, the other a placebo. Participants also will have MRIs before and at the end of treatment to determine whether rosiglitazone slows the rate of atrophy in brain structures that support memory. This trial will provide valuable data about the effects of improved insulin sensitivity, reduced insulin levels in the body, and reduced inflammation on cognitive function and biomarkers in MCI with memory loss.

AD Prevention Trials

NIH is currently conducting AD prevention clinical trials. Some prevention trials are exploring the potential of drugs and other compounds that already have been tested as treatments in people with established AD. Even when results have indicated that the compounds are not effective treatments for people who already have AD, enough laboratory, animal, and epidemiologic evidence exists to suggest that they may still have a potentially useful preventive function. Here are highlights from a few AD prevention studies.

The multiple outcomes of Raloxifene evaluation. This clinical trial, conducted with nearly 5,400 postmenopausal women with osteoporosis, was designed to determine whether treatment with raloxifene (Evista), a selective estrogen receptor modulator (SERM) that is used to treat osteoporosis, affects the risk of developing AD and cognitive impairment (Yaffe et al., 2005). The women were divided into three groups: one group received a placebo, one group received 60 mg of the drug every day, and the third group received 120 mg daily. After three years of treatment, the 60 mg group and the placebo group did not differ. However, women who took 120 mg had a statistically significantly lower risk of developing MCI and a somewhat lower risk of developing AD and any cognitive impairment than did the women who took the placebo. Additional clinical trials are needed to confirm these results.

The memory impairment study: Over the course of three years, this study compared the effectiveness of vitamin E, donepezil (Aricept), and a placebo in delaying the onset of a diagnosis of AD in 769 people with amnestic MCI. Results indicated that participants taking donepezil were at reduced risk of progressing to AD during the first 12 months of the study, but this benefit disappeared by 18 months (Petersen et al., 2005). However, in the subset of patients who carried the ApoE-ε4 allele, donepezil appeared to decrease the risk of progression to a diagnosis of AD for the full 36 months of the study. Vitamin E did not appear to slow the progression to AD. The investigators are conducting additional analyses to determine why donepezil's effect dropped off over time and to assess the practical and clinical implications of this complex study.

This landmark MCI trial, which took place in 69 sites in the U.S. and Canada, represents a major advance in clinical trial methodology, as it demonstrated that investigators could use standardized criteria in a multi-center trial to define and differentiate individuals with amnestic MCI, healthy people, and those with AD. Future clinical trials in people with this type of MCI should be instrumental in research to detect, treat, and delay AD (Grundman et al., 2004).

NSAIDs and inflammation: Some epidemiologic studies have suggested that NSAIDs might help slow the progression of AD, but clinical trials thus far have not demonstrated a benefit from these drugs. A clinical trial studying two of these drugs, rofecoxib (Vioxx) and naproxen (Aleve) showed that they did not delay the progression of AD in people who already have the disease. Treatment in another trial, testing whether the NSAIDs celecoxib (Celebrex) and naproxen could prevent AD in healthy older people at risk of the disease, was suspended after some participants showed indications of increased cardiovascular risk with long-term use of these drugs. Investigators are examining data about possible cardiovascular risk and continue to assess the participants' health periodically. However, researchers are continuing to look for ways to test how other anti-inflammatory drugs might affect the development or progression of AD.

The prevention of Alzheimer disease with Vitamin E and Selenium (PREADVISE) trial. This trial is NIA's add-on to the National Cancer Institute (NCI)'s Selenium and Vitamin E Cancer Prevention Trial (SELECT), which is evaluating whether taking selenium and/or vitamin E supplements can prevent prostate cancer in healthy men older than 60. PREADVISE is evaluating whether these agents can help prevent memory loss and dementia, such as that found in AD. Studies show that increased oxidative stress may damage brain cells and is linked with AD. Animal and tissue culture studies of vitamin E and selenium suggest that they can protect brain cells from oxidative damage.

Ginkgo biloba: Extracts of leaves from the ginkgo tree are thought to have beneficial effects on brain function, especially those related to dementia and AD. NIA is co-funding a National Center for Complementary and Alternative Medicine prevention trial comparing ginkgo to placebo in more than 3,000 people older than 70 who are cognitively healthy at the beginning of the trial. The study's results should indicate whether ginkgo is helpful in preventing or delaying the onset of dementia. As part of this trial, University of Pittsburgh investigators have used brain imaging techniques to determine whether cognitively healthy individuals and those with amnestic MCI show any differences in activation in specific parts of the brain that are normally related to an aspect of cognitive function called attentional control (Rosano et al., 2005). They have been able to detect differences in activation in these brain regions between the two groups, and these changes are likely to be related to early changes in cognitive impairment.

Lifestyle Modifications

We now know that exercise, a healthy diet, and not smoking can help people stay healthy as they grow older. Research has shown that several chronic diseases and conditions that commonly affect people as they age—including diabetes, heart disease, stroke, and high blood pressure—are heavily influenced by lifestyle factors. Investigators are realizing that AD also may share some of these risk factors and have even begun to examine how lifestyle might contribute to the overall emotional health and cognitive abilities of older adults. A number of studies have shed light on this important topic.

Lessons Learned from Couch Mice, Marathon Mice, and Men and Women Who Like to Walk

These days, exercise and physical activity are big buzz words. People are physically active—or know they should be—because they've heard the message: Exercise is good for everyone, whether we are young children or older adults. Exercise builds muscles, improves heart and lung function, helps prevent osteoporosis, and improves mood and overall well-being. So, it is not surprising that scientists began to think that if exercise benefited all parts of the body from the neck down, it surely must benefit the brain as well.

Epidemiologic studies have examined whether exercise and physical activity are associated with beneficial effects on cognitive performance. For example, in an NIA-funded study, researchers at the Harvard School of Public Health analyzed data from almost 19,000 women aged 70–81 who participated in the Nurses' Health Study, a large study funded by the National Heart, Lung, and Blood Institute (NHLBI) in which nearly 122,000 nurses are asked questions every two years about their health, illnesses, diet, and lifestyles (Weuve et al., 2004). Comparing women at various levels of long-term (over several years) physical activity, they found that women at higher activity levels had better cognitive performance and reduced cognitive decline than women at lower activity levels. The cognitive benefit was similar to being about three years younger in age. And the association wasn't confined only to the vigorous exercisers. Walking the equivalent of at least 1½ hours per week at a 21–30 minute-per-mile pace also was associated with better cognitive performance. NIA supports several clinical trials to explore issues related to exercise, cognitive function, and dementia risk.

A Healthy Diet May Be Important to Brain Health

A nutritious diet rich in fruits, vegetables, and whole grains and that is low in fat and added sugar can reduce the risks of many chronic conditions, including heart disease, diabetes, obesity, and some forms of cancer. In recent years, investigators have used epidemiologic, animal, and test tube studies and clinical trials to explore whether diet can play a role in preserving cognitive function or even reducing risk of AD.

A long-held theory about aging suggests that, over time, damage from free radicals (molecules that chemically react easily with other molecules) can build up in neurons, causing loss of function. This damage is called oxidative damage. The brain's unique characteristics, including its high rate of metabolism and its long-lived neurons, may make it particularly vulnerable to oxidative damage. Previous epidemiologic and laboratory studies have suggested that fruits and vegetables that are high in antioxidants might protect the brain against this kind of damage.

A group of Harvard Medical School researchers explored this possibility (Kang et al., 2005). They found that the women who ate the most vegetables—especially green leafy vegetables (like spinach and romaine lettuce) and cruciferous vegetables (like broccoli and cauliflower)—experienced a slower rate of cognitive decline than did women who ate the least vegetables. The scientists were careful to account for other factors that might influence the results, such as use of vitamin supplements, physical activity, smoking and alcohol use, and educational attainment. Interestingly, fruit consumption did not appear to be associated with any change in cognitive ability. The scientists speculate that the abundant antioxidant and folate (a nutrient that appears to be important for proper neural activity and cognitive function) content of the green leafy and cruciferous vegetables was responsible for these results.

This and other studies have provided intriguing hints about possible associations between various dietary elements, oxidative damage, and inflammation in brain tissues, and AD pathology. To confirm these results, scientists have turned to clinical trials to study fish oil, alpha-lipoic acid, vitamin E, a high-potency supplement consisting of two cellular antioxidants (vitamins E and C) and a mitochondrial antioxidant (alpha-lipoic acid), and soy isoflavones (a class of chemicals found in plants that act like estrogen in the body).

Managing Chronic Illness

As we've seen with exercise and diet, evidence suggests that what may be good for the heart may be good for the brain. Moreover, metabolic changes that occur in a variety of chronic diseases of aging, such as heart disease, stroke, high blood pressure, and diabetes, may contribute to the development of AD, affect the severity of AD, or cause vascular dementia (Luchsinger et al., 2005; Curb, 2005).

However, it has been difficult to untangle the association between AD and these chronic diseases. Scientists have offered several possible explanations. For example, many believe that atherosclerosis, which may or may not be clinically apparent as heart disease or stroke, may add to or accelerate cognitive decline in people who already have AD. Or, it is possible that metabolic changes related to chronic disease, such as elevated insulin levels in diabetes, may actually increase the amount of AD pathology that accumulates in brain tissue and directly contribute to the development of AD. Other possibilities or a combination of factors also may explain the associations. As we develop new strategies to treat AD, it will be important to know whether the metabolic changes related to chronic vascular disease actually increase the amount of AD pathology or whether they independently cause dementia.

These relationships need to be sorted out because heart disease and stroke are major causes of illness and death. Diabetes, high blood pressure, and other risk factors for these chronic diseases can, to a large extent, be modified by diet, exercise, and other lifestyle changes, so it is important to know whether reducing risks of or controlling diabetes and high blood pressure also may reduce AD risk.

References

Curb JD. The tangled story of plaques and arteries. *Journal of the American Geriatrics Society* 2005;53(7):1257-1258.

Grundman M, Petersen RC, Ferris SH, Thomas RG, Aisen PS, Bennett DA, Foster NL, Jack CR Jr, Galasko DR, Doody R, Kaye J, Sano M, Mohs R, Gauthier S, Kim HT, Jin S, Schultz AN, Schafer K, Mulnard R, van Dyck CH, Mintzer J, Zamrini EY, Cahn-Weiner D, Thal LJ, Alzheimer's Disease Cooperative Study. Mild cognitive impairment can be distinguished from Alzheimer disease and normal aging for clinical trials. *Archives of Neurology* 2004;61(1):59-66.

Kang JH, Ascherio A, Grodstein F. Fruit and vegetable consumption and cognitive decline in aging women. *Annals of Neurology* 2005;57(5):713-720.

Luchsinger JA, Reitz C, Honig LS, Tang MX, Shea S, Mayeux R. Aggregation of vascular risk factors and risk of incident Alzheimer disease. *Neurology* 2005;65(4):545-551.

Petersen RC, Thomas RG, Grundman M, Bennett D, Doody R, Ferris S, Galasko D, Jin S, Kaye J, Levey A, Pfeiffer E, Sano M, van Dyck CH, Thal LJ, Alzheimer's Disease Cooperative Study Group. Vitamin E and donepezil for the treatment of mild cognitive impairment. *New England Journal of Medicine* 2005b;352(23):2379-2388.

Rosano C, Aizenstein HJ, Cochran JL, Saxton JA, DeKosky ST, Newman AB, Kuller LH, Lopez OL, Carter CS. Event-related functional magnetic resonance imaging investigation of executive control in very old individuals with mild cognitive impairment. *Biological Psychiatry* 2005;57(7):761-767.

Weuve J, Kang JH, Manson JE, Breteler MM, Ware JH, Grodstein F. Physical activity, including walking, and cognitive function in older women. *JAMA* 2004;292(12):1454-1461.

Yaffe K, Krueger K, Cummings SR, Blackwell T, Henderson VW, Sarkar S, Ensrud K, Grady D. Effect of raloxifene on prevention of dementia and cognitive impairment in older women: the Multiple Outcomes of Raloxifene Evaluation (MORE) randomized trial. *American Journal of Psychiatry* 2005;162(4):683-690.

Part Two

Other Dementias and Related Disorders

Chapter 9

Dementia: An Overview

A woman in her early 50s was admitted to a hospital because of increasingly odd behavior. Her family reported that she had been showing memory problems and strong feelings of jealousy. She also had become disoriented at home and was hiding objects. During a doctor's examination, the woman was unable to remember her husband's name, the year, or how long she had been at the hospital. She could read but did not seem to understand what she read, and she stressed the words in an unusual way. She sometimes became agitated and seemed to have hallucinations and irrational fears.

This woman, known as Auguste D., was the first person reported to have the disease now known as Alzheimer disease (AD) after Alois Alzheimer, the German doctor who first described it. After Auguste D. died in 1906, doctors examined her brain and found that it appeared shrunken and contained several unusual features, including strange clumps of protein called plaques and tangled fibers inside the nerve cells. Memory impairments and other symptoms of dementia, which means "deprived of mind," had been described in older adults since ancient times. However, because Auguste D. began to show symptoms at a relatively early age, doctors did not think her disease could be related to what was then called "senile dementia." The word senile is derived from a Latin term that means, roughly, "old age."

It is now clear that AD is a major cause of dementia in elderly people as well as in relatively young adults. Furthermore, we know that

"Dementia: Hope through Research," National Institute of Neurological Disorders and Stroke, April 2007.

it is only one of many disorders that can lead to dementia. The U.S. Congress Office of Technology Assessment estimates that as many as 6.8 million people in the United States have dementia, and at least 1.8 million of those are severely affected. Studies in some communities have found that almost half of all people age 85 and older have some form of dementia. Although it is common in very elderly individuals, dementia is not a normal part of the aging process. Many people live into their 90s and even 100s without any symptoms of dementia.

Besides senile dementia, other terms often used to describe dementia include senility and organic brain syndrome. Senility and senile dementia are outdated terms that reflect the formerly widespread belief that dementia was a normal part of aging. Organic brain syndrome is a general term that refers to physical disorders (not psychiatric in origin) that impair mental functions.

Research in the last 30 years has led to a greatly improved understanding of what dementia is, who gets it, and how it develops and affects the brain. This work is beginning to pay off with better diagnostic techniques, improved treatments, and even potential ways of preventing these diseases.

What is dementia?

Dementia is not a specific disease. It is a descriptive term for a collection of symptoms that can be caused by a number of disorders that affect the brain. People with dementia have significantly impaired intellectual functioning that interferes with normal activities and relationships. They also lose their ability to solve problems and maintain emotional control, and they may experience personality changes and behavioral problems such as agitation, delusions, and hallucinations. While memory loss is a common symptom of dementia, memory loss by itself does not mean that a person has dementia. Doctors diagnose dementia only if two or more brain functions—such as memory, language skills, perception, or cognitive skills including reasoning and judgment—are significantly impaired without loss of consciousness.

There are many disorders that can cause dementia. Some, such as AD, lead to a progressive loss of mental functions. But other types of dementia can be halted or reversed with appropriate treatment.

With AD and many other types of dementia, disease processes cause many nerve cells to stop functioning, lose connections with other neurons, and die. In contrast, normal aging does not result in the loss of large numbers of neurons in the brain.

What are the different kinds of dementia?

Dementing disorders can be classified many different ways. These classification schemes attempt to group disorders that have particular features in common, such as whether they are progressive or what parts of the brain are affected. Some frequently used classifications include the following:

- **Cortical dementia:** dementia where the brain damage primarily affects the brain's cortex, or outer layer. Cortical dementias tend to cause problems with memory, language, thinking, and social behavior.

- **Subcortical dementia:** dementia that affects parts of the brain below the cortex. Subcortical dementia tends to cause changes in emotions and movement in addition to problems with memory.

- **Progressive dementia:** dementia that gets worse over time, gradually interfering with more and more cognitive abilities.

- **Primary dementia:** dementia such as AD that does not result from any other disease.

- **Secondary dementia:** dementia that occurs as a result of a physical disease or injury.

Some types of dementia fit into more than one of these classifications. For example, AD is considered both a progressive and a cortical dementia.

Alzheimer disease is the most common cause of dementia in people aged 65 and older. Experts believe that up to 4 million people in the United States are currently living with the disease: one in ten people over the age of 65 and nearly half of those over 85 have AD. At least 360,000 Americans are diagnosed with AD each year and about 50,000 are reported to die from it.

In most people, symptoms of AD appear after age 60. However, there are some early-onset forms of the disease, usually linked to a specific gene defect, which may appear as early as age 30. AD usually causes a gradual decline in cognitive abilities, usually during a span of 7 to 10 years. Nearly all brain functions, including memory, movement, language, judgment, behavior, and abstract thinking, are eventually affected.

AD is characterized by two abnormalities in the brain: amyloid plaques and neurofibrillary tangles. Amyloid plaques, which are found in the tissue between the nerve cells, are unusual clumps of a protein called beta amyloid along with degenerating bits of neurons and other cells.

Neurofibrillary tangles are bundles of twisted filaments found within neurons. These tangles are largely made up of a protein called tau. In healthy neurons, the tau protein helps the functioning of microtubules, which are part of the cell's structural support and deliver substances throughout the nerve cell. However, in AD, tau is changed in a way that causes it to twist into pairs of helical filaments that collect into tangles. When this happens, the microtubules cannot function correctly and they disintegrate. This collapse of the neuron's transport system may impair communication between nerve cells and cause them to die.

Researchers do not know if amyloid plaques and neurofibrillary tangles are harmful or if they are merely side effects of the disease process that damages neurons and leads to the symptoms of AD. They do know that plaques and tangles usually increase in the brain as AD progresses.

In the early stages of AD, patients may experience memory impairment, lapses of judgment, and subtle changes in personality. As the disorder progresses, memory and language problems worsen and patients begin to have difficulty performing activities of daily living, such as balancing a checkbook or remembering to take medications. They also may have visuospatial problems, such as difficulty navigating an unfamiliar route. They may become disoriented about places and times, may suffer delusions (such as the idea that someone is stealing from them or that their spouse is being unfaithful), and may become short-tempered and hostile. During the late stages of the disease, patients begin to lose the ability to control motor functions. They may have difficulty swallowing and lose bowel and bladder control. They eventually lose the ability to recognize family members and to speak. As AD progresses, it begins to affect the person's emotions and behavior. Most people with AD eventually develop symptoms such as aggression, agitation, depression, sleeplessness, or delusions.

On average, patients with AD live for 8 to 10 years after they are diagnosed. However, some people live as long as 20 years. Patients with AD often die of aspiration pneumonia because they lose the ability to swallow late in the course of the disease.

Vascular dementia is the second most common cause of dementia, after AD. It accounts for up to 20 percent of all dementias and is caused by brain damage from cerebrovascular or cardiovascular problems—usually strokes. It also may result from genetic diseases, endocarditis (infection of a heart valve), or amyloid angiopathy (a process in which amyloid protein builds up in the brain's blood vessels, sometimes causing hemorrhagic or "bleeding" strokes). In many cases, it may coexist with AD. The incidence of vascular dementia increases with advancing age and is similar in men and women.

Symptoms of vascular dementia often begin suddenly, frequently after a stroke. Patients may have a history of high blood pressure, vascular disease, or previous strokes or heart attacks. Vascular dementia may or may not get worse with time, depending on whether the person has additional strokes. In some cases, symptoms may get better with time. When the disease does get worse, it often progresses in a stepwise manner, with sudden changes in ability. Vascular dementia with brain damage to the mid-brain regions, however, may cause a gradual, progressive cognitive impairment that may look much like AD. Unlike people with AD, people with vascular dementia often maintain their personality and normal levels of emotional responsiveness until the later stages of the disease.

People with vascular dementia frequently wander at night and often have other problems commonly found in people who have had a stroke, including depression and incontinence.

There are several types of vascular dementia, which vary slightly in their causes and symptoms. One type, called multi-infarct dementia (MID), is caused by numerous small strokes in the brain. MID typically includes multiple damaged areas, called infarcts, along with extensive lesions in the white matter, or nerve fibers, of the brain.

Because the infarcts in MID affect isolated areas of the brain, the symptoms are often limited to one side of the body or they may affect just one or a few specific functions, such as language. Neurologists call these "local" or "focal" symptoms, as opposed to the "global" symptoms seen in AD, which affect many functions and are not restricted to one side of the body.

Although not all strokes cause dementia, in some cases a single stroke can damage the brain enough to cause dementia. This condition is called single-infarct dementia. Dementia is more common when the stroke takes place on the left side (hemisphere) of the brain or when it involves the hippocampus, a brain structure important for memory.

Another type of vascular dementia is called Binswanger disease. This rare form of dementia is characterized by damage to small blood vessels in the white matter of the brain (white matter is found in the inner layers of the brain and contains many nerve fibers coated with a whitish, fatty substance called myelin). Binswanger disease leads to brain lesions, loss of memory, disordered cognition, and mood changes. Patients with this disease often show signs of abnormal blood pressure, stroke, blood abnormalities, disease of the large blood vessels in the neck, or disease of the heart valves. Other prominent features include urinary incontinence, difficulty walking, clumsiness, slowness, lack of facial expression, and speech difficulty. These symptoms, which usually begin after the age of 60, are not always present in all patients and may sometimes appear only temporarily. Treatment of Binswanger disease is symptomatic, and may include the use of medications to control high blood pressure, depression, heart arrhythmias, and low blood pressure. The disorder often includes episodes of partial recovery.

Another type of vascular dementia is linked to a rare hereditary disorder called CADASIL, which stands for cerebral autosomal dominant arteriopathy with subcortical infarct and leukoencephalopathy. CADASIL is linked to abnormalities of a specific gene, Notch3, which is located on chromosome 19. This condition causes multi-infarct dementia as well as stroke, migraine with aura, and mood disorders. The first symptoms usually appear in people who are in their twenties, thirties, or forties and affected individuals often die by age 65. Researchers believe most people with CADASIL go undiagnosed, and the actual prevalence of the disease is not yet known.

Other causes of vascular dementia include vasculitis, an inflammation of the blood vessel system; profound hypotension (low blood pressure); and lesions caused by brain hemorrhage. The autoimmune disease lupus erythematosus and the inflammatory disease temporal arteritis can also damage blood vessels in a way that leads to vascular dementia.

Lewy body dementia (LBD) is one of the most common types of progressive dementia. LBD usually occurs sporadically, in people with no known family history of the disease. However, rare familial cases have occasionally been reported.

In LBD, cells die in the brain's cortex, or outer layer, and in a part of the mid-brain called the substantia nigra. Many of the remaining nerve cells in the substantia nigra contain abnormal structures called Lewy bodies that are the hallmark of the disease. Lewy bodies may also appear in the brain's cortex, or outer layer. Lewy bodies contain a protein called alpha-synuclein that has been linked to Parkinson disease and several other disorders. Researchers, who sometimes refer to these disorders collectively as "synucleinopathies," do not yet know why this protein accumulates inside nerve cells in LBD.

The symptoms of LBD overlap with AD in many ways, and may include memory impairment, poor judgment, and confusion. However,

LBD typically also includes visual hallucinations, parkinsonian symptoms such as a shuffling gait and flexed posture, and day-to-day fluctuations in the severity of symptoms. Patients with LBD live an average of seven years after symptoms begin.

There is no cure for LBD, and treatments are aimed at controlling the parkinsonian and psychiatric symptoms of the disorder. Patients sometimes respond dramatically to treatment with antiparkinsonian drugs or cholinesterase inhibitors, such as those used for AD. Some studies indicate that neuroleptic drugs, such as clozapine and olanzapine, also can reduce the psychiatric symptoms of this disease. But neuroleptic drugs may cause severe adverse reactions, so other therapies should be tried first and patients using these drugs should be closely monitored.

Lewy bodies are often found in the brains of people with Parkinson disease and AD. These findings suggest that either LBD is related to these other causes of dementia or that the diseases sometimes coexist in the same person.

Frontotemporal dementia (FTD), sometimes called frontal lobe dementia, describes a group of diseases characterized by degeneration of nerve cells—especially those in the frontal and temporal lobes of the brain. Unlike AD, FTD usually does not include formation of amyloid plaques. In many people with FTD, there is an abnormal form of tau protein in the brain, which accumulates into neurofibrillary tangles. This disrupts normal cell activities and may cause the cells to die.

Experts believe FTD accounts for 2 to 10 percent of all cases of dementia. Symptoms of FTD usually appear between the ages of 40 and 65. In many cases, people with FTD have a family history of dementia, suggesting that there is a strong genetic factor in the disease. The duration of FTD varies, with some patients declining rapidly over two to three years and others showing only minimal changes for many years. People with FTD live with the disease for an average of five to ten years after diagnosis.

Because structures found in the frontal and temporal lobes of the brain control judgment and social behavior, people with FTD often have problems maintaining normal interactions and following social conventions. They may steal or exhibit impolite and socially inappropriate behavior, and they may neglect their normal responsibilities. Other common symptoms include loss of speech and language, compulsive or repetitive behavior, increased appetite, and motor problems such as stiffness and balance problems. Memory loss also may occur, although it typically appears late in the disease.

In one type of FTD called Pick disease, certain nerve cells become abnormal and swollen before they die. These swollen, or ballooned, neurons are one hallmark of the disease. The brains of people with Pick disease also have abnormal structures called Pick bodies, composed largely of the protein tau, inside the neurons. The cause of Pick disease is unknown, but it runs in some families and thus it is probably due at least in part to a faulty gene or genes. The disease usually begins after age 50 and causes changes in personality and behavior that gradually worsen over time. The symptoms of Pick disease are very similar to those of AD, and may include inappropriate social behavior, loss of mental flexibility, language problems, and difficulty with thinking and concentration. There is currently no way to slow the progressive degeneration found in Pick disease. However, medication may be helpful in reducing aggression and other behavioral problems, and in treating depression.

In some cases, familial FTD is linked to a mutation in the tau gene. This disorder, called frontotemporal dementia with parkinsonism linked to chromosome 17 (FTDP-17), is much like other types of FTD but often includes psychiatric symptoms such as delusions and hallucinations.

Primary progressive aphasia (PPA) is a type of FTD that may begin in people as early as their forties. "Aphasia" is a general term used to refer to deficits in language functions, such as speaking, understanding what others are saying, and naming common objects. In PPA one or more of these functions can become impaired. Symptoms often begin gradually and progress slowly over a period of years. As the disease progresses, memory and attention may also be impaired and patients may show personality and behavior changes. Many, but not all, people with PPA eventually develop symptoms of dementia.

HIV-associated dementia (HAD) results from infection with the human immunodeficiency virus (HIV) that causes AIDS. HAD can cause widespread destruction of the brain's white matter. This leads to a type of dementia that generally includes impaired memory, apathy, social withdrawal, and difficulty concentrating. People with HAD often develop movement problems as well. There is no specific treatment for HAD, but AIDS drugs can delay onset of the disease and may help to reduce symptoms.

Huntington disease (HD) is a hereditary disorder caused by a faulty gene for a protein called huntingtin. The children of people with the disorder have a 50 percent chance of inheriting it. The disease causes degeneration in many regions of the brain and spinal cord. Symptoms of HD usually begin when patients are in their thirties or forties, and the average life expectancy after diagnosis is about 15 years.

Cognitive symptoms of HD typically begin with mild personality changes, such as irritability, anxiety, and depression, and progress to severe dementia. Many patients also show psychotic behavior. HD causes chorea—involuntary jerky, arrhythmic movements of the body—as well as muscle weakness, clumsiness, and gait disturbances.

Dementia pugilistica, also called chronic traumatic encephalopathy or Boxer's syndrome, is caused by head trauma, such as that experienced by people who have been punched many times in the head during boxing. The most common symptoms of the condition are dementia and parkinsonism, which can appear many years after the trauma ends. Affected individuals may also develop poor coordination and slurred speech. A single traumatic brain injury may also lead to a disorder called post-traumatic dementia (PTD). PTD is much like dementia pugilistica but usually also includes long-term memory problems. Other symptoms vary depending on which part of the brain was damaged by the injury.

Corticobasal degeneration (CBD) is a progressive disorder characterized by nerve cell loss and atrophy of multiple areas of the brain. Brain cells from people with CBD often have abnormal accumulations of the protein tau. CBD usually progresses gradually over the course of 6 to 8 years. Initial symptoms, which typically begin at or around age 60, may first appear on one side of the body but eventually will affect both sides. Some of the symptoms, such as poor coordination and rigidity, are similar to those found in Parkinson disease. Other symptoms may include memory loss, dementia, visual-spatial problems, apraxia (loss of the ability to make familiar, purposeful movements), hesitant and halting speech, myoclonus (involuntary muscular jerks), and dysphagia (difficulty swallowing). Death is often caused by pneumonia or other secondary problems such as sepsis (severe infection of the blood) or pulmonary embolism (a blood clot in the lungs).

There are no specific treatments available for CBD. Drugs such as clonazepam may help with myoclonus, however, and occupational, physical, and speech therapy can help in managing the disabilities associated with this disease. The symptoms of the disease often do not respond to Parkinson disease medications or other drugs.

Creutzfeldt-Jakob disease (CJD) is a rare, degenerative, fatal brain disorder that affects about one in every million people per year worldwide. Symptoms usually begin after age 60 and most patients die within one year. Many researchers believe CJD results from an abnormal form of a protein called a prion. Most cases of CJD occur sporadically—that is, in people who have no known risk factors for the disease. However, about 5 to 10 percent of cases of CJD in the United

States are hereditary, caused by a mutation in the gene for the prion protein. In rare cases, CJD can also be acquired through exposure to diseased brain or nervous system tissue, usually through certain medical procedures. There is no evidence that CJD is contagious through the air or through casual contact with a CJD patient.

Patients with CJD may initially experience problems with muscular coordination; personality changes, including impaired memory, judgment, and thinking; and impaired vision. Other symptoms may include insomnia and depression. As the illness progresses, mental impairment becomes severe. Patients often develop myoclonus and they may go blind. They eventually lose the ability to move and speak, and go into a coma. Pneumonia and other infections often occur in these patients and can lead to death.

CJD belongs to a family of human and animal diseases known as the transmissible spongiform encephalopathies (TSEs). Spongiform refers to the characteristic appearance of infected brains, which become filled with holes until they resemble sponges when viewed under a microscope. CJD is the most common of the known human TSEs. Others include fatal familial insomnia and Gerstmann-Straussler-Scheinker disease.

In recent years, a new type of CJD, called variant CJD (vCJD), has been found in Great Britain and several other European countries. The initial symptoms of vCJD are different from those of classic CJD and the disorder typically occurs in younger patients. Research suggests that vCJD may have resulted from human consumption of beef from cattle with a TSE disease called bovine spongiform encephalopathy (BSE), also known as "mad cow disease."

Other rare hereditary dementias include Gerstmann-Straussler-Scheinker (GSS) disease, fatal familial insomnia, familial British dementia, and familial Danish dementia. Symptoms of GSS typically include ataxia and progressive dementia that begins when people are between 50 and 60 years old. The disease may last for several years before patients eventually die. Fatal familial insomnia causes degeneration of a brain region called the thalamus, which is partially responsible for controlling sleep. It causes a progressive insomnia that eventually leads to a complete inability to sleep. Other symptoms may include poor reflexes, dementia, hallucinations, and eventually coma. It can be fatal within 7 to 13 months after symptoms begin but may last longer. Familial British dementia and familial Danish dementia have been linked to two different defects in a gene found on chromosome 13. The symptoms of both diseases include progressive dementia, paralysis, and loss of balance.

Secondary dementias: Dementia may occur in patients who have other disorders that primarily affect movement or other functions. These cases are often referred to as secondary dementias. The relationship between these disorders and the primary dementias is not always clear. For instance, people with advanced Parkinson disease, which is primarily a movement disorder, sometimes develop symptoms of dementia. Many Parkinson patients also have amyloid plaques and neurofibrillary tangles like those found in AD. The two diseases may be linked in a yet-unknown way, or they may simply coexist in some people. People with Parkinson and associated dementia sometimes show signs of Lewy body dementia or progressive supranuclear palsy at autopsy, suggesting that these diseases may also overlap with Parkinson or that Parkinson is sometimes misdiagnosed.

Other disorders that may include symptoms of dementia include multiple sclerosis; presenile dementia with motor neuron disease, also called ALS dementia; olivopontocerebellar atrophy (OPCA); Wilson disease; and normal pressure hydrocephalus (NPH).

Dementias in children: While it is usually found in adults, dementia can also occur in children. For example, infections and poisoning can lead to dementia in people of any age. In addition, some disorders unique to children can cause dementia.

Niemann-Pick disease is a group of inherited disorders that affect metabolism and are caused by specific genetic mutations. Patients with Niemann-Pick disease cannot properly metabolize cholesterol and other lipids. Consequently, excessive amounts of cholesterol accumulate in the liver and spleen and excessive amounts of other lipids accumulate in the brain. Symptoms may include dementia, confusion, and problems with learning and memory. These diseases usually begin in young school-age children but may also appear during the teen years or early adulthood.

Batten disease is a fatal, hereditary disorder of the nervous system that begins in childhood. Symptoms are linked to a buildup of substances called lipopigments in the body's tissues. The early symptoms include personality and behavior changes, slow learning, clumsiness, or stumbling. Over time, affected children suffer mental impairment, seizures, and progressive loss of sight and motor skills. Eventually, children with Batten disease develop dementia and become blind and bedridden. The disease is often fatal by the late teens or twenties.

Lafora body disease is a rare genetic disease that causes seizures, rapidly progressive dementia, and movement problems. These problems usually begin in late childhood or the early teens. Children with

107

Lafora body disease have microscopic structures called Lafora bodies in the brain, skin, liver, and muscles. Most affected children die within 2 to 10 years after the onset of symptoms.

A number of other childhood-onset disorders can include symptoms of dementia. Among these are mitochondrial myopathies, Rasmussen encephalitis, mucopolysaccharidosis III (Sanfilippo syndrome), neurodegeneration with brain iron accumulation, and leukodystrophies such as Alexander disease, Schilder disease, and metachromatic leukodystrophy.

What other conditions can cause dementia?

Doctors have identified many other conditions that can cause dementia or dementia-like symptoms. Many of these conditions are reversible with appropriate treatment.

Reactions to medications: Medications can sometimes lead to reactions or side effects that mimic dementia. These dementia-like effects can occur in reaction to just one drug or they can result from drug interactions. They may have a rapid onset or they may develop slowly over time.

Metabolic problems and endocrine abnormalities: Thyroid problems can lead to apathy, depression, or dementia. Hypoglycemia, a condition in which there is not enough sugar in the bloodstream, can cause confusion or personality changes. Too little or too much sodium or calcium can also trigger mental changes. Some people have an impaired ability to absorb vitamin B_{12}, which creates a condition called pernicious anemia that can cause personality changes, irritability, or depression. Tests can determine if any of these problems are present.

Nutritional deficiencies: Deficiencies of thiamine (vitamin B_1) frequently result from chronic alcoholism and can seriously impair mental abilities, in particular memories of recent events. Severe deficiency of vitamin B_6 can cause a neurological illness called pellagra that may include dementia. Deficiencies of vitamin B_{12} also have been linked to dementia in some cases. Dehydration can also cause mental impairment that can resemble dementia.

Infections: Many infections can cause neurological symptoms, including confusion or delirium, due to fever or other side effects of the body's fight to overcome the infection. Meningitis and encephalitis, which are infections of the brain or the membrane that covers it, can cause confusion, sudden severe dementia, withdrawal from social interaction, impaired judgment, or memory loss. Untreated syphilis also can damage the nervous system and cause dementia. In rare cases, Lyme disease can cause memory or thinking difficulties. People in the advanced stages of AIDS also may develop a form of dementia. People with compromised immune systems, such as those with leukemia and AIDS, may also develop an infection called progressive multifocal leukoencephalopathy (PML). PML is caused by a common human polyomavirus, JC virus, and leads to damage or destruction of the myelin sheath that covers nerve cells. PML can lead to confusion, difficulty with thinking or speaking, and other mental problems.

Subdural hematomas: Subdural hematomas, or bleeding between the brain's surface and its outer covering (the dura), can cause dementia-like symptoms and changes in mental function.

Poisoning: Exposure to lead, other heavy metals, or other poisonous substances can lead to symptoms of dementia. These symptoms may or may not resolve after treatment, depending on how badly the brain is damaged. People who have abused substances such as alcohol and recreational drugs sometimes display signs of dementia even after the substance abuse has ended. This condition is known as substance-induced persisting dementia.

Brain tumors: In rare cases, people with brain tumors may develop dementia because of damage to their brains. Symptoms may include changes in personality, psychotic episodes, or problems with speech, language, thinking, and memory.

Anoxia: Anoxia and a related term, hypoxia, are often used interchangeably to describe a state in which there is a diminished supply of oxygen to an organ's tissues. Anoxia may be caused by many different problems, including heart attack, heart surgery, severe asthma, smoke or carbon monoxide inhalation, high-altitude exposure, strangulation, or an overdose of anesthesia. In severe cases of anoxia the patient may be in a stupor or a coma for periods ranging from hours to days, weeks, or months. Recovery depends on the severity of the oxygen deprivation. As recovery proceeds, a variety of psychological and neurological abnormalities, such as dementia or psychosis, may occur. The person also may experience confusion, personality changes, hallucinations, or memory loss.

Heart and lung problems: The brain requires a high level of oxygen in order to carry out its normal functions. Therefore, problems such as chronic lung disease or heart problems that prevent the brain from receiving adequate oxygen can starve brain cells and lead to the symptoms of dementia.

What conditions are not dementia?

Age-related cognitive decline: As people age, they usually experience slower information processing and mild memory impairment. In addition, their brains frequently decrease in volume and some nerve cells, or neurons, are lost. These changes, called age-related cognitive decline, are normal and are not considered signs of dementia.

Mild cognitive impairment: Some people develop cognitive and memory problems that are not severe enough to be diagnosed as dementia but are more pronounced than the cognitive changes associated with normal aging. This condition is called mild cognitive impairment. Although many patients with this condition later develop dementia, some do not. Many researchers are studying mild cognitive impairment to find ways to treat it or prevent it from progressing to dementia.

Depression: People with depression are frequently passive or unresponsive, and they may appear slow, confused, or forgetful. Other emotional problems can also cause symptoms that sometimes mimic dementia.

Delirium: Delirium is characterized by confusion and rapidly altering mental states. The person may also be disoriented, drowsy, or incoherent, and may exhibit personality changes. Delirium is usually caused by a treatable physical or psychiatric illness, such as poisoning or infections. Patients with delirium often, though not always, make a full recovery after their underlying illness is treated.

What causes dementia?

All forms of dementia result from the death of nerve cells or the loss of communication among these cells. The human brain is a very complex and intricate machine and many factors can interfere with its functioning. Researchers have uncovered many of these factors, but they have not yet been able to fit these puzzle pieces together in order to form a complete picture of how dementias develop.

Many types of dementia, including AD, Lewy body dementia, Parkinson dementia, and Pick disease, are characterized by abnormal structures called inclusions in the brain. Because these inclusions, which contain abnormal proteins, are so common in people with dementia, researchers suspect that they play a role in the development of symptoms. However, that role is unknown, and in some cases the inclusions may simply be a side effect of the disease process that leads to the dementia.

Genes clearly play a role in the development of some kinds of dementia. However, in AD and many other disorders, the dementia usually cannot be tied to a single abnormal gene. Instead, these forms of dementia appear to result from a complex interaction of genes, lifestyle factors, and other environmental influences.

Researchers have identified several genes that influence susceptibility to AD. Mutations in three of the known genes for AD—genes that control the production of proteins such as amyloid precursor protein (APP), presenilin 1, and presenilin 2—are linked to early-onset forms of the disease.

Variations in another gene, called apolipoprotein E (ApoE), have been linked to an increased risk of late-onset AD. The ApoE gene does not cause the disease by itself, but one version of the gene, called ApoE epsilon4 (ApoE ε4), appears to increase the risk of AD. People with two copies of the ApoE ε4 gene have about ten times the risk of developing AD compared to people without ApoE ε4. This gene variant seems to encourage amyloid deposition in the brain. One study also found that this gene is associated with shorter survival in men with AD. In contrast, another version of the ApoE gene, called ApoE ε2, appears to protect against AD.

Studies have suggested that mutations in another gene, called CYP46, may contribute to an increased risk of developing late-onset sporadic AD. This gene normally produces a protein that helps the brain metabolize cholesterol.

Scientists are trying to determine how beta amyloid influences the development of AD. A number of studies indicate that the buildup of this protein initiates a complex chain of events that culminates in dementia. One study found that beta amyloid buildup in the brain triggers cells called microglia, which act like janitors that mop up potentially harmful substances in the brain, to release a potent neurotoxin called peroxynitrite. This may contribute to nerve cell death in AD. Another study found that beta amyloid causes a protein called p35 to be split into two proteins. One of the resulting proteins triggers changes in the tau protein that lead to formation of neurofibrillary tangles. A third study found that beta amyloid activates cell-death enzymes called caspases that alter the tau protein in a way that causes it to form tangles. Researchers believe these tangles may contribute to the neuron death in AD.

Vascular dementia can be caused by cerebrovascular disease or any other condition that prevents normal blood flow to the brain. Without a normal supply of blood, brain cells cannot obtain the oxygen they need to work correctly, and they often become so deprived that they die.

The causes of other types of dementias vary. Some, such as CJD and GSS, have been tied to abnormal forms of specific proteins. Others, including Huntington disease and FTDP-17, have been linked to defects in a single gene. Post-traumatic dementia is directly related to brain cell death after injury. HIV-associated dementia is clearly tied to infection by the HIV virus, although the exact way the virus causes damage is not yet certain. For other dementias, such as corticobasal degeneration and most types of frontotemporal dementia, the underlying causes have not yet been identified.

What are the risk factors for dementia?

Researchers have identified several risk factors that affect the likelihood of developing one or more kinds of dementia. Some of these factors are modifiable, while others are not.

Age: The risk of AD, vascular dementia, and several other dementias goes up significantly with advancing age.

Genetics/family history: Researchers have discovered a number of genes that increase the risk of developing AD. Although people with a family history of AD are generally considered to be at heightened risk of developing the disease themselves, many people with a family history never develop the disease, and many without a family history of the disease do get it. In most cases, it is still impossible to predict a specific person's risk of the disorder based on family history alone. Some families with CJD, GSS, or fatal familial insomnia have mutations in the prion protein gene, although these disorders can also occur in people without the gene mutation. Individuals with these mutations are at significantly higher risk of developing these forms of dementia. Abnormal genes are also clearly implicated as risk factors in Huntington disease, FTDP-17, and several other kinds of dementia.

Smoking and alcohol use: Several recent studies have found that smoking significantly increases the risk of mental decline and dementia. People who smoke have a higher risk of atherosclerosis and other types of vascular disease, which may be the underlying causes for the increased dementia risk. Studies also have found that drinking large amounts of alcohol appears to increase the risk of dementia. However, other studies have suggested that people who drink moderately have a lower risk of dementia than either those who drink heavily or those who completely abstain from drinking.

Atherosclerosis: Atherosclerosis is the buildup of plaque—deposits of fatty substances, cholesterol, and other matter—in the inner lining of an artery. Atherosclerosis is a significant risk factor for vascular dementia, because it interferes with the delivery of blood to the brain and can lead to stroke. Studies have also found a possible link between atherosclerosis and AD.

Cholesterol: High levels of low-density lipoprotein (LDL), the so-called bad form of cholesterol, appear to significantly increase a person's risk of developing vascular dementia. Some research has also linked high cholesterol to an increased risk of AD.

Plasma homocysteine: Research has shown that a higher-than-average blood level of homocysteine—a type of amino acid—is a strong risk factor for the development of AD and vascular dementia.

Diabetes: Diabetes is a risk factor for both AD and vascular dementia. It is also a known risk factor for atherosclerosis and stroke, both of which contribute to vascular dementia.

Mild cognitive impairment: While not all people with mild cognitive impairment develop dementia, people with this condition do have a significantly increased risk of dementia compared to the rest of the population. One study found that approximately 40 percent of people over age 65 who were diagnosed with mild cognitive impairment developed dementia within three years.

Down syndrome: Studies have found that most people with Down syndrome develop characteristic AD plaques and neurofibrillary tangles by the time they reach middle age. Many, but not all, of these individuals also develop symptoms of dementia.

How is dementia diagnosed?

Doctors employ a number of strategies to diagnose dementia. It is important that they rule out any treatable conditions, such as depression, normal pressure hydrocephalus, or vitamin B_{12} deficiency, which can cause similar symptoms.

Early, accurate diagnosis of dementia is important for patients and their families because it allows early treatment of symptoms. For people with AD or other progressive dementias, early diagnosis may allow them to plan for the future while they can still help to make decisions. These people also may benefit from drug treatment.

The "gold standard" for diagnosing dementia, autopsy, does not help the patient or caregivers. Therefore, doctors have devised a number of techniques to help identify dementia with reasonable accuracy while the patient is still alive.

Patient history: Doctors often begin their examination of a patient suspected of having dementia by asking questions about the patient's history. For example, they may ask how and when symptoms developed and about the patient's overall medical condition. They also may try to evaluate the patient's emotional state, although patients with dementia often may be unaware of or in denial about how their disease is affecting them. Family members also may deny the existence of the disease because they do not want to accept the diagnosis and because, at least in the beginning, AD and other forms of dementia can resemble normal aging. Therefore additional steps are necessary to confirm or rule out a diagnosis of dementia.

Physical examination: A physical examination can help rule out treatable causes of dementia and identify signs of stroke or other disorders that can contribute to dementia. It can also identify signs of other illnesses, such as heart disease or kidney failure, that can overlap with dementia. If a patient is taking medications that may be causing or contributing to his or her symptoms, the doctor may suggest stopping or replacing some medications to see if the symptoms go away.

Neurological evaluations: Doctors will perform a neurological examination, looking at balance, sensory function, reflexes, and other functions, to identify signs of conditions—for example movement disorders or stroke—that may affect the patient's diagnosis or are treatable with drugs.

Cognitive and neuropsychological tests: Doctors use tests that measure memory, language skills, math skills, and other abilities related to mental functioning to help them diagnose a patient's condition accurately. For example, people with AD often show changes in so-called executive functions (such as problem-solving), memory, and the ability to perform once-automatic tasks.

Doctors often use a test called the Mini-Mental State Examination (MMSE) to assess cognitive skills in people with suspected dementia. This test examines orientation, memory, and attention, as well as the ability to name objects, follow verbal and written commands, write a sentence spontaneously, and copy a complex shape. Doctors also use a variety of other tests and rating scales to identify specific types of cognitive problems and abilities.

Brain scans: Doctors may use brain scans to identify strokes, tumors, or other problems that can cause dementia. Also, cortical atrophy—degeneration of the brain's cortex (outer layer)—is common in many forms of dementia and may be visible on a brain scan. The brain's cortex normally appears very wrinkled, with ridges of tissue (called gyri) separated by "valleys" called sulci. In individuals with cortical atrophy, the progressive loss of neurons causes the ridges to become thinner and the sulci to grow wider. As brain cells die, the ventricles (or fluid-filled cavities in the middle of the brain) expand to fill the available space, becoming much larger than normal. Brain scans also can identify changes in the brain's structure and function that suggest AD.

The most common types of brain scans are computed tomographic (CT) scans and magnetic resonance imaging (MRI). Doctors frequently request a CT scan of the brain when they are examining a patient with suspected dementia. These scans, which use x-rays to detect brain structures, can show evidence of brain atrophy, strokes and transient ischemic attacks (TIAs), changes to the blood vessels, and other problems such as hydrocephalus and subdural hematomas. MRI scans use magnetic fields and focused radio waves to detect hydrogen atoms in tissues within the body. They can detect the same problems as CT scans but they are better for identifying certain conditions, such as brain atrophy and damage from small TIAs.

Doctors also may use electroencephalograms (EEGs) in people with suspected dementia. In an EEG, electrodes are placed on the scalp over several parts of the brain in order to detect and record patterns of electrical activity and check for abnormalities. This electrical activity can indicate cognitive dysfunction in part or all of the brain. Many patients with moderately severe to severe AD have abnormal EEGs. An EEG may also be used to detect seizures, which occur in about 10 percent of AD patients as well as in many other disorders. EEGs also can help diagnose CJD.

Several other types of brain scans allow researchers to watch the brain as it functions. These scans, called functional brain imaging, are not often used as diagnostic tools, but they are important in research and they may ultimately help identify people with dementia earlier than is currently possible. Functional brain scans include functional MRI (fMRI), single photon-emission computed tomography (SPECT), positron emission tomography (PET), and magnetoencephalography (MEG). fMRI uses radio waves and a strong magnetic field to measure the metabolic changes that take place in active parts of the brain. SPECT shows the distribution of blood in the brain, which generally increases with brain activity. PET scans can detect changes in glucose metabolism, oxygen metabolism, and blood flow, all of which can reveal abnormalities of brain function. MEG shows the electromagnetic fields produced by the brain's neuronal activity.

Laboratory tests: Doctors may use a variety of laboratory tests to help diagnose dementia or rule out other conditions, such as kidney failure, that can contribute to symptoms. A partial list of these tests includes a complete blood count, blood glucose test, urinalysis, drug and alcohol tests (toxicology screen), cerebrospinal fluid analysis (to rule out specific infections that can affect the brain), and analysis of thyroid and thyroid-stimulating hormone levels. A doctor will order only the tests that he or she feels are necessary or likely to improve the accuracy of a diagnosis.

Psychiatric evaluation: A psychiatric evaluation may be obtained to determine if depression or another psychiatric disorder may be causing or contributing to a person's symptoms.

Presymptomatic testing: Testing people before symptoms begin to determine if they will develop dementia is not possible in most cases. However, in disorders such as Huntington where a known gene defect is clearly linked to the risk of the disease, a genetic test can help identify people who are likely to develop the disease. Since this type of genetic information can be devastating, people should carefully consider whether they want to undergo such testing.

Researchers are examining whether a series of simple cognitive tests, such as matching words with pictures, can predict who will develop dementia. One study suggested that a combination of a verbal learning test and an odor-identification test can help identify AD before symptoms become obvious. Other studies are looking at whether memory tests and brain scans can be useful indicators of future dementia.

Is there any treatment?

While treatments to reverse or halt disease progression are not available for most of the dementias, patients can benefit to some extent from treatment with available medications and other measures, such as cognitive training.

Drugs to specifically treat AD and some other progressive dementias are now available and are prescribed for many patients. Although these drugs do not halt the disease or reverse existing brain damage, they can improve symptoms and slow the progression of the disease. This may improve the patient's quality of life, ease the burden on caregivers, and/or delay admission to a nursing home. Many researchers are also examining whether these drugs may be useful for treating other types of dementia.

Many people with dementia, particularly those in the early stages, may benefit from practicing tasks designed to improve performance in specific aspects of cognitive functioning. For example, people can sometimes be taught to use memory aids, such as mnemonics, computerized recall devices, or note taking.

Behavior modification—rewarding appropriate or positive behavior and ignoring inappropriate behavior—also may help control unacceptable or dangerous behaviors.

Alzheimer disease: Most of the drugs currently approved by the U. S. Food and Drug Administration (FDA) for AD fall into a category called cholinesterase inhibitors. These drugs slow the breakdown of the neurotransmitter acetylcholine, which is reduced in the brains of people with AD. Acetylcholine is important for the formation of memories and it is used in the hippocampus and the cerebral cortex, two brain regions that are affected by AD. There are currently four cholinesterase inhibitors approved for use in the United States: tacrine (Cognex), donepezil (Aricept), rivastigmine (Exelon), and galantamine (Reminyl). These drugs temporarily improve or stabilize memory and thinking skills in some individuals. Many studies have shown that cholinesterase inhibitors help to slow the decline in mental functions associated with AD, and that they can help reduce behavioral problems and improve the ability to perform everyday tasks. However, none of these drugs can stop or reverse the course of AD.

A fifth drug, memantine (Namenda), is also approved for use in the United States. Unlike other drugs for AD, which affect acetylcholine levels, memantine works by regulating the activity of a neurotransmitter called glutamate that plays a role in learning and memory. Glutamate activity is often disrupted in AD. Because this drug works differently from cholinesterase inhibitors, combining memantine with other AD drugs may be more effective than any single therapy. One controlled clinical trial found that patients receiving donepezil plus memantine had better cognition and other functions than patients receiving donepezil alone.

Doctors may also prescribe other drugs, such as anticonvulsants, sedatives, and antidepressants, to treat seizures, depression, agitation, sleep disorders, and other specific problems that can be associated with dementia. In 2005, research showed that use of "atypical" antipsychotic drugs such as olanzapine and risperidone to treat behavioral problems in elderly people with dementia was associated with an elevated risk of death in these patients. Most of the deaths were caused by heart problems or infections. The FDA has issued a public health advisory to alert patients and their caregivers to this safety issue.

Vascular dementia: There is no standard drug treatment for vascular dementia, although some of the symptoms, such as depression, can be treated. Most other treatments aim to reduce the risk factors for further brain damage. However, some studies have found that cholinesterase inhibitors, such as galantamine and other AD drugs, can improve cognitive function and behavioral symptoms in patients with early vascular dementia.

The progression of vascular dementia can often be slowed significantly or halted if the underlying vascular risk factors for the disease are treated. To prevent strokes and TIAs, doctors may prescribe medicines to control high blood pressure, high cholesterol, heart disease, and diabetes. Doctors also sometimes prescribe aspirin, warfarin, or other drugs to prevent clots from forming in small blood vessels. When patients have blockages in blood vessels, doctors may recommend surgical procedures, such as carotid endarterectomy, stenting, or angioplasty, to restore the normal blood supply. Medications to relieve restlessness or depression or to help patients sleep better may also be prescribed.

Other dementias: Some studies have suggested that cholinesterase inhibitors, such as donepezil (Aricept), can reduce behavioral symptoms in some patients with Parkinson dementia.

At present, no medications are approved specifically to treat or prevent FTD and most other types of progressive dementia. However, sedatives, antidepressants, and other medications may be useful in treating specific symptoms and behavioral problems associated with these diseases.

Scientists continue to search for specific treatments to help people with Lewy body dementia. Current treatment is symptomatic, often involving the use of medication to control the parkinsonian and psychiatric symptoms. Although antiparkinsonian medication may help reduce tremor and loss of muscle movement, it may worsen symptoms such as hallucinations and delusions. Also, drugs prescribed for psychiatric symptoms may make the movement problems worse. Several studies have suggested that cholinesterase inhibitors may be able to improve cognitive function and behavioral symptoms in patients with Lewy body disease.

There is no known treatment that can cure or control CJD. Current treatment is aimed at alleviating symptoms and making the patient as comfortable as possible. Opiate drugs can help relieve pain, and the drugs clonazepam and sodium valproate may help relieve myoclonus. During later stages of the disease, treatment focuses on supportive care, such as administering intravenous fluids and changing the person's position frequently to prevent bedsores.

Can dementia be prevented?

Research has revealed a number of factors that may be able to prevent or delay the onset of dementia in some people. For example, studies have shown that people who maintain tight control over their glucose levels tend to score better on tests of cognitive function than those with poorly controlled diabetes. Several studies also have suggested that people who engage in intellectually stimulating activities, such as social interactions, chess, crossword puzzles, and playing a musical instrument, significantly lower their risk of developing AD and other forms of dementia. Scientists believe mental activities may stimulate the brain in a way that increases the person's "cognitive reserve"—the ability to cope with or compensate for the pathologic changes associated with dementia.

Researchers are studying other steps people can take that may help prevent AD in some cases. So far, none of these factors has been definitively proven to make a difference in the risk of developing the disease. Moreover, most of the studies addressed only AD, and the results may or may not apply to other forms of dementia. Nevertheless, scientists are encouraged by the results of these early studies and many believe it will eventually become possible to prevent some forms of dementia. Possible preventive actions include:

- **Lowering homocysteine:** In one study, elevated blood levels of the amino acid homocysteine were associated with a 2.9 times greater risk of AD and a 4.9 times greater risk of vascular dementia. A preliminary study has shown that high doses of three B vitamins that help lower homocysteine levels—folic acid, B_{12}, and B_6—appear to slow the progression of AD. Researchers are conducting a multi-center clinical trial to test this effect in a larger group of patients.

- **Lowering cholesterol levels:** Research has suggested that people with high cholesterol levels have an increased risk of developing AD. Cholesterol is involved in formation of amyloid plaques in the brain. Mutations in a gene called CYP46 and the ApoE ε4 gene variant, both of which have been linked to an increased risk of AD, are also involved in cholesterol metabolism. Several studies have also found that the use of drugs called statins, which lower cholesterol levels, is associated with a lower likelihood of cognitive impairment.

- **Lowering blood pressure:** Several studies have shown that antihypertensive medicine reduces the odds of cognitive impairment in elderly people with high blood pressure. One large European study found a 55 percent lower risk of dementia in people over 60 who received drug treatment for hypertension. These people had a reduced risk of both AD and vascular dementia.

- **Exercise:** Regular exercise stimulates production of chemicals called growth factors that help neurons survive and adapt to new situations. These gains may help to delay the onset of dementia symptoms. Exercise also may reduce the risk of brain damage from atherosclerosis.

- **Education:** Researchers have found evidence that formal education may help protect people against the effects of AD. In one study, researchers found that people with more years of formal education had relatively less mental decline than people with less schooling, regardless of the number of amyloid plaques and neurofibrillary tangles each person had in his or her brain. The researchers think education may cause the brain to develop robust nerve cell networks that can help compensate for the cell damage caused by AD.

- **Controlling inflammation:** Many studies have suggested that inflammation may contribute to AD. Moreover, autopsies of people who died with AD have shown widespread inflammation in the brain that appeared to be caused by the accumulation of beta amyloid. Another study found that men with high levels of C-reactive protein, a general marker of inflammation, had a significantly increased risk of AD and other kinds of dementia.

- **Nonsteroidal anti-inflammatory drugs (NSAIDs):** Research indicates that long-term use of NSAIDs—ibuprofen, naproxen, and similar drugs—may prevent or delay the onset of AD. Researchers are not sure how these drugs may protect against the disease, but some or all of the effect may be due to reduced inflammation. A 2003 study showed that these drugs also bind to amyloid plaques and may help to dissolve them and prevent formation of new plaques.

The risk of vascular dementia is strongly correlated with risk factors for stroke, including high blood pressure, diabetes, elevated cholesterol levels, and smoking. This type of dementia may be prevented in many cases by changing lifestyle factors, such as excessive weight and high blood pressure, which are associated with an increased risk of cerebrovascular disease. One European study found that treating isolated systolic hypertension (high blood pressure in which only the systolic or top number is high) in people age 60 and older reduced the risk of dementia by 50 percent. These studies strongly suggest that effective use of current treatments can prevent many future cases of vascular dementia.

A study published in 2005 found that people with mild cognitive impairment who took 10 mg/day of the drug donepezil had a significantly reduced risk of developing AD during the first two years of treatment, compared to people who received vitamin E or a placebo. By the end of the third year, however, the rate of AD was just as high in the people treated with donepezil as it was in the other two groups.

What kind of care does a person with dementia need?

People with moderate and advanced dementia typically need round-the-clock care and supervision to prevent them from harming themselves or others. They also may need assistance with daily activities such as eating, bathing, and dressing. Meeting these needs takes patience, understanding, and careful thought by the person's caregivers.

A typical home environment can present many dangers and obstacles to a person with dementia, but simple changes can overcome many of these problems. For example, sharp knives, dangerous chemicals, tools, and other hazards should be removed or locked away. Other safety measures include installing bed and bathroom safety rails, removing locks from bedroom and bathroom doors, and lowering the hot water temperature to 120°F (48.9°C) or less to reduce the risk of accidental scalding. People with dementia also should wear some form of identification at all times in case they wander away or become lost. Caregivers can help prevent unsupervised wandering by adding locks or alarms to outside doors.

People with dementia often develop behavior problems because of frustration with specific situations. Understanding and modifying or preventing the situations that trigger these behaviors may help to make life more pleasant for the person with dementia as well as his or her caregivers. For instance, the person may be confused or frustrated by the level of activity or noise in the surrounding environment. Reducing unnecessary activity and noise (such as limiting the number of visitors and turning off the television when it's not in use) may make it easier for the person to understand requests and perform simple tasks. Confusion also may be reduced by simplifying home decorations, removing clutter, keeping familiar objects nearby, and following a predictable routine throughout the day. Calendars and clocks also may help patients orient themselves.

People with dementia should be encouraged to continue their normal leisure activities as long as they are safe and do not cause frustration. Activities such as crafts, games, and music can provide important mental stimulation and improve mood. Some studies have suggested that participating in exercise and intellectually stimulating activities may slow the decline of cognitive function in some people.

Many studies have found that driving is unsafe for people with dementia. They often get lost and they may have problems remembering or following rules of the road. They also may have difficulty processing information quickly and dealing with unexpected circumstances. Even a second of confusion while driving can lead to an accident. Driving with impaired cognitive functions can also endanger others. Some experts have suggested that regular screening for changes in cognition might help to reduce the number of driving accidents among elderly people, and some states now require that doctors report people with AD to their state motor vehicle department. However, in many cases, it is up to the person's family and friends to ensure that the person does not drive.

The emotional and physical burden of caring for someone with dementia can be overwhelming. Support groups can often help caregivers deal with these demands and they can also offer helpful information about the disease and its treatment. It is important that caregivers occasionally have time off from round-the-clock nursing demands. Some communities provide respite facilities or adult day care centers that will care for dementia patients for a period of time, giving the primary caregivers a break. Eventually, many patients with dementia require the services of a full-time nursing home.

What research is being done?

Current research focuses on many different aspects of dementia. This research promises to improve the lives of people affected by the dementias and may eventually lead to ways of preventing or curing these disorders.

Causes and prevention: Research on the causes of AD and other dementias includes studies of genetic factors, neurotransmitters, inflammation, factors that influence programmed cell death in the brain, and the roles of tau, beta amyloid, and the associated neurofibrillary tangles and plaques in AD. Some other researchers are trying to determine the possible roles of cholesterol metabolism, oxidative stress (chemical reactions that can damage proteins, DNA, and lipids inside cells), and microglia in the development of AD. Scientists also are investigating the role of aging-related proteins such as the enzyme telomerase.

Since many dementias and other neurodegenerative diseases have been linked to abnormal clumps of proteins in cells, researchers are trying to learn how these clumps develop, how they affect cells, and how the clumping can be prevented.

Some studies are examining whether changes in white matter—nerve fibers lined with myelin—may play a role in the onset of AD. Myelin may erode in AD patients before other changes occur. This may be due to a problem with oligodendrocytes, the cells that produce myelin.

Researchers are searching for additional genes that may contribute to AD, and they have identified a number of gene regions that may be involved. Some researchers suggest that people will eventually be screened for a number of genes that contribute to AD and that they will be able to receive treatments that specifically address their individual genetic risks. However, such individualized screening and treatment is still years away.

Insulin resistance is common in people with AD, but it is not clear whether the insulin resistance contributes to the development of the disease or if it is merely a side effect.

Several studies have found a reduced risk of dementia in people who take cholesterol-lowering drugs called statins. However, it is not yet clear if the apparent effect is due to the drugs or to other factors.

Early studies of estrogen suggested that it might help prevent AD in older women. However, a clinical study of several thousand postmenopausal women aged 65 or older found that combination therapy with estrogen and progestin substantially increased the risk of AD. Estrogen alone also appeared to slightly increase the risk of dementia in this study.

A 2003 study found that people with HIV-associated dementia have different levels of activity for more than 30 different proteins, compared to people who have HIV but no signs of dementia. The study suggests a possible way to screen HIV patients for the first signs of cognitive impairment, and it may lead to ways of intervening to prevent this form of dementia.

Diagnosis: Improving early diagnosis of AD and other types of dementia is important not only for patients and families, but also for researchers who seek to better understand the causes of dementing diseases and find ways to reverse or halt them at early stages. Improved diagnosis can also reduce the risk that people will receive inappropriate treatments.

Some researchers are investigating whether three-dimensional computer models of PET and MRI images can identify brain changes typical of early AD, before any symptoms appear. This research may lead to ways of preventing the symptoms of the disease.

One study found that levels of beta amyloid and tau in spinal fluid can be used to diagnose AD with a sensitivity of 92 percent. If other studies confirm the validity of this test, it may allow doctors to identify people who are beginning to develop the disorder before they start to show symptoms. This would allow treatment at very early stages of the disorder, and may help in testing new treatments to prevent or delay symptoms of the disease. Other researchers have identified factors in the skin and blood of AD patients that are different from those in healthy people. They are trying to determine if these factors can be used to diagnose the disease.

Treatment: Researchers are continually working to develop new drugs for AD and other types of dementia. Many researchers believe a vaccine that reduces the number of amyloid plaques in the brain might ultimately prove to be the most effective treatment for AD. In 2001, researchers began one clinical trial of a vaccine called AN-1792. The study was halted after a number of people developed inflammation of the brain and spinal cord. Despite these problems, one patient appeared to have reduced numbers of amyloid plaques in the brain. Other patients showed little or no cognitive decline during the course of the study, suggesting that the vaccine may slow or halt the disease. Researchers are now trying to find safer and more effective vaccines for AD.

Researchers are also investigating possible methods of gene therapy for AD. In one case, researchers used cells genetically engineered to produce nerve growth factor and transplanted them into monkeys' forebrains. The transplanted cells boosted the amount of nerve growth factors in the brain and seemed to prevent degeneration of acetylcholine-producing neurons in the animals. This suggests that gene therapy might help to reduce or delay symptoms of the disease. Researchers are now testing a similar therapy in a small number of patients. Other researchers have experimented with gene therapy that adds a gene called neprilysin in a mouse model that produces human beta amyloid. They found that increasing the level of neprilysin greatly reduced the amount of beta amyloid in the mice and halted the amyloid-related brain degeneration. They are now trying to determine whether neprilysin gene therapy can improve cognition in mice.

A clinical trial called the Vitamins to Slow Alzheimer's Disease (VITAL) study is testing whether high doses of three common B vitamins—folic acid, B_{12}, and B_6—can reduce homocysteine levels and slow the rate of cognitive decline in AD.

Since many studies have found evidence of brain inflammation in AD, some researchers have proposed that drugs that control inflammation, such as NSAIDs, might prevent the disease or slow its progression. Studies in mice have suggested that these drugs can limit production of amyloid plaques in the brain. Early studies of these drugs in humans have shown promising results. However, a large NIH-funded clinical trial of two NSAIDs (naproxen and celecoxib) to prevent AD was stopped in late 2004 because of an increase in stroke and heart attack in people taking naproxen, and an unrelated study that linked celecoxib to an increased risk of heart attack.

Some studies have suggested that two drugs, pentoxifylline and propentofylline, may be useful in treating vascular dementia. Pentoxifylline improves blood flow, while propentofylline appears to interfere with some of the processes that cause cell death in the brain.

One study is testing the safety and effectiveness of donepezil (Aricept) for treating mild dementia in patients with Parkinson dementia, while another is investigating whether skin patches with the drug selegiline can improve mental function in patients with cognitive problems related to HIV.

How can I help research?

People with dementia and others who wish to help research on dementing disorders may be able to do so by participating in clinical studies designed to learn more about the disorders or to test potential new therapies. Information about many such studies is available free of charge from the Federal government's database of clinical trials, available online at http://clinicaltrials.gov.

Information about clinical trials specific to AD is available from the Alzheimer's Disease Clinical Trials Database (www.alzheimers .org/trials), a joint project of the U. S. Food and Drug Administration and the National Institute on Aging (NIA) that is maintained by the NIA's Alzheimer's Disease Education and Referral Center.

For clinical trials taking place at the National Institutes of Health, additional information is available from the following office:

Patient Recruitment and Public Liaison Office
Clinical Center
National Institutes of Health
Building 61, 10 Cloister Court
Bethesda, MD 20892-4754
Phone: 800-411-1222
TTY: 301-594-9774 (local); 866-411-1010 (toll free)
Website: www.cc.nih.gov/ccc/prpl

Voluntary health organizations may be able to provide information about additional clinical studies.

Another important way that people can help dementia research is by arranging to donate their brains to brain and tissue banks after they die. Tissue from these banks is made available to qualified researchers so that they can continue their studies of how these diseases develop and how they affect the brain. A list of brain banks can be found in Chapter 62.

People who have more than one family member affected by AD also may be able to help research by contributing blood samples to a gene bank. A large initiative to collect such samples was announced in 2003. This large gene bank should accelerate research efforts to identify genes that play a role in AD. People interested in participating in this gene bank can learn more about it at the address and telephone numbers below:

Alzheimer's Disease Genetics Initiative
National Cell Repository for Alzheimer's Disease (NCRAD)
Indiana University
Indianapolis, IN 46202-5251
Toll-Free: 800-526-2839
Phone: 317-274-7360
Website: http://ncrad.iu.edu
E-mail: alzstudy@iupui.edu

Chapter 10

Delirium Versus Dementia

Delirium, or acute confusion, is a sudden change in mental function. Minor problems with memory and understanding, such as forgetting a name or taking more time to figure out directions, are a normal part of aging for everyone. However, some older adults develop extreme problems with remembering, understanding, or thinking. For example, they can "get lost" walking to the bathroom, become confused by simple tasks, forget the names of loved ones, and have difficulty speaking logically. These problems can be very difficult for people to cope with, and they also strongly affect family, friends, and other caregivers.

The most common problems are dementia and delirium. These two conditions share several characteristics that sometimes make it difficult to tell them apart. In addition, dementia and delirium also commonly occur at the same time.

Delirium is one of the most common complications of medical illness or recovery from surgery among older adults in the hospital. Delirium has also been called acute confusional state, toxic psychosis, metabolic encephalopathy, or acute organic brain syndrome.

Delirium has been described in the medical literature for more than 2,000 years, and it is still quite common today. One-third of older

"Delirium (Sudden Confusion)," reprinted with permission from the American Geriatrics Society Foundation for Health in Aging (http://www .healthinaging.org) from the Aging in the Know website (http://www .healthinaging.org/agingintheknow). For more information visit the AGS online at www.americangeriatrics.org.

adults arriving at hospital emergency departments are delirious. Similarly, approximately one-third of patients aged 70 or older admitted to the hospital for general medical care experience delirium. Delirium is even more common among older adults admitted to intensive care units. Delirium is present in half of hospital patients transferred to a nursing home.

Delirium is traditionally viewed as a short-term, temporary problem, but evidence is growing that it may persist for weeks to months in a substantial number of people. Very old people with pre-existing mental difficulties seem to be at highest risk of long-term delirium. In general, all types of delirium appear strongly associated with poor outcomes among hospitalized patients. These include increased chance of death, complications, long hospital stays, and nursing home care after discharge. Poor outcomes are particularly common among older adults who have long-term delirium.

Diagnosis

When people hear the term delirium, many think it means that someone is wildly agitated. However, the type, number, and severity of symptoms vary quite a bit. Only about one-quarter of people with delirium are agitated. Most people with delirium have "quiet" delirium, or delirium with a mix of symptoms (e.g., agitated at times and quiet

Table 10.1. Characteristics of Dementia and Delirium

Dementia	Delirium
Slow onset over months to years	Sudden onset over hours to days
Normal speech	Slurred speech
Conscious and attentive	In and out of consciousness, inattentive, easily distracted
Memory loss	Memory loss
Language difficulties	Language difficulties
Hallucinations possible	Hallucinations common
Listless or apathetic mood most common; agitation also possible	Can be anxious, fearful, suspicious, agitated, or can seem to care less and react less
Often no other signs of illness	Signs of medical illness (e.g., fever, chills, pain on urinating, etc.) or drug side effects common

at times). The prognosis for quiet delirium is that same as that for agitated delirium, but it is recognized and treated less frequently.

A diagnosis of delirium is based on careful observation, awareness of changes in the person's usual mental state, and knowledge of the current physical problems. Usually, trying to talk to the person shows that his or her attention wanders and that he or she is distracted easily and has a hard time following directions. The person may speak in a disorganized way that does not make much sense. He or she may also appear restless and move a lot, and may "nod in and out." During the night, sometimes the muscles jerk and twitch and, rarely, the hands "flap."

The person's difficulty in thinking may not be obvious. Healthcare professionals sometimes use a series of simple standardized questions to try to evaluate mental function. Using standardized questions makes it possible to monitor future improvement or decline to some extent. Types of standardized questions include the following:

- Perform a simple math calculation

- Spell a short word backward

- Repeat a series of four or five numbers, in order and then in reverse order

- Name the days of the week backward

More formal and extensive testing may be able to better identify and monitor key symptoms, such as lack of attention.

When a medical condition(s) that is causing delirium is not apparent, a complete history and physical examination are necessary. The history should include a review of all drugs being taken, including over-the-counter medications, herbal remedies, etc. The healthcare provider may also recommend diagnostic laboratory tests such as blood tests, a urinalysis, a brain imaging study (e.g., a CAT scan or MRI), or an electroencephalogram (EEG). An EEG monitors brain waves through electrodes placed on the scalp. Although an EEG may not determine the reason for delirium, it is a good test for ruling out delirium. In other words, if the EEG is normal, the person does not have delirium.

Causes

We don't yet know all the mechanisms that can cause delirium, but some causes are known. A key goal of treatment is to identify any causes and correct those that are reversible. Reversible causes of delirium include the following:

- **Drugs**, including any new medications, increased dosages, drug interactions, over-the-counter drugs, alcohol, etc.

- **Electrolyte** disturbances, especially dehydration, sodium (sodium) imbalance, and thyroid problems

- **Lack of drugs**, such as stopping use of long-term sedatives (including alcohol and sleeping pills) or having pain that is poorly controlled

- **Infection**, especially urinary or respiratory tract infection

- **Reduced** sensory input, such as poor vision or hearing

- **Intracranial**, such as a brain infection, hemorrhage, stroke, or tumor (rare)

- **Urinary** or fecal problems, such as not being able to urinate or have a bowel movement

- **Myocardial** (heart) and lungs, e.g., heart attack, problems with heart rhythm, worsening of heart failure or chronic obstructive lung disease

Delirium can reflect changes in a chemical in the brain called acetylcholine, which transmits signals between nerves. Levels of acetylcholine can be affected in many ways. If oxygen or glucose levels in the brain go down, even by a small amount, the amount of acetylcholine can go down significantly. Brain damage in people with Alzheimer disease can kill the cells in the brain that produce acetylcholine, making the brain more prone to delirium when supplies of oxygen or glucose become limited. Medications that block acetylcholine can also produce delirium. In fact, side effects of medication are the most common and most treatable cause of delirium.

Drugs

Many common drugs can trigger delirium in older adults. These include narcotics (and other pain relievers), sedatives, corticosteroids, and drugs that specifically affect acetylcholine levels in the brain (e.g., atropine). Drugs are a leading cause of delirium in the hospital. In addition, nearly 60% of nursing-home residents and about 25% of older adults living in the community take drugs that block at least some acetylcholine transmission, which could lead to delirium.

Alcohol abuse is frequently overlooked as a cause of delirium in older adults. Delirium can be result from either intoxication or a sudden withdrawal from alcohol. Delirium caused by withdrawal of alcohol (i.e., the "DTs") appears to be as common in older adults with alcoholism as in their younger counterparts. However, the death rate after withdrawal is higher in older alcoholics than in younger ones. Delirium can also be caused by withdrawal from sedatives that have been taken for a long time.

Medical Conditions

Virtually any medical condition can potentially cause delirium. For example, delirium may be the first sign of a serious, life-threatening illness such as a heart attack. Often, a person has more than one potential medical cause. The most common causes among people in the hospital include problems in bodily fluids, drug reactions, infections, low blood pressure, and low levels of oxygen in the blood. Delirium caused by a sudden change in the nervous system, such as a stroke, brain tumor, or brain infection, is seen in only a small number of people.

Delirium can also result from too little stimulation of the senses, especially in people who already have some degree of mental impairment. In one study, delirium after an operation occurred twice as often in patients in intensive care units without windows as in patients in similar units with windows. In addition, a form of delirium that occurs at night (i.e., sundowning) may be partly due to sensory deprivation. Vision and hearing loss may make it more difficult for the person to perceive reality and increase the chances of delusions or hallucinations.

Delirium after Surgery

Delirium may be the most common complication after surgery in older adults. Delirium after surgery in older adults leads to longer hospital stays, a higher death rate, and a greater need for nursing-home care after discharge. Delirium may be the first sign of medical complications after surgery, such as infection, heart problems, or drug toxicities.

Several personal or medical risk factors seem to increase the chances of delirium after surgery. These include advanced age, pre-existing dementia, pre-existing physical disability, history of alcohol abuse, and very abnormal results of certain blood tests. The type of anesthesia (e.g., general, spinal, or epidural) does not seem to affect the risk of delirium, but the type of operation does. For example, delirium is much more common after hip surgery and chest surgery.

Differentiating Delirium from Look-Alike Conditions

Delirium can be mistaken for dementia or for psychiatric diseases such as schizophrenia. Certain rare forms of epilepsy can also closely resemble delirium. However, in epilepsy there is usually a history of seizures before the episode of sudden confusion.

The best way to differentiate delirium from psychiatric problems is by considering age and the rate of onset of symptoms. Any sudden change in an older person's behavior should be considered as possible delirium until examination or testing proves otherwise. Other features that may help separate psychiatric disease from delirium are the types of hallucinations that the person experiences. Psychotic patients typically hear voices or sounds, while people with delirium usually see things. In addition, physical characteristics that are typical of delirium (e.g., hand flapping and EEG changes), or evidence of a sudden underlying medical illness, are generally absent in psychiatric disorders.

Dementia also produces memory and thinking problems, just like delirium. However, dementia has a much longer onset, and mental abilities vary much less over the course of hours or days. In addition, people with dementia generally remain aware of their environment until very late in the illness. It is important to remember that dementia and delirium can be seen together, and that delirium develops commonly in people with dementia. Whenever the behavior or thinking of a person with dementia deteriorates suddenly, particularly when the person is sick or hospitalized, the cause is likely to be delirium.

Treatment

The best way to treat delirium is first to prevent it, by careful attention to underlying causes and triggers (e.g., medications). However, when delirium does occur, it is a true medical emergency that requires immediate evaluation and treatment. The cornerstones of medical management include promptly identifying the condition and the specific cause, managing any agitation or disruptive behavior, and providing general supportive care. Because delirium can be caused by so many different things, there is no simple strategy for evaluation.

The main goal of treatment is to identify and correct the underlying cause of delirium. Generally, a comprehensive medical evaluation is needed, including specific laboratory tests. These may include simple blood tests and more sophisticated tests like brain imaging studies (e.g., CAT scan and MRI). Unless they are absolutely necessary, all drugs are generally stopped.

Supportive care for people with delirium includes careful attention to medical, environmental, and social situations. People with delirium are particularly vulnerable to complications and poor outcomes and must be given special hospital care. Medical complications include problems with bodily fluids, inhaling secretions or vomit, malnutrition, pressure ulcers, joint stiffness, and other conditions such as constipation or wetting oneself that might result from not being able to move around much or from reduced consciousness.

Management of the environment involves continually helping the person feel oriented, avoiding unnecessary moves from one room or space to another. Leaving on dim lights at night can help decrease delusions or hallucinations. Things like clocks, calendars, and window views can help with orientation. Eyeglasses or hearing aids can improve a person's link to reality. Family members, close friends, or even paid assistants to be with the person can reduce the fear and anxiety seen in delirium.

Professionals in social work and nursing are often quite skilled at helping people with delirium. A person's hospital behavior while he or she is in the hospital may not accurately predict how well he or she will do at home in a familiar, stable environment. This should be kept in mind so that the decision to place someone in a nursing home is not made prematurely.

Drug treatment is often not necessary, or desirable, in cases of delirium. However, sometimes, drug treatment is needed to control highly agitated or disruptive behaviors that could cause injury. Most often, antipsychotic drugs are used, but cautiously. Sedatives can actually trigger delirium, so they are used for only a short time and only in cases of serious agitation. Sedatives are never used in people who are already drowsy or who cannot be easily wakened.

Physical restraints should rarely, if ever, be used in delirium. There is no evidence that they reduce falls or other accidents. In addition, they prevent movement, which increases the risk of developing pneumonia or pressure ulcers. Accidental strangling is even a possibility. Also, restraints and very strong medications are considered a form of involuntary treatment and may violate the rights of an agitated person.

Outlook

Family members need to understand that delirium is usually not a permanent condition, and that it improves over time, although it may take weeks or months. Slow recovery is more common if delirium is severe or if the person already has dementia or is 85 years old or older. Careful supportive care and monitoring of mental status during this period are crucial to recovery.

Family members can play an important role by providing appropriate orientation, support, and assistance. More and more, hospitals are allowing family members to sleep overnight with relatives who are already delirious or at high risk of becoming delirious. Families should seek prompt medical attention if the patient's mental status worsens suddenly.

Chapter 11

Mild Cognitive Impairment

Mild cognitive impairment (MCI) is a general term most commonly defined as a subtle but measurable memory disorder. A person with MCI experiences memory problems greater than normally expected with aging, but does not show other symptoms of dementia, such as impaired judgment or reasoning.

Compared with the large body of information about Alzheimer disease, research about MCI is at a relatively early stage. Because scientists are still answering basic questions about this disorder, it is important to note that the definition of MCI is itself a "work in progress."

Defining MCI

In 2001, the American Academy of Neurology (AAN) published practice guidelines for the early detection of memory problems. The AAN workgroup of specialists identified the following criteria for an MCI diagnosis:

- An individual's report of his or her own memory problems, preferably confirmed by another person

- Measurable, greater-than-normal memory impairment detected with standard memory assessment tests

137

- Normal general thinking and reasoning skills

- Ability to perform normal daily activities

These criteria do not settle all debate about MCI. Key questions that researchers continue to investigate include the following:

- How much memory impairment is too much to be considered more than normal?

- How much memory impairment is significant enough to be considered a symptom of mild dementia?

- How hard should one look for subtle abnormalities in other areas of thinking?

- How do we know if these other changes are normal aging or worse?

Because researchers are still investigating these questions, other details about MCI remain unclear. For example, some research suggests that essentially all cases of MCI progress to Alzheimer disease or another form of dementia. This would mean that MCI is simply a very early sign of dementia. Other studies suggest that some people with MCI may not develop dementia, but that many are at a very high risk of developing the disorder. Still other studies indicate that a significant number of people diagnosed with MCI may "revert" to normal.

The Need for Further Research about MCI

The differences in these conclusions are the result, at least in part, of significant inconsistencies in definitions of MCI. For example, some definitions involve problems with aspects of thinking other than memory. The different findings also point to the need for long-term studies that follow the progression of symptoms in people with differently defined MCI. More work is also needed on the biological changes associated with normal aging, MCI, and Alzheimer disease and other dementias.

In the December 2001 *Archives of Neurology*, a team of specialists recommended further research to define subcategories of MCI. For example, a problem primarily with language rather than memory might be considered a type of mild cognitive impairment that is an early sign of a dementia other than Alzheimer disease.

Are There Treatment Options for MCI?

Because there is a lack of agreement about a definition, any two individuals with a diagnosis of MCI may have relatively significant differences in symptoms. Physicians' recommendations for treatment will also vary. At this time, there is no widely accepted professional guideline for treatment of MCI and there is not enough evidence to recommend a standard approach. In most cases, if a person is diagnosed with MCI, the physician will regularly monitor the individual for changes in memory and thinking skills that indicate a worsening of symptoms or a development of mild dementia.

A large study reported at the April 2005 annual meeting of the American Academy of Neurology and published online in the April 14, 2005, *New England Journal of Medicine*, was the first clinical trial ever to demonstrate that a treatment could delay transition from MCI to Alzheimer disease. That three-year study enrolled more than 750 older adults with "amnestic MCI," the type whose chief feature is memory difficulties greater than would be expected for an individual's age and education. Participants were randomly assigned to one of three daily regimens: 10 milligrams of donepezil (Aricept), 2,000 international units of vitamin E, or a placebo.

Participants receiving donepezil had a reduced risk of developing Alzheimer disease during the first year of the trial, but by the end of the three-year study their risk was the same as those taking vitamin E or the placebo. Vitamin E showed no significant benefit at any time.

Study authors said the results were not strong enough to support a clear recommendation to treat MCI with donepezil, but could prompt a discussion between a physician and a patient on an individual basis. Donepezil is currently approved by the U.S. Food and Drug Administration (FDA) to treat mild to moderate Alzheimer disease.

Most experts saw the most positive outcome of this study as an important proof of concept in treating MCI, setting the stage for testing future drugs with potentially greater effect. Results also demonstrated success in the clinically challenging process of identifying individuals with MCI and monitoring their status in a large, multisite clinical trial.

Two other clinical trials have evaluated the Alzheimer drug galantamine (Razadyne, formerly Reminyl) as a possible treatment for MCI. Neither of these trials found any statistically significant benefit for galantamine in improving function or preventing transition to Alzheimer disease. However, investigators did note a significantly greater number of deaths in the galantamine treatment groups than in those

receiving the placebo. In April 2005, the FDA and its European equivalent mandated a labeling change reflecting this imbalance in the number of deaths. Data from these MCI galantamine studies have not been
published, but are posted online.

Sources

R. C. Petersen, M.D., Ph.D.; J. C. Stevens, M.D.; M. Ganguli, M.D.,
M.P.H.; E. G. Tangalos, M.D.; J. L. Cummings, M.D.; and S. T. DeKosky,
M.D. "Practice parameter: Early Detection of dementia: Mild cogni-
tive impairment (an evidence-based review). Report of the Quality
Standards Subcommittee of the American Academy of Neurology."
Neurology 2001; 56: 1133–1142. (Available online at http://aan.com/
professionals/practice/pdfs/gl0070.pdf)

R. C. Petersen, R. Doody, A. Kurz, R. C. Mohs, J. C. Morris, P. V. Rabins,
K. Ritchie, M. Rossor, L. Thal, B. Winblad. "Current concepts in mild
cognitive impairment." *Archives of Neurology* 2001; 58 (12): 1985–1992.

Petersen, R.C. et al. "Vitamin E and Donepezil for the Treatment of
Mild Cognitive Impairment." *New England Journal of Medicine* online
release April 14, 2005. Also scheduled for publication in the New England Journal print version June 9, 2005.

Synopsis and data from the MCI trials of galantamine:

- GAL-INT-11: http://www.clinicalstudyresults.org/documents/
  company-study_96_1.pdf
- GAL-INT-18: http://www.clinicalstudyresults.org/documents/
  company-study_96_2.pdf

Chapter 12

Vascular Cognitive Impairment and Multi-Infarct Dementia

The number of people affected by dementia in the U.S. is expected to increase three-fold in the next 50 years to a total of over 13 million. The best-known form of dementia is Alzheimer disease (AD), however, a large portion of dementia cases in the elderly population are not due to AD, but rather to cerebrovascular disease. Dementia due to cerebrovascular disease is referred to as "vascular dementia" and can occur in the absence of AD pathology. In recent years, the term "vascular dementia" [is sometimes] replaced by the term "vascular cognitive impairment (VCI)."

Vascular Dementia

Vascular dementia has been estimated to account for 15% to 20% of all dementias among older adults and is precipitated by some form of cerebrovascular disease. Most commonly, blockage of blood vessels in the brain yields the death of tissues, or infarction, in the affected region. Infarction underlying dementia may involve a single strategic

This chapter begins with an excerpt from "Funding News: Research Sought on Genetics and Pathobiology of Vascular Cognitive Impairment," National Institute of Neurological Disorders and Stroke, June 2006. It continues with "Vascular Dementia," excerpted from "Dementia and Its Implications for Public Health," by D.P. Chapman, et al., *Preventing Chronic Disease* [serial online, Centers for Disease Control and Prevention] April 2006 [cited July 26, 2007], available from http://www.cdc.gov/pcd/issues/2006/apr/05_0167.htm. "Multi-Infarct Dementia," is a Fact Sheet from the National Institute on Aging (http://www.nia.nih.gov), August 2006.

141

blood vessel or numerous smaller ones (multi-infarct dementia). Traditionally, vascular dementia has been characterized by sudden onset, stepwise progression, and focal neurological deficits associated with the region of the brain affected. However, results of research undertaken during the last decade have revealed that an estimated 20% of cases of vascular dementia are characterized by an insidious onset and a steadily progressive course. Postmortem examinations of the brains of individuals with dementia have suggested that the coexistence of vascular dementia with AD is not uncommon.

Laboratory tests and brain imaging techniques can be used in the diagnosis of vascular dementia. Hypertension, diabetes, age, atherosclerosis, and male sex are probable risk factors for vascular dementia. Because several of these factors have also been associated with an increased risk of AD, recognition of potential vascular components of AD is growing.

Multi-Infarct Dementia

Multi-infarct dementia is the most common form of vascular dementia and accounts for 10–20% of all cases of progressive, or gradually worsening, dementia. It usually affects people between the ages of 60–75 and is more likely to occur in men than women.

Multi-infarct dementia is caused by a series of strokes that disrupt blood flow and damage or destroy brain tissue. A stroke occurs when blood cannot get to part of the brain. Strokes can be caused when a blood clot or fatty deposit (called plaque) blocks the vessels that supply blood to the brain. A stroke also can happen when a blood vessel in the brain bursts.

Some of the main causes of strokes include the following:

- Untreated high blood pressure (hypertension)
- Diabetes
- High cholesterol
- Heart disease

Of these, the most important risk factor for multi-infarct dementia is high blood pressure.

Because strokes occur suddenly, loss of thinking and remembering skills—the symptoms of dementia—also occurs quickly and often in a stepwise pattern. People with multi-infarct dementia may even appear to improve for short periods of time, then decline again after having more strokes.

Symptoms

Sudden onset of any of the following symptoms may be a sign of multi-infarct dementia:

- Confusion and problems with recent memory
- Wandering or getting lost in familiar places
- Moving with rapid, shuffling steps
- Loss of bladder or bowel control
- Laughing or crying inappropriately
- Difficulty following instructions
- Problems handling money

Multi-infarct dementia is often the result of a series of small strokes. Some of these small strokes produce no obvious symptoms and are noticed only on brain imaging studies, so they are sometimes called "silent strokes." A person may have several small strokes before noticing serious changes in memory or other signs of multi-infarct dementia.

Transient ischemic attacks, or TIAs, are caused by a temporary blockage of blood flow. Symptoms of TIAs are similar to symptoms of stroke and include mild weakness in an arm or leg, slurred speech, and dizziness. Symptoms generally do not last for more than 20 minutes. A recent history of TIAs greatly increases a person's chance of suffering permanent brain damage from a stroke. Prompt medical attention is required to determine what may be causing the blockage in blood flow and to start proper treatment (such as aspirin or warfarin).

If you believe someone is having a stroke—if a person experiences sudden weakness or numbness on one or both sides of the body, or difficulty speaking, seeing, or walking—call 911 immediately. If the physician believes the symptoms are caused by a blocked blood vessel, treatment with a "clot buster," such as t-PA (tissue plasminogen activator), within three hours can reopen the vessel and may reduce the severity of the stroke.

Diagnosis

People who show signs of dementia and who have a history of strokes should be evaluated for possible multi-infarct dementia. The doctor usually will ask the patient and the family about the person's diet, medications, sleep patterns, personal habits, past strokes, and other risk factors (such as high blood pressure, diabetes, high cholesterol, and heart disease). The doctor also may ask about recent illnesses or stressful events, like the death of someone close or problems at home or work, which may account for the symptoms. To look for signs of stroke, the doctor will check for weakness or numbness in the arms and legs, difficulty with speech, or dizziness. To check for other health problems that could cause symptoms of dementia, the doctor may order office or laboratory tests. These tests may include a blood pressure reading, an electroencephalogram (EEG), a test of thyroid function, or blood tests.

The doctor also may ask for x-rays or special tests such as a computerized tomography (CT) scan or a magnetic resonance imaging (MRI) scan. Both CT scans and MRI scans take pictures of sections of the brain. The pictures are displayed on a computer screen to allow the doctor to see inside the brain and check for signs of stroke, tumors, or other sources of brain injury. Specialists called radiologists and neurologists interpret these scans. In addition, the doctor may send the patient to a psychologist or psychiatrist to assess reasoning, learning ability, memory, and attention span.

Sometimes multi-infarct dementia is difficult to distinguish from AD because their symptoms can be very similar. It is possible for a person to have both diseases, making it hard for the doctor to diagnose either.

Treatment

While no treatment can reverse brain damage that has already been caused by a stroke, treatment to prevent further strokes is very important. For example, high blood pressure, the primary risk factor for multi-infarct dementia, and diabetes are treatable. To prevent more strokes, doctors may prescribe medicines to control high blood pressure, high cholesterol, heart disease, and diabetes. They will counsel patients about good health habits such as exercising, avoiding smoking and drinking alcohol, and eating a low-fat diet.

To reduce symptoms of dementia, doctors may change or stop medications that can cause confusion, such as sedatives, antihistamines, strong painkillers, and other medications. Some patients also may have to be treated for additional medical conditions that can increase confusion, such as heart failure, thyroid disorders, anemia, or infections.

Doctors sometimes prescribe aspirin, warfarin, or other drugs to prevent clots from forming in small blood vessels. Medications also can be prescribed to relieve restlessness or depression or to help patients sleep better.

To improve blood flow or remove blockages in blood vessels, doctors may recommend surgical procedures, such as carotid endarterectomy, angioplasty, or stenting. Studies are under way to see how well these treatments work for patients with multi-infarct dementia. Scientists are also studying drugs that can improve blood flow to the brain, such as anti-platelet and anti-coagulant medications; drugs to treat symptoms of dementia, including Alzheimer disease medications; as well as drugs to reduce the risk of TIAs and stroke, such as cholesterol-lowering statins and blood pressure medications.

Helping Someone with Multi-Infarct Dementia

Family members and friends can help someone with multi-infarct dementia cope with mental and physical problems. They can encourage individuals to maintain their daily routines and regular social and physical activities. By talking with them about events and daily experiences, family members can help their loved ones use their mental abilities as much as possible. Some families find it helpful to use reminders such as lists, alarm clocks, and calendars to help the patient remember important times and dates.

A person with multi-infarct dementia should see their primary care doctor regularly. Health problems such as high blood pressure, diabetes, high cholesterol, and heart disease should be carefully monitored. If a person has additional medical conditions, such as depression, mental health experts may be consulted as well.

Help for home caregivers is available from a variety of sources, including nurses, family doctors, social workers, and physical and occupational therapists. Home health care and respite or neighborhood day care services can provide much-needed relief to caregivers. Support groups offer emotional support for family members caring for a person with dementia. A state or local health department, a local hospital, or the patient's doctor may be able to provide telephone numbers for such services.

Chapter 13

Subcortical Dementia (Binswanger Disease)

What is Binswanger Disease?

Binswanger disease (BD), also called subcortical vascular dementia, is a type of dementia caused by widespread, microscopic areas of damage to the deep layers of white matter in the brain. The damage is the result of the thickening and narrowing (atherosclerosis) of arteries that feed the subcortical areas of the brain. Atherosclerosis (commonly known as "hardening of the arteries") is a systemic process that affects blood vessels throughout the body. It begins late in the fourth decade of life and increases in severity with age. As the arteries become more and more narrowed, the blood supplied by those arteries decreases and brain tissue dies. A characteristic pattern of BD-damaged brain tissue can be seen with modern brain imaging techniques such as CT scans or magnetic resonance imaging (MRI). The symptoms associated with BD are related to the disruption of subcortical neural circuits that control what neuroscientists call executive cognitive functioning: short-term memory, organization, mood, the regulation of attention, the ability to act or make decisions, and appropriate behavior. The most characteristic feature of BD is psychomotor slowness—an increase in the length of time it takes, for example, for the fingers to turn the thought of a letter into the shape of a letter on a piece of paper. Other symptoms include forgetfulness

"NINDS Binswanger's Disease Information Page," National Institute of Neurological Disorders and Stroke (NINDS), April 2007.

147

(but not as severe as the forgetfulness of Alzheimer disease), changes in speech, an unsteady gait, clumsiness or frequent falls, changes in personality or mood (most likely in the form of apathy, irritability, and depression), and urinary symptoms that aren't caused by urological disease. Brain imaging, which reveals the characteristic brain lesions of BD, is essential for a positive diagnosis.

Is there any treatment?

There is no specific course of treatment for BD. Treatment is symptomatic. People with depression or anxiety may require antidepressant medications such as the serotonin-specific reuptake inhibitors (SSRI) sertraline or citalopram. Atypical antipsychotic drugs, such as risperidone and olanzapine, can be useful in individuals with agitation and disruptive behavior. Recent drug trials with the drug memantine have shown improved cognition and stabilization of global functioning and behavior. The successful management of hypertension and diabetes can slow the progression of atherosclerosis, and subsequently slow the progress of BD. Because there is no cure, the best treatment is preventive, early in the adult years, by controlling risk factors such as hypertension, diabetes, and smoking.

What is the prognosis?

BD is a progressive disease; there is no cure. Changes may be sudden or gradual and then progress in a stepwise manner. BD can often coexist with Alzheimer disease. Behaviors that slow the progression of high blood pressure, diabetes, and atherosclerosis—such as eating a healthy diet and keeping healthy wake/sleep schedules, exercising, and not smoking or drinking too much alcohol—can also slow the progression of BD.

What research is being done?

The National Institute of Neurological Disorders and Stroke (NINDS) conducts research related to BD in its laboratories at the National Institutes of Health (NIH), and also supports additional research through grants to major medical institutions across the country. Much of this research focuses on finding better ways to prevent, treat, and ultimately cure neurological disorders, such as BD.

Chapter 14

Lewy Body Dementia

What Is Lewy Body Dementia?

Lewy body dementia (LBD) is a progressive brain disease and the second leading cause of degenerative dementia in the elderly. The clinical name, "dementia with Lewy bodies" (DLB), accounts for up to 20% of all dementia cases, or 800,000 patients in the U.S. Over 50% of Parkinson disease patients develop "Parkinson disease dementia" (PDD), which accounts for at least 750,000 patients. (PDD is also a Lewy body dementia.)

Other names for the Lewy body dementias are:

- Lewy body disease (LBD);

- Diffuse Lewy body disease (DLBD);

- Cortical Lewy body disease (CLBD);

- Lewy body variant of Alzheimer disease (LBV) (LBVA);

- Parkinson disease with dementia (PDD).

In the early 1900s, while researching Parkinson disease, the scientist Friederich H. Lewy discovered abnormal protein deposits that disrupt the brain's normal functioning. These Lewy body proteins are

"What is Lewy Body Dementia?" "LBD Symptoms," and "Diagnosing Lewy Body Dementia," © 2007 Lewy Body Dementia Association. Reprinted with permission.

149

found in an area of the brain stem where they deplete the neurotransmitter dopamine, causing Parkinsonian symptoms. In Lewy body dementia, these abnormal proteins are diffuse throughout other areas of the brain, including the cerebral cortex. The brain chemical acetylcholine is depleted, causing disruption of perception, thinking, and behavior. Lewy body dementia exists either in pure form, or in conjunction with other brain changes, including those typically seen in Alzheimer disease and Parkinson disease.

LBD Symptoms

Lewy Body Dementia Symptoms and Diagnostic Criteria

Every person with LBD is different and will manifest different degrees of the following symptoms. Some will show no signs of certain features, especially in the early stages of the disease. Symptoms may fluctuate as often as moment-to-moment, hour-to-hour or day-to-day. Please note that some patients meet the criteria for LBD yet score in the normal range of some cognitive assessment tools. The Mini-Mental State Examination (MMSE), for example, cannot be relied upon to distinguish LBD from other common syndromes.

The latest clinical diagnostic criteria for LBD groups symptoms into three types:

Central Feature

Progressive dementia: Deficits in attention and executive function are typical. Prominent memory impairment may not be evident in the early stages.

Core features:

- Fluctuating cognition with pronounced variations in attention and alertness.

- Recurrent complex visual hallucinations, typically well formed and detailed.

- Spontaneous features of parkinsonism.

Suggestive features:

- Rapid eye movement (REM) sleep behavior disorder (RBD), which can appear years before the onset of dementia and parkinsonism.

- Severe sensitivity to neuroleptics occurs in up to 50% of LBD patients who take them.

- Low dopamine transporter uptake in the brain's basal ganglia as seen on single photon emission computerized tomography (SPECT) and positron emission tomography (PET) imaging scans. (These scans are not yet available outside of research settings.)

Supportive features:

- Repeated falls and syncope (fainting)

- Transient, unexplained loss of consciousness

- Autonomic dysfunction

- Hallucinations of other modalities

- Visuospatial abnormalities

- Other psychiatric disturbances

A clinical diagnosis of LBD can be probable or possible based on different symptom combinations.

A probable LBD diagnosis requires either:

- Dementia plus two or more core features, or

- Dementia plus one core feature and one or more suggestive features.

A possible LBD diagnosis requires:

- Dementia plus one core feature, or

- Dementia plus one or more suggestive features.

Symptoms Explained

In this section we'll discuss each of the symptoms, starting with the key word: dementia. Dementia is a process whereby the person becomes progressively confused. The earliest signs are usually memory problems, changes in their way of speaking, such as forgetting words, and personality problems. Cognitive symptoms of dementia include poor problem solving, difficulty with learning new skills, and impaired decision making.

Other causes of dementia should be ruled out first, such as alcoholism, overuse of medication, thyroid, or metabolic problems. Strokes can also cause dementia. If these reasons are ruled out then the person is said to have a degenerative dementia. Lewy body dementia is second only to Alzheimer disease as the most common form of dementia.

Fluctuations in cognition will be noticeable to those who are close to the person with LBD, such as their partner. At times the person will be alert and then suddenly have acute episodes of confusion. These may last hours or days. Because of these fluctuations, it is not uncommon for it to be thought that the person is "faking". This fluctuation is not related to the well-known "sundowning" of Alzheimer disease. In other words, there is no specific time of day when confusion can be seen to occur.

Hallucinations are usually, but not always, visual and often are more pronounced when the person is most confused. They are not necessarily frightening to the person. Other modalities of hallucinations include sound, taste, smell, and touch.

Parkinsonism or Parkinson disease symptoms, take the form of changes in gait; the person may shuffle or walk stiffly. There may also be frequent falls. Body stiffness in the arms or legs, or tremors may also occur. Parkinson mask (blank stare, emotionless look on face), stooped posture, drooling, and runny nose may be present.

REM sleep behavior disorder (RBD) is often noted in persons with Lewy body dementia. During periods of REM sleep, the person will move, gesture or speak. There may be more pronounced confusion between the dream and waking reality when the person awakens. RBD may actually be the earliest symptom of LBD in some patients, and is now considered a significant risk factor for developing LBD. (One recent study found that nearly two-thirds of patients diagnosed with RBD developed degenerative brain diseases, including Lewy body dementia, Parkinson disease, and multiple system atrophy, after an average of 11 years of receiving an RBD diagnosis. All three diseases are called synucleinopathies, due to the presence of a mis-folded protein in the brain called alpha-synuclein.)

Sensitivity to neuroleptic (anti-psychotic) drugs is another significant symptom that may occur. These medications can worsen the Parkinsonism or decrease the cognition or increase the hallucinations. Neuroleptic malignancy syndrome, a life-threatening illness, has been reported in persons with Lewy body dementia. For this reason, it is very important that the proper diagnosis is made and that healthcare providers are educated about the disease.

Other Symptoms

Visuospatial difficulties, including depth perception, object orientation, directional sense, and illusions may occur.

Autonomic dysfunction, including blood pressure fluctuations (e.g., postural/orthostatic hypotension) heart rate variability (HRV), sexual disturbances/impotence, constipation, urinary problems, hyperhidrosis (excessive sweating), decreased sweating/heat intolerance, syncope (fainting), dry eyes/mouth, and difficulty swallowing which may lead to aspiration pneumonia.

Other psychiatric disturbances may include systematized delusions, aggression, and depression. The onset of aggression in LBD may have a variety of causes, including infections (e.g., UTI), medications, misinterpretation of the environment or personal interactions, and the natural progression of the disease.

Diagnosing LBD

Diagnosis

An experienced clinician within the medical community should perform a diagnostic evaluation. If one is not available, the neurology department of the nearest medical university should be able to recommend appropriate resources or may even provide an experienced diagnostic team skilled in Lewy body dementia.

A thorough dementia diagnostic evaluation includes physical and neurological examinations, patient and family interviews (including a detailed lifestyle and medical history), and neuro-psychological and mental status tests. The patient's functional ability, attention, language, visuospatial skills, memory, and executive functioning are assessed. In addition, brain imaging (CT or MRI scans), blood tests, and other laboratory studies may be performed. The evaluation will provide a clinical diagnosis. Currently, a conclusive diagnosis of LBD can be obtained only from a postmortem autopsy for which arrangements should be made in advance. Some research studies may offer brain autopsies as part of their protocols. Participating in research studies is a good way to benefit others with Lewy body dementia.

Medications

Medications are one of the most controversial subjects in dealing with LBD. A medication that doesn't work for one person may work for another person.

Prescribing should only be done by a physician who is thoroughly knowledgeable about LBD. With new medications and even "over-the-counter," the patient should be closely monitored. At the first sign of an adverse reaction, consult with the patient's physician. Consider joining the online caregiver support groups to see what others have observed with prescription and over-the-counter medicines.

Risk Factors

Advanced age is considered to be the greatest risk factor for Lewy body dementia, with onset typically, but not always, between the ages of 50 and 85. Some cases have been reported much earlier. It appears to affect slightly more men than women. Having a family member with Lewy body dementia may increase a person's risk. Observational studies suggest that adopting a healthy lifestyle (exercise, mental stimulation, and nutrition) might delay age-associated dementias.

Clinical Trials

The recruitment of LBD patients for participation in clinical trials for studies on LBD, other dementias and Parkinsonian studies is now steadily increasing.

Prognosis and Stages

No cure or definitive treatment for Lewy body dementia has been discovered as yet. The disease has an average duration of five to seven years. It is possible, though, for the time span to be anywhere from 2 to 20 years, depending on several factors, including the person's overall health, age, and severity of symptoms.

Defining the stages of disease progression for LBD is difficult. The symptoms, medicine management, and duration of LBD vary greatly from person to person. To further complicate the stages assessment, LBD has a progressive but vacillating clinical course. It is typical to observe a significance progression, followed by regression back to a higher functioning level. Downward fluctuations are often caused by medications, infections, or other compromises to the immune system, but may also be due to the natural course of the disease.

Chapter 15

Frontotemporal Dementia

What Is Frontotemporal Dementia?

There is a type of dementia called "frontotemporal" which typically affects patients at a very early age. In this type of dementia, there is no true memory loss in the early stages of the type that is seen in Alzheimer dementia. Instead, there are changes in personality, ability to concentrate, social skills, motivation, and reasoning. Because of their nature, these symptoms are often confused with psychiatric disorders. There are gradual changes in one's customary ways of behaving and responding emotionally to others. Memory, language, and visual perception are usually not impaired for the first two years, yet as the disease progresses and spreads to other areas of the brain, they too may become affected. Typically, the disorder affects females more than males.

The symptoms reflect the fact that the brain degeneration is not initially widespread and settles in the parts of the brain that are important for social skills, reasoning, judgment, and the ability to take initiative.

When the brains of individuals with frontal lobe dementia are studied after death, the types of microscopic abnormalities that are seen are typically of two kinds. The first type is called non-specific focal degeneration and the second is labeled Pick disease. Non-specific focal degeneration accounts for 80% of cases of frontal lobe dementia. It is called "non specific" because there are no abnormal particles that are identifiable—only evidence that brain cells have been eliminated. Pick disease, which accounts for 20% of cases of frontal lobe dementia, is identified under the microscope by abnormal particles called "Pick bodies," named after the neurologist who first observed them.

Comportment, Insight, and Reasoning

Frontotemporal dementia affects the part of the brain that regulates comportment, insight, and reasoning. "Comportment" is a term that refers to social behavior, insight, and "appropriateness" in different social contexts. Normal comportment involves having insight and the ability to recognize what behavior is appropriate in a particular social situation and to adapt one's behavior to the situation. For example, a funeral is a solemn event requiring certain types of behavior and decorum. Similarly, while it may be perfectly natural and acceptable to take one's shoes and socks off at home, it is probably not the thing to do while in a restaurant. Comportment also refers to the style and content of a person's language. Certain types of language are acceptable in some situations or with friends and family, and not acceptable in others.

Insight, an important aspect of comportment, has to do with the ability to "see" oneself as others do. Insight is necessary in order to determine whether one is behaving in a socially acceptable or in a reasonable manner. Insight is also necessary for the patient to recognize his/her deficits and illness. Changes in comportment may be manifested as "personality" alterations. A generally active, involved person could become apathetic and disinterested. The opposite may also occur. A usually quiet individual may become more outgoing, boisterous, and disinhibited. Personality changes can also involve increased irritability, anger, and even verbal or physical outbursts toward others (usually the caregiver). Comportment is assessed by observing the patient's behavior throughout the examination and interviewing other people (family and friends) who have information about the patient's "characteristic" behavior.

Individuals with frontotemporal dementia frequently have executive function and reasoning deficits. "Reasoning" refers to mental activities that promote decision-making. Being able to categorize information and to move from one perspective of a problem to another are examples of reasoning. "Executive functions" is a term that refers to yet another group of mental activities that organize and plan the flow of behavior. A good example of executive functions is what might happen if one were driving a car, talking with the passenger and suddenly having to respond to a child running into traffic. The ability to handle all the stimulation and to quickly plan a course of action is accomplished via executive functions. Individuals with frontal lobe dementia often lack flexibility in thinking and are unable to carry a project through to completion. Failure of executive functions may increase safety risk since they may not be able to plan appropriate actions or inhibit inappropriate actions.

Symptoms of Frontotemporal Dementia

- Impairments in social skills
  - inappropriate or bizarre social behavior (eating with one's fingers in public, doing sit-ups in a public restroom, being overly familiar with strangers)
  - "loosening" of normal social restraints (using obscene language or making inappropriate sexual remarks)
- Change in activity level
  - apathy, withdrawal, loss of interest, lack of motivation, and initiative which may appear to be depression but the patient does not experience sad feelings
  - in some instances there is an increase in purposeless activity (pacing, constant cleaning, or agitation)
- Decreased judgment
  - impairments in financial decision-making (impulsive spending)
  - difficulty recognizing consequences of behavior
  - lack of appreciation for threats to safety (inviting strangers into home)
- Changes in personal habits
  - lack of concern over personal appearance
  - irresponsibility
  - compulsiveness (need to carry out repeated actions that are inappropriate or not relevant to the situation at hand

- Alterations in personality and mood
  - increased irritability, decreased ability to tolerate frustration
- Changes is one's customary emotional responsiveness
  - a lack of sympathy or compassion in someone who was typically responsive to others' distress
  - heightened emotionality in someone who was typically less emotionally responsive

Persons with this form of dementia may look like they have problems in almost all areas of mental function. This is because all mental activity requires attention, concentration, and the ability to organize information, all of which are impaired in frontal lobe dementia. Careful testing, however, usually shows that most of the problems stem from a lack of persistence and increased inertia.

Psychosocial Issues

The psychological, social, family, and financial issues that affect individuals with frontotemporal dementia are drastically different from those that affect individuals with Alzheimer type dementia. When dementia occurs earlier in life, issues such as working, teenage children, and financial stress are different from the issues dealt with by individuals who are older and most likely retired. Planning for the family's financial security and for the education of children becomes a difficult prospect when an individual is faced with a dementing illness in the prime of his/her working career. The nature of the symptoms themselves are often embarrassing to family members and there may be loss of friends and other sources of social support. Finally, most adult day programs and residential care facilities are not equipped to address the special needs of the younger patient, especially if the behavioral symptoms are difficult to manage. As more is known about the disease, more policy changes may come into effect. Some residential care and adult day programs are recognizing the needs of the younger dementia patient and are beginning to offer services to meet their needs. Before making any decisions, it is best to investigate your options.

Depending on severity, a patient with impaired comportment may not be able to manage their daily activities without supervision. They may be at risk for harming themselves or being victimized because they would not be able to recognize their limitations or use proper judgment. Driving is usually unsafe for persons with this diagnosis.

Fortunately, there are steps that can be taken to provide a secure environment for the diagnosed person and obtain help for family:

- Obtain a psychiatric evaluation from an individual with experience treating people with dementia. Certain medications can help with behavior problems such as agitation and hostility.

- Share information with family and friends. This will help them better understand the patient's behavior and provide an opportunity for them to offer the diagnosed persona and their family some support and respite.

- Encourage the person to attend an early stage support group. Even if the support group is geared toward the person with early Alzheimer disease, much information will also be relevant to frontal lobe dementia.

- Meet with an attorney or financial consultant. Make sure Durable Power of Attorney forms have been completed for both health care and finances. Give copies to your doctor. An "elder law" attorney who is well-versed in these issues is still an appropriate choice to help you draft these documents or you may obtain the forms at many stationary stores and complete them on your own.

- Attend a caregiver support group. Listening to others who are going through similar experiences can be very comforting. They may also aid you in developing new caregiver techniques and learn about different resources within your community.

- Try to remain physically and mentally healthy. Be sure to get regular health check-ups for both the diagnosed person and family. Exercise and eat nutritious meals. Build in time for things that allow you to rejuvenate.

- Obtain a driving evaluation: Contact your local Alzheimer's Association for the driving evaluation program near you.

Important Contacts

If the patient is working and needs to file for disability, it is best to speak to their employer as well as the local social security office. Disability benefits are usually obtained as long as your impairment does not medically improve and you cannot work.

Social Security's Toll-Free Number: 800-772-1213
Internet address: http://www.ssa.gov

Chapter 16

AIDS Dementia Complex

Dementia is a brain disorder that affects a person's ability to think clearly and can impact his or her daily activities. AIDS dementia complex (ADC)—dementia caused by HIV infection—is a complicated syndrome made up of different nervous system and mental symptoms. These symptoms are somewhat common in people with HIV disease.

The frequency of ADC increases with advancing HIV disease and as CD4+ cell counts decrease. It is fairly uncommon in people with early HIV disease, but it's more common in people with severely weakened immune systems and symptoms of advanced disease. Severe ADC is almost exclusively seen only in people with advanced HIV disease.

ADC consists of many conditions that can be of varying degrees and may progressively worsen. These conditions can easily be mistaken for symptoms of other common HIV-associated problems including depression, drug side effects, or opportunistic infections that affect the brain like toxoplasmosis or lymphoma. Symptoms of ADC may include poor concentration, forgetfulness, loss of short- or long-term memory, social

"AIDS Dementia Complex," © 2007 Project Inform. For more information, contact the National HIV/AIDS Treatment Infoline, 1-800-822-7422, or visit the Project Inform website at www.projectinform.org. This material has been produced as a result of a collaboration between Project Inform and Gay Men's Health Crisis. For more information about Project Inform, call the Project Inform Infoline at 1-800-822-7422. For more information about Gay Men's Health Crisis in New York, call 212-367-1451. Special thanks goes to Dr. Richard Price of University of California's San Francisco General Hospital, Neurology Services and Dr. Justin McArthur, Professor of Neurology and Epidemiology at Johns Hopkins University in Baltimore for their editorial support.

withdrawal, slowed thinking, short attention span, irritability, apathy (lack of caring or concern for oneself or others), weakness, poor coordination, impaired judgment, problems with vision, and personality change.

Because ADC varies so much from person to person, it is poorly understood and has been reported and described in many conflicting ways. This information will shed light on some of these issues as well as the available treatments for ADC.

Possible symptoms of early stage ADC:

- Difficulty concentrating
- Difficulty remembering phone numbers or appointments
- Slowed thinking
- Longer time needed to complete complicated tasks
- Reliance on list keeping to help track daily activities
- Mental status tests and other mental capabilities may be normal
- Irritability
- Unsteady gait (walk) or difficulty keeping balance
- Poor hand coordination and change in writing
- Depression

Possible symptoms of middle stage ADC:

- Symptoms of motor dysfunction, like muscle weakness
- Poor performance on regular tasks
- More concentration and attention required
- Slow responses and frequently dropping objects
- General feelings of indifference or apathy
- Slowness in normal activities, like eating and writing
- Walking, balance, and coordination require a great deal of effort

Possible symptoms of late stage ADC:

- Loss of bladder or bowel control
- Spastic gait, making walking more difficult
- Loss of initiative or interest
- Withdrawing from life
- Psychosis or mania
- Confinement to bed

What is ADC?

ADC is characterized by severe changes in four areas: a person's ability to understand, process, and remember information (cognition); behavior; ability to coordinate muscles and movement (motor coordination); or emotions (mood). These changes are called ADC when they're believed to be related to HIV itself rather than other factors that might cause them, like other brain infections, drug side effects, etc.

In ADC, cognitive impairment is often characterized by memory loss, speech problems, inability to concentrate and poor judgment. Cognitive problems are often the first symptoms a person with ADC will notice. These include the need to make lists in order to remember routine tasks or forgetting, in mid-sentence, what one was talking about.

Behavioral changes in ADC are the least understood and defined. They can be described as impairments in one's ability to perform common tasks and activities of daily living. These changes are found in 30–40% of people with early ADC.

Motor impairment is often characterized by a loss of control of the bladder; loss of feeling in and loss of control of the legs; and stiff, awkward or obviously slowed movements. Motor impairment is not common in early ADC. Early symptoms may include a change in handwriting.

Mood impairments are defined as changes in emotional responses. In ADC, this impairment is associated with conditions, such as severe depression, severe personality changes (psychosis), and, less commonly, intense excitability (mania).

The Symptoms of ADC

Properly diagnosing ADC is heavily dependent on the keen judgment of doctors, often together with specialists like psychiatric, brain, or neurology experts. It's easy to imagine how difficult it is to determine impairments in mood and behavior since there's no standard or common course of ADC. In one person it may be very mild with periods of varying severity of symptoms. In another it can be abrupt, severe, and progressive. Currently, there is no way to tell how a person will progress with ADC.

Sometimes symptoms of ADC are overlooked or dismissed by caregivers, who may believe the symptoms are due to advanced HIV disease. In fact, people with advanced disease generally do not have symptoms of ADC but do have fairly normal mental functioning as long as they also have no other neurological problems. At the other end of the spectrum, ADC should be carefully distinguished from severe depression—common among people with HIV that may result in symptoms similar to ADC.

ADC occurs more commonly in children with HIV than with adults. It presents similarly and is often more severe and progressive.

How does HIV cause ADC?

While it is clear that HIV can cause serious nervous system disease, how it causes ADC is unclear. In general, nervous system and mental disorders are caused by the death of nerve cells. While HIV does not directly infect nerve cells, it's thought that HIV can somehow kill them indirectly.

Macrophages—white cells that are prevalent in the brain and act as large reservoirs for HIV—appear to be HIV's first target in the central nervous system. HIV-infected macrophages can carry HIV into the brain from the bloodstream. Test tube studies offer these hypotheses about how macrophages may help destroy nerve cells:

- An infected macrophage in the brain may shed a particle on HIV's outer coat (called gp120), causing damage to nerve cells.

- HIV's TAT gene, which helps produce new virus, detaches from HIV and circulates in the blood, causing toxic effects in nerve cells.

- The macrophage itself releases a number of substances that, in excess, can be toxic to the brain. Some examples are quinolinic acid and nitric oxide, among an array of other signal molecules. These can bind to nerve cells and cause cell dysfunction or death. Research has found higher levels of quinolinic acid and other markers of cell activation in the CSF [cerebrospinal fluid] of people with ADC.

- HIV infection of other brain cells, including astrocytes.

Incidence

Anecdotal reports indicate that there are fewer people with ADC since anti-HIV therapy became standard. People who develop ADC today tend to be "sicker" than those who developed it before the use of anti-HIV therapy. One early study from England supports this theory.

The British study found that only 2% of people with AIDS taking AZT [azidothymidine; zidovudine] developed ADC from 1982–1988, compared to 20% of those not on AZT. The incidence of ADC dropped from 53% in 1987 (before the arrival of AZT) to 3% in 1988 (after the arrival of AZT).

Early in the epidemic, many new AIDS cases were attributed to ADC. These newly-diagnosed people often had ADC but no other AIDS-related condition. Many doctors report that they are no longer seeing people who have just ADC. It has increasingly become a disease of late-stage AIDS when people suffer from multiple infections.

Diagnosing ADC

Three tests are required to diagnose ADC accurately: a mental status exam, one of the standard scans (CT [computed tomography] and/or (MRI [magnetic resonance imaging]), and a spinal tap. These may also help tell ADC apart from other brain disorders like toxoplasmosis, PML (progressive multifocal leukoencephalopathy), or lymphoma. Care should be taken, however, as ADC may occur along with the symptoms of other brain disorders. Diagnosing both conditions at the same time can be more difficult.

The main way to detect and evaluate ADC is through a mental status exam. The examination is designed to reveal problems like short- or long-term memory loss, problems with orientation, concentration and abstract thinking, as well as swings in mood. Imaging of the brain with scans (like an x-ray) is also used. Certain lab tests can also be useful like examining cerebrospinal fluid (CSF) obtained by a spinal tap (also called lumbar puncture).

CT and MRI scans are routinely used in the detection of ADC. CT scans are x-rays that use special beams to produce detailed images of organs and structures within the body. In people with ADC these scans usually show signs of destroyed brain tissue. MRI, or magnetic resonance imaging, is a sensitive brain scan that is used when CT findings are not conclusive. Results from both of these tests are helpful in ruling out other causes for the symptoms.

Tests of CSF may help determine if someone has ADC, but they are not conclusive. Mostly they're used to rule out other causes of the symptoms of ADC, and that's why they're important. Many people with ADC have higher levels of certain proteins or white blood cells in their CSF. However, not everyone with these levels turns out to have ADC. Also, people with advanced ADC are generally more likely to have higher HIV levels in their CSF, although people with no symptoms of brain disorders sometimes have high HIV levels in their CSF.

What if I think I have ADC?

• Don't be afraid to tell your doctor or any other providers that you suspect something is wrong. If you don't have a doctor or need help finding one, contact local AIDS organizations for help in getting one. They can also help you find a doctor for a second opinion if you need one.

• Keep a small notepad with you and write down your symptoms whenever they occur. This information will greatly help your doctor to help you.

• Build as much support as possible, including friends, family, and professionals. Although it's possible to treat ADC successfully, it may take awhile for some symptoms to go away.

Treating ADC

The best therapies to treat ADC appear to be anti-HIV drugs, and high-dose AZT is the most studied drug for it. However, many specialists contend that how well a potent regimen controls HIV reproduction overall is more important than the actual drugs used in the regimen. This may or may not include using standard, or even high-dose, AZT as part of the regimen.

Generally speaking, creating an anti-HIV regimen with the extra goal of treating ADC follows three basic principals:

1. Start a potent regimen (usually three drugs) to decrease HIV levels to below the limit of detection of viral load tests;

2. In people who have used anti-HIV therapy before, consider the prior therapy history as well as information from anti-HIV resistance tests;

3. If possible, use anti-HIV drugs that cross the blood-brain barrier as part of a combination therapy regimen.

It's believed—based on findings that high-dose AZT (1,000–1,200mg/daily) can cross the blood-brain barrier and effectively treat ADC—that an anti-HIV drug that crosses the blood-brain barrier might help prevent or treat ADC. To date, AZT is the best understood treatment available for ADC. Several groups have reported improvements in cognitive functions with AZT as well as prevention of HIV infection of the brain. Larger doses (1,000 mg compared to the now-standard 600 mg per day) of AZT appear to be necessary for treating ADC.

However, high-dose AZT may present problems since many people with HIV, particularly those who are the sickest, are often unable to tolerate its side effects.

While AZT may be the most researched drug for treating ADC, other anti-HIV drugs that cross the blood-brain barrier may be equally useful. These include—in addition to AZT—d4T, abacavir, nevirapine, amprenavir, atazanavir, and, to a lesser degree, indinavir and 3TC. Efavirenz has not been shown to cross this barrier to a significant degree, but some experts speculate that it may be useful in treating ADC.

Anti-HIV therapies are best used in combinations. It may also be important to consider a drug's ability to cross into the brain when constructing an effective regimen. For information on developing long-term strategies and creating potent anti-HIV therapy regimen, call Project Inform's Infoline (1-800-822-7422).

Treating the Symptoms of ADC

Psychoactive drugs are often used to treat the symptoms of ADC. These include antipsychotics, antidepressants, anxiolytics, psychostimulants, antimanics, and anticonvulsants. These drugs do not treat the underlying cause of ADC, or even stop its progression. However, they may ease some of its symptoms. Haloperidol (Haldol) is often used for easing ADC symptoms, though it has many side effects. People with ADC are sensitive to Haldol, so small doses of 5–10 mg daily should be used to avoid severe side effects.

Ritalin (methylphenidate) has been used with success in people with ADC to ease apathy and to increase energy, concentration, and appetite. Daily doses of 5–10 mg are often sufficient.

In cases of severe behavior disorders, antipsychotics like Thorazine and Mellaril can be used to control agitation. Lorazepam (Ativan) and diazepam (Valium) may also be used for sedation and controlling anxiety. Other drugs include perphenazine (Trilafon), thiothixene (Navane), molindone (Moban), and fluoxetine (Prozac) with bupropion (Wellbutrin).

Many of the therapies listed here may have potential drug interaction with commonly used anti-HIV therapies as well as therapies to treat or prevent HIV-related conditions. For more information about drug interactions, call Project Inform's Infoline (1-800-822-7422).

What if someone I care for has symptoms or was diagnosed with ADC?

- Help them access the proper diagnosis and treatment.

- Understand that loss of mental and emotional control is terribly frightening for most people, even if it's only moderate or short-term. However, be honest about their symptoms as you offer support and encouragement to establish trust.

- Because mood changes and memory problems are common with ADC, you may encounter resistance while trying to help. Helping the person you care for to write down their symptoms in their own handwriting, as they experience them, can sometimes encourage them to seek medical care.

- Professional caregivers, like home health aides, are sometimes needed to care for people with severe ADC or ADC that doesn't respond to treatment. Seeking this kind of support is sometimes the best way to help those you love.

- Caregiving for someone with memory and behavioral problems can be overwhelming, especially if it's over a long period of time. There are support services in many cities for those who care for others with life-threatening illnesses.

Conclusion

New treatments for ADC are desperately needed. It's also important that new anti-HIV drugs be fully evaluated for their usefulness in treating ADC. At the same time, promising drugs that may work to treat the underlying causes of ADC also need to be investigated.

Chapter 17

Creutzfeldt-Jakob Disease

What is Creutzfeldt-Jakob disease?

Creutzfeldt-Jakob disease (CJD) is a rare, degenerative, invariably fatal brain disorder. It affects about one person in every one million people per year worldwide; in the United States there are about 200 cases per year. CJD usually appears in later life and runs a rapid course. Typically, onset of symptoms occurs about age 60, and about 90 percent of patients die within one year. In the early stages of disease, patients may have failing memory, behavioral changes, lack of coordination and visual disturbances. As the illness progresses, mental deterioration becomes pronounced and involuntary movements, blindness, weakness of extremities, and coma may occur.

There are three major categories of CJD:

- In sporadic CJD, the disease appears even though the person has no known risk factors for the disease. This is by far the most common type of CJD and accounts for at least 85 percent of cases.

- In hereditary CJD, the person has a family history of the disease or tests positive for a genetic mutation associated with CJD. About 5 to 10 percent of cases of CJD in the United States are hereditary.

- In acquired CJD, the disease is transmitted by exposure to brain or nervous system tissue, usually through certain medical

"Creutzfeldt-Jakob Disease Fact Sheet," National Institute of Neurological Disorders and Stroke (http://www.ninds.nih.gov), April 2007.

procedures. There is no evidence that CJD is contagious through casual contact with a CJD patient. Since CJD was first described in 1920, fewer than one percent of cases have been acquired CJD.

CJD belongs to a family of human and animal diseases known as the transmissible spongiform encephalopathies (TSEs). Spongiform refers to the characteristic appearance of infected brains, which become filled with holes until they resemble sponges under a microscope. CJD is the most common of the known human TSEs. Other human TSEs include kuru, fatal familial insomnia (FFI), and Gerstmann-Straussler-Scheinker disease (GSS). Kuru was identified in people of an isolated tribe in Papua New Guinea and has now almost disappeared. FFI and GSS are extremely rare hereditary diseases, found in just a few families around the world. Other TSEs are found in specific kinds of animals. These include bovine spongiform encephalopathy (BSE), which is found in cows and is often referred to as "mad cow" disease; scrapie, which affects sheep and goats; mink encephalopathy; and feline encephalopathy. Similar diseases have occurred in elk, deer, and exotic zoo animals.

What are the symptoms of the disease?

CJD is characterized by rapidly progressive dementia. Initially, patients experience problems with muscular coordination; personality changes, including impaired memory, judgment, and thinking; and impaired vision. People with the disease also may experience insomnia, depression, or unusual sensations. CJD does not cause a fever or other flu-like symptoms. As the illness progresses, the patients' mental impairment becomes severe. They often develop involuntary muscle jerks called myoclonus, and they may go blind. They eventually lose the ability to move and speak and enter a coma. Pneumonia and other infections often occur in these patients and can lead to death.

There are several known variants of CJD. These variants differ somewhat in the symptoms and course of the disease. For example, a variant form of the disease-called new variant or variant (nvCJD, vCJD), described in Great Britain and France-begins primarily with psychiatric symptoms, affects younger patients than other types of CJD, and has a longer than usual duration from onset of symptoms to death. Another variant, called the panencephalopathic form, occurs primarily in Japan and has a relatively long course, with symptoms often progressing for several years. Scientists are trying to learn what causes these variations in the symptoms and course of the disease.

Some symptoms of CJD can be similar to symptoms of other progressive neurological disorders, such as Alzheimer or Huntington disease. However, CJD causes unique changes in brain tissue which can be seen at autopsy. It also tends to cause more rapid deterioration of a person's abilities than Alzheimer disease or most other types of dementia.

How is CJD diagnosed?

There is currently no single diagnostic test for CJD. When a doctor suspects CJD, the first concern is to rule out treatable forms of dementia such as encephalitis (inflammation of the brain) or chronic meningitis. A neurological examination will be performed and the doctor may seek consultation with other physicians. Standard diagnostic tests will include a spinal tap to rule out more common causes of dementia and an electroencephalogram (EEG) to record the brain's electrical pattern, which can be particularly valuable because it shows a specific type of abnormality in CJD. Computerized tomography of the brain can help rule out the possibility that the symptoms result from other problems such as stroke or a brain tumor. Magnetic resonance imaging (MRI) brain scans also can reveal characteristic patterns of brain degeneration that can help diagnose CJD.

The only way to confirm a diagnosis of CJD is by brain biopsy or autopsy. In a brain biopsy, a neurosurgeon removes a small piece of tissue from the patient's brain so that it can be examined by a neuropathologist. This procedure may be dangerous for the patient, and the operation does not always obtain tissue from the affected part of the brain. Because a correct diagnosis of CJD does not help the patient, a brain biopsy is discouraged unless it is needed to rule out a treatable disorder. In an autopsy, the whole brain is examined after death. Both brain biopsy and autopsy pose a small, but definite, risk that the surgeon or others who handle the brain tissue may become accidentally infected by self-inoculation. Special surgical and disinfection procedures can minimize this risk.

Scientists are working to develop laboratory tests for CJD. One such test, developed at the National Institute of Neurological Disorders and Stroke (NINDS), is performed on a person's cerebrospinal fluid and detects a protein marker that indicates neuronal degeneration. This can help diagnose CJD in people who already show the clinical symptoms of the disease. This test is much easier and safer than a brain biopsy. The false positive rate is about five to ten percent. Scientists are working to develop this test for use in commercial laboratories. They are also working to develop other tests for this disorder.

How is the disease treated?

There is no treatment that can cure or control CJD. Researchers have tested many drugs, including amantadine, steroids, interferon, acyclovir, antiviral agents, and antibiotics. Studies of a variety of other drugs are now in progress. However, so far none of these treatments has shown any consistent benefit in humans.

Current treatment for CJD is aimed at alleviating symptoms and making the patient as comfortable as possible. Opiate drugs can help relieve pain if it occurs, and the drugs clonazepam and sodium valproate may help relieve myoclonus. During later stages of the disease, changing the person's position frequently can keep him or her comfortable and helps prevent bedsores. A catheter can be used to drain urine if the patient cannot control bladder function, and intravenous fluids and artificial feeding also may be used.

What causes Creutzfeldt-Jakob disease?

Some researchers believe an unusual "slow virus" or another organism causes CJD. However, they have never been able to isolate a virus or other organism in people with the disease. Furthermore, the agent that causes CJD has several characteristics that are unusual for known organisms such as viruses and bacteria. It is difficult to kill, it does not appear to contain any genetic information in the form of nucleic acids (DNA or RNA), and it usually has a long incubation period before symptoms appear. In some cases, the incubation period may be as long as 40 years. The leading scientific theory at this time maintains that CJD and the other TSEs are caused by a type of protein called a prion.

Prion proteins occur in both a normal form, which is a harmless protein found in the body's cells, and in an infectious form, which causes disease. The harmless and infectious forms of the prion protein have the same sequence of amino acids (the "building blocks" of proteins) but the infectious form of the protein takes a different folded shape than the normal protein. Sporadic CJD may develop because some of a person's normal prions spontaneously change into the infectious form of the protein and then alter the prions in other cells in a chain reaction.

Once they appear, abnormal prion proteins aggregate, or clump together. Investigators think these protein aggregates may lead to the neuron loss and other brain damage seen in CJD. However, they do not know exactly how this damage occurs.

About five to ten percent of all CJD cases are inherited. These cases arise from a mutation, or change, in the gene that controls formation of the normal prion protein. While prions themselves do not contain genetic information and do not require genes to reproduce themselves, infectious prions can arise if a mutation occurs in the gene for the body's normal prion protein. If the prion protein gene is altered in a person's sperm or egg cells, the mutation can be transmitted to the person's offspring. Several different mutations in the prion gene have been identified. The particular mutation found in each family affects how frequently the disease appears and what symptoms are most noticeable. However, not all people with mutations in the prion protein gene develop CJD.

How is CJD transmitted?

CJD cannot be transmitted through the air or through touching or most other forms of casual contact. Spouses and other household members of sporadic CJD patients have no higher risk of contracting the disease than the general population. However, exposure to brain tissue and spinal cord fluid from infected patients should be avoided to prevent transmission of the disease through these materials.

In some cases, CJD has spread to other people from grafts of dura mater (a tissue that covers the brain), transplanted corneas, implantation of inadequately sterilized electrodes in the brain, and injections of contaminated pituitary growth hormone derived from human pituitary glands taken from cadavers. Doctors call these cases that are linked to medical procedures iatrogenic cases. Since 1985, all human growth hormone used in the United States has been synthesized by recombinant DNA procedures, which eliminates the risk of transmitting CJD by this route.

The appearance of the new variant of CJD (nvCJD or vCJD) in several younger than average people in Great Britain and France has led to concern that BSE may be transmitted to humans through consumption of contaminated beef. Although laboratory tests have shown a strong similarity between the prions causing BSE and v-CJD, there is no direct proof to support this theory.

Many people are concerned that it may be possible to transmit CJD through blood and related blood products such as plasma. Some animal studies suggest that contaminated blood and related products may transmit the disease, although this has never been shown in humans. If there are infectious agents in these fluids, they are probably in very low concentrations. Scientists do not know how many abnormal prions a person must receive before he or she develops CJD, so they do not know whether these fluids are potentially infectious or not. They do know that, even though millions of people receive blood transfusions each year, there are no reported cases of someone contracting CJD from a transfusion. Even among people with hemophilia, who sometimes receive blood plasma concentrated from thousands of donors, there are no reported cases of CJD.

While there is no evidence that blood from people with sporadic CJD is infectious, studies have found that infectious prions from BSE and vCJD may accumulate in the lymph nodes (which produce white blood cells), the spleen, and the tonsils. These findings suggest that blood transfusions from people with vCJD might transmit the disease. The possibility that blood from people with vCJD may be infectious has led to a policy preventing people in the United States from donating blood if they have resided for more than three months in a country or countries where BSE is common.

How can people avoid spreading the disease?

To reduce the already very low risk of CJD transmission from one person to another, people should never donate blood, tissues, or organs if they have suspected or confirmed CJD, or if they are at increased risk because of a family history of the disease, a dura mater graft, or other factor.

Normal sterilization procedures such as cooking, washing, and boiling do not destroy prions. Caregivers, health care workers, and undertakers should take the following precautions when they are working with a person with CJD:

- Wash hands and exposed skin before eating, drinking, or smoking.

- Cover cuts and abrasions with waterproof dressings.

- Wear surgical gloves when handling a patient's tissues and fluids or dressing the patient's wounds.

- Avoid cutting or sticking themselves with instruments contaminated by the patient's blood or other tissues.

- Use face protection if there is a risk of splashing contaminated material such as blood or cerebrospinal fluid.

- Soak instruments that have come in contact with the patient in undiluted chlorine bleach for an hour or more, then use an autoclave (pressure cooker) to sterilize them in distilled water for at least one hour at 132–134 degrees Centigrade.

What research is taking place?

Many researchers are studying CJD. They are examining whether the transmissible agent is, in fact, a prion or a product of the infection, and are trying to discover factors that influence prion infectivity and how the disorder damages the brain. Using rodent models of the disease and brain tissue from autopsies, they are also trying to identify factors that influence susceptibility to the disease and that govern when in life the disease appears. They hope to use this knowledge to develop improved tests for CJD and to learn what changes ultimately kill the neurons so that effective treatments can be developed.

How can I help research?

Scientists are conducting biochemical analyses of brain tissue, blood, spinal fluid, urine, and serum in hope of determining the nature of the transmissible agent or agents causing Creutzfeldt-Jakob disease. To help with this research, they are seeking biopsy and autopsy tissue, blood, and cerebrospinal fluid from patients with CJD and related diseases. The following investigators have expressed an interest in receiving such material:

Dr. Pierluigi Gambetti, Director
National Prion Disease Pathology Surveillance Center
Institute of Pathology
Room 419, Case Western Reserve University
2085 Adelbert Road
Cleveland, OH 44106
Telephone: 216-368-058; Fax: 216-368-4090
E-mail: cjdsurv@cwru.edu
Website: http://www.cjdsurveillance.com

Dr. Laura Manuelidis
Yale University School of Medicine
Section of Neuropathology
310 Cedar Street
New Haven, CT 06510
Telephone: 203-785-4442

Dr. Stephen DeArmond or Dr. Stanley Prusiner
Department of Pathology/Neuropathology Unit, HSW 430
University of California, San Francisco
San Francisco, CA 94143
Telephone: 415-476-5236

Chapter 18

Huntington Disease

In 1872, the American physician George Huntington wrote about an illness that he called "an heirloom from generations away back in the dim past." He was not the first to describe the disorder, which has been traced back to the Middle Ages at least. One of its earliest names was chorea, which, as in "choreography," is the Greek word for dance. The term chorea describes how people affected with the disorder writhe, twist, and turn in a constant, uncontrollable dance-like motion. Later, other descriptive names evolved. "Hereditary chorea" emphasizes how the disease is passed from parent to child. "Chronic progressive chorea" stresses how symptoms of the disease worsen over time. Today, physicians commonly use the simple term Huntington disease (HD) to describe this highly complex disorder that causes untold suffering for thousands of families.

In the United States alone, about 30,000 people have HD; estimates of its prevalence are about one in every 10,000 persons. At least 150,000 others have a 50 percent risk of developing the disease and thousands more of their relatives live with the possibility that they, too, might develop HD.

Until recently, scientists understood very little about HD and could only watch as the disease continued to pass from generation to generation. Families saw the disease destroy their loved ones' ability to feel, think, and move. In the last several years, scientists working with

"Huntington's Disease: Hope through Research," National Institute of Neurological Disorders and Stroke, April 2007.

support from the National Institute of Neurological Disorders and Stroke (NINDS) have made several breakthroughs in the area of HD research. With these advances, our understanding of the disease continues to improve.

This chapter presents information about HD, and about current research progress, to health professionals, scientists, caregivers, and, most important, to those already too familiar with the disorder: the many families who are affected by HD.

What causes Huntington disease?

HD results from genetically programmed degeneration of nerve cells, called neurons, in certain areas of the brain. This degeneration causes uncontrolled movements, loss of intellectual faculties, and emotional disturbance. Specifically affected are cells of the basal ganglia, structures deep within the brain that have many important functions, including coordinating movement. Within the basal ganglia, HD especially targets neurons of the striatum, particularly those in the caudate nuclei and the pallidum. Also affected is the brain's outer surface, or cortex, which controls thought, perception, and memory.

How is HD inherited?

HD is found in every country of the world. It is a familial disease, passed from parent to child through a mutation or misspelling in the normal gene.

A single abnormal gene, the basic biological unit of heredity, produces HD. Genes are composed of deoxyribonucleic acid (DNA), a molecule shaped like a spiral ladder. Each rung of this ladder is composed of two paired chemicals called bases. There are four types of bases—adenine, thymine, cytosine, and guanine—each abbreviated by the first letter of its name: A, T, C, and G. Certain bases always "pair" together, and different combinations of base pairs join to form coded messages. A gene is a long string of this DNA in various combinations of A, T, C, and G. These unique combinations determine the gene's function, much like letters join together to form words. Each person has about 30,000 genes—a billion base pairs of DNA or bits of information repeated in the nuclei of human cells—which determine individual characteristics or traits.

Genes are arranged in precise locations along 23 rod-like pairs of chromosomes. One chromosome from each pair comes from an individual's mother, the other from the father. Each half of a chromosome pair is similar to the other, except for one pair, which determines the sex of the individual. This pair has two X chromosomes in females and one X and one Y chromosome in males. The gene that produces HD lies on chromosome 4, one of the 22 non-sex-linked, or "autosomal," pairs of chromosomes, placing men and women at equal risk of acquiring the disease.

The impact of a gene depends partly on whether it is dominant or recessive. If a gene is dominant, then only one of the paired chromosomes is required to produce its called-for effect. If the gene is recessive, both parents must provide chromosomal copies for the trait to be present. HD is called an autosomal dominant disorder because only one copy of the defective gene, inherited from one parent, is necessary to produce the disease.

The genetic defect responsible for HD is a small sequence of DNA on chromosome 4 in which several base pairs are repeated many, many times. The normal gene has three DNA bases, composed of the sequence CAG. In people with HD, the sequence abnormally repeats itself dozens of times. Over time—and with each successive generation—the number of CAG repeats may expand further.

Each parent has two copies of every chromosome but gives only one copy to each child. Each child of an HD parent has a 50-50 chance of inheriting the HD gene. If a child does not inherit the HD gene, he or she will not develop the disease and cannot pass it to subsequent generations. A person who inherits the HD gene, and survives long enough, will sooner or later develop the disease. In some families, all the children may inherit the HD gene; in others, none do. Whether one child inherits the gene has no bearing on whether others will or will not share the same fate.

A small number of cases of HD are sporadic, that is, they occur even though there is no family history of the disorder. These cases are thought to be caused by a new genetic mutation—an alteration in the gene that occurs during sperm development and that brings the number of CAG repeats into the range that causes disease.

What are the major effects of the disease?

Early signs of the disease vary greatly from person to person. A common observation is that the earlier the symptoms appear, the faster the disease progresses.

Family members may first notice that the individual experiences mood swings or becomes uncharacteristically irritable, apathetic, passive, depressed, or angry. These symptoms may lessen as the disease progresses or, in some individuals, may continue and include hostile outbursts or deep bouts of depression.

HD may affect the individual's judgment, memory, and other cognitive functions. Early signs might include having trouble driving, learning new things, remembering a fact, answering a question, or making a decision. Some may even display changes in handwriting. As the disease progresses, concentration on intellectual tasks becomes increasingly difficult.

In some individuals, the disease may begin with uncontrolled movements in the fingers, feet, face, or trunk. These movements—which are signs of chorea—often intensify when the person is anxious. HD can also begin with mild clumsiness or problems with balance. Some people develop choreic movements later, after the disease has progressed. They may stumble or appear uncoordinated. Chorea often creates serious problems with walking, increasing the likelihood of falls.

The disease can reach the point where speech is slurred and vital functions, such as swallowing, eating, speaking, and especially walking, continue to decline. Some individuals cannot recognize other family members. Many, however, remain aware of their environment and are able to express emotions.

Some physicians have employed a recently developed Unified HD Rating Scale, or UHDRS, to assess the clinical features, stages, and course of HD. In general, the duration of the illness ranges from 10 to 30 years. The most common causes of death are infection (most often pneumonia), injuries related to a fall, or other complications.

At what age does HD appear?

The rate of disease progression and the age at onset vary from person to person. Adult-onset HD, with its disabling, uncontrolled movements, most often begins in middle age. There are, however, other variations of HD distinguished not just by age at onset but by a distinct array of symptoms. For example, some persons develop the disease as adults, but without chorea. They may appear rigid and move very little, or not at all, a condition called akinesia.

Some individuals develop symptoms of HD when they are very young—before age 20. The terms "early-onset" or "juvenile" HD are often used to describe HD that appears in a young person. A common sign of HD in a younger individual is a rapid decline in school performance. Symptoms can also include subtle changes in handwriting and slight problems with movement, such as slowness, rigidity, tremor, and rapid muscular twitching, called myoclonus. Several of these symptoms are similar to those seen in Parkinson disease, and they differ from the chorea seen in individuals who develop the disease as adults. These young individuals are said to have "akinetic-rigid" HD or the Westphal variant of HD. People with juvenile HD may also have seizures and mental disabilities. The earlier the onset, the faster the disease seems to progress. The disease progresses most rapidly in individuals with juvenile or early-onset HD, and death often follows within 10 years.

Individuals with juvenile HD usually inherit the disease from their fathers. These individuals also tend to have the largest number of CAG repeats. The reason for this may be found in the process of sperm production. Unlike eggs, sperm are produced in the millions. Because DNA is copied millions of times during this process, there is an increased possibility for genetic mistakes to occur. To verify the link between the number of CAG repeats in the HD gene and the age at onset of symptoms, scientists studied a boy who developed HD symptoms at the age of two, one of the youngest and most severe cases ever recorded. They found that he had the largest number of CAG repeats of anyone studied so far—nearly 100. The boy's case was central to the identification of the HD gene and at the same time helped confirm that juveniles with HD have the longest segments of CAG repeats, the only proven correlation between repeat length and age at onset.

A few individuals develop HD after age 55. Diagnosis in these people can be very difficult. The symptoms of HD may be masked by other health problems, or the person may not display the severity of symptoms seen in individuals with HD of earlier onset. These individuals may also show symptoms of depression rather than anger or irritability, or they may retain sharp control over their intellectual functions, such as memory, reasoning, and problem-solving.

There is also a related disorder called senile chorea. Some elderly individuals display the symptoms of HD, especially choreic movements, but do not become demented, have a normal gene, and lack a family history of the disorder. Some scientists believe that a different gene mutation may account for this small number of cases, but this has not been proven.

How is HD diagnosed?

The great American folk singer and composer Woody Guthrie died on October 3, 1967, after suffering from HD for 13 years. He had been misdiagnosed, considered an alcoholic, and shuttled in and out of mental institutions and hospitals for years before being properly diagnosed. His case, sadly, is not extraordinary, although the diagnosis can be made easily by experienced neurologists.

A neurologist will interview the individual intensively to obtain the medical history and rule out other conditions. A tool used by physicians to diagnose HD is to take the family history, sometimes called a pedigree or genealogy. It is extremely important for family members to be candid and truthful with a doctor who is taking a family history.

The doctor will also ask about recent intellectual or emotional problems, which may be indications of HD, and will test the person's hearing, eye movements, strength, coordination, involuntary movements (chorea), sensation, reflexes, balance, movement, and mental status, and will probably order a number of laboratory tests as well.

People with HD commonly have impairments in the way the eye follows or fixes on a moving target. Abnormalities of eye movements vary from person to person and differ, depending on the stage and duration of the illness.

The discovery of the HD gene in 1993 resulted in a direct genetic test to make or confirm a diagnosis of HD in an individual who is exhibiting HD-like symptoms. Using a blood sample, the genetic test analyzes DNA for the HD mutation by counting the number of repeats in the HD gene region. Individuals who do not have HD usually have 28 or fewer CAG repeats. Individuals with HD usually have 40 or more repeats. A small percentage of individuals, however, have a number of repeats that fall within a borderline region.

The physician may ask the individual to undergo a brain imaging test. Computed tomography (CT) and magnetic resonance imaging (MRI) provide excellent images of brain structures with little if any discomfort. Those with HD may show shrinkage of some parts of the

Table 18.1. CAG Repeats and Outcome

No. of CAG Repeats	Outcome
Less than 28	Normal range; individual will not develop HD
29–34	Individual will not develop HD but the next generation is at risk
35–39	Some, but not all, individuals in this range will develop HD; next generation is also at risk
More than 40	Individual will develop HD

brain—particularly two areas known as the caudate nuclei and puta-men—and enlargement of fluid-filled cavities within the brain called ventricles. These changes do not definitely indicate HD, however, be-cause they can also occur in other disorders. In addition, a person can have early symptoms of HD and still have a normal CT scan. When used in conjunction with a family history and record of clinical symp-toms, however, CT can be an important diagnostic tool.

Another technology for brain imaging includes positron emission tomography (PET,) which is important in HD research efforts but is not often needed for diagnosis.

What is presymptomatic testing?

Presymptomatic testing is used for people who have a family his-tory of HD but have no symptoms themselves. If either parent had HD, the person's chance would be 50-50. In the past, no laboratory test could positively identify people carrying the HD gene—or those fated to develop HD—before the onset of symptoms. That situation changed in 1983, when a team of scientists supported by the NINDS located the first genetic marker for HD—the initial step in develop-ing a laboratory test for the disease.

A marker is a piece of DNA that lies near a gene and is usually inherited with it. Discovery of the first HD marker allowed scientists to locate the HD gene on chromosome 4. The marker discovery quickly led to the development of a presymptomatic test for some individu-als, but this test required blood or tissue samples from both affected and unaffected family members in order to identify markers unique to that particular family. For this reason, adopted individuals, orphans, and people who had few living family members were unable to use the test.

Discovery of the HD gene has led to a less expensive, scientifically simpler, and far more accurate presymptomatic test that is applicable to the majority of at-risk people. The new test uses CAG repeat length to detect the presence of the HD mutation in blood. This is discussed further later.

There are many complicating factors that reflect the complexity of diagnosing HD. In a small number of individuals with HD—one to three percent—no family history of HD can be found. Some individuals may not be aware of their genetic legacy, or a family member may conceal a genetic disorder from fear of social stigma. A parent may not want to worry children, scare them, or deter them from marrying. In other cases, a family member may die of another cause before he or she begins to show signs of HD. Sometimes, the cause of death for a relative may not be known, or the family is not aware of a relative's death. Adopted children may not know their genetic heritage, or early symptoms in an individual may be too slight to attract attention.

How is the presymptomatic test conducted?

An individual who wishes to be tested should contact the nearest testing center. (A list of such centers can be obtained from the Huntington Disease Society of America at 800-345-HDSA.) The testing process should include several components. Most testing programs include a neurological examination, pretest counseling, and follow-up. The purpose of the neurological examination is to determine whether or not the person requesting testing is showing any clinical symptoms of HD. It is important to remember that if an individual is showing even slight symptoms of HD, he or she risks being diagnosed with the disease during the neurological examination, even before the genetic test. During pretest counseling, the individual will learn about HD, and about his or her own level of risk, about the testing procedure. The person will be told about the test's limitations, the accuracy of the test, and possible outcomes. He or she can then weigh the risks and benefits of testing and may even decide at that time against pursuing further testing.

If a person decides to be tested, a team of highly trained specialists will be involved, which may include neurologists, genetic counselors, social workers, psychiatrists, and psychologists. This team of professionals helps the at-risk person decide if testing is the right thing to do and carefully prepares the person for a negative, positive, or inconclusive test result.

Individuals who decide to continue the testing process should be accompanied to counseling sessions by a spouse, a friend, or a relative who is not at risk. Other interested family members may participate in the counseling sessions if the individual being tested so desires.

The genetic testing itself involves donating a small sample of blood that is screened in the laboratory for the presence or absence of the HD mutation. Testing may require a sample of DNA from a closely related affected relative, preferably a parent, for the purpose of confirming the diagnosis of HD in the family. This is especially important if the family history for HD is unclear or unusual in some way.

Results of the test should be given only in person and only to the individual being tested. Test results are confidential. Regardless of test results, follow-up is recommended.

In order to protect the interests of minors, including confidentiality, testing is not recommended for those under the age of 18 unless there is a compelling medical reason (for example, the child is exhibiting symptoms).

Testing of a fetus (prenatal testing) presents special challenges and risks; in fact some centers do not perform genetic testing on fetuses. Because a positive test result using direct genetic testing means the at-risk parent is also a gene carrier, at-risk individuals who are considering a pregnancy are advised to seek genetic counseling prior to conception.

Some at-risk parents may wish to know the risk to their fetus but not their own. In this situation, parents may opt for prenatal testing using linked DNA markers rather than direct gene testing. In this case, testing does not look for the HD gene itself but instead indicates whether or not the fetus has inherited a chromosome 4 from the affected grandparent or from the unaffected grandparent on the side of the family with HD. If the test shows that the fetus has inherited a chromosome 4 from the affected grandparent, the parents then learn that the fetus's risk is the same as the parent (50-50), but they learn nothing new about the parent's risk. If the test shows that the fetus has inherited a chromosome 4 from the unaffected grandparent, the risk to the fetus is very low (less than 1%) in most cases.

Another option open to parents is in vitro fertilization with pre-implantation screening. In this procedure, embryos are screened to determine which ones carry the HD mutation. Embryos determined not to have the HD gene mutation are then implanted in the woman's uterus.

In terms of emotional and practical consequences, not only for the individual taking the test but for his or her entire family, testing is enormously complex and has been surrounded by considerable controversy. For example, people with a positive test result may risk losing health and life insurance, suffer loss of employment, and other liabilities. People undergoing testing may wish to cover the cost themselves, since coverage by an insurer may lead to loss of health insurance in the event of a positive result, although this may change in the future.

With the participation of health professionals and people from families with HD, scientists have developed testing guidelines. All individuals seeking a genetic test should obtain a copy of these guidelines from their testing center. These organizations have information on sites that perform testing using the established procedures and they strongly recommend that individuals avoid testing that does not adhere to these guidelines.

How does a person decide whether to be tested?

The anxiety that comes from living with a 50 percent risk for HD can be overwhelming. How does a young person make important choices about long-term education, marriage, and children? How do older parents of adult children cope with their fears about children and grandchildren? How do people come to terms with the ambiguity and uncertainty of living at risk?

Some individuals choose to undergo the test out of a desire for greater certainty about their genetic status. They believe the test will enable them to make more informed decisions about the future. Others choose not to take the test. They are able to make peace with the uncertainty of being at risk, preferring to forego the emotional consequences of a positive result, as well as possible losses of insurance and employment. There is no right or wrong decision, as each choice is highly individual. The guidelines for genetic testing for HD, discussed in the previous section, were developed to help people with this life-changing choice.

Whatever the results of genetic testing, the at-risk individual and family members can expect powerful and complex emotional responses. The health and happiness of spouses, brothers and sisters, children, parents, and grandparents are affected by a positive test result, as are an individual's friends, work associates, neighbors, and others. Because receiving test results may prove to be devastating, testing guidelines call for continued counseling even after the test is complete and the results are known.

Is there a treatment for HD?

Physicians may prescribe a number of medications to help control emotional and movement problems associated with HD. It is important to remember however, that while medicines may help keep these clinical symptoms under control, there is no treatment to stop or reverse the course of the disease.

Antipsychotic drugs, such as haloperidol, or other drugs, such as clonazepam, may help to alleviate choreic movements and may also be used to help control hallucinations, delusions, and violent outbursts. Antipsychotic drugs, however, are not prescribed for another form of muscle contraction associated with HD, called dystonia, and may in fact worsen the condition, causing stiffness and rigidity. These medications may also have severe side effects, including sedation, and for that reason should be used in the lowest possible doses.

For depression, physicians may prescribe fluoxetine, sertraline, nortriptyline, or other compounds. Tranquilizers can help control anxiety and lithium may be prescribed to combat pathological excitement and severe mood swings. Medications may also be needed to treat the severe obsessive-compulsive rituals of some individuals with HD.

Most drugs used to treat the symptoms of HD have side effects such as fatigue, restlessness, or hyperexcitability. Sometimes it may be difficult to tell if a particular symptom, such as apathy or incontinence, is a sign of the disease or a reaction to medication.

What kind of care does the individual with HD need?

Although a psychologist or psychiatrist, a genetic counselor, and other specialists may be needed at different stages of the illness, usually the first step in diagnosis and in finding treatment is to see a neurologist. While the family doctor may be able to diagnose HD, and may continue to monitor the individual's status, it is better to consult with a neurologist about management of the varied symptoms.

Problems may arise when individuals try to express complex thoughts in words they can no longer pronounce intelligibly. It can be helpful to repeat words back to the person with HD so that he or she knows that some thoughts are understood. Sometimes people mistakenly assume that if individuals do not talk, they also do not understand. Never isolate individuals by not talking, and try to keep their environment as normal as possible. Speech therapy may improve the individual's ability to communicate.

It is extremely important for the person with HD to maintain physical fitness as much as his or her condition and the course of the disease allows. Individuals who exercise and keep active tend to do better than those who do not. A daily regimen of exercise can help the person feel better physically and mentally. Although their coordination may be poor, individuals should continue walking, with assistance if necessary. Those who want to walk independently should be allowed to do so as long as possible, and careful attention should be given to keeping their environment free of hard, sharp objects. This will help ensure maximal independence while minimizing the risk of injury from a fall. Individuals can also wear special padding during walks to help protect against injury from falls. Some people have found that small weights around the ankles can help stability. Wearing sturdy shoes that fit well can help too, especially shoes without laces that can be slipped on or off easily.

Impaired coordination may make it difficult for people with HD to feed themselves and to swallow. As the disease progresses, persons with HD may even choke. In helping individuals to eat, caregivers should allow plenty of time for meals. Food can be cut into small pieces, softened, or pureed to ease swallowing and prevent choking. While some foods may require the addition of thickeners, other foods may need to be thinned. Dairy products, in particular, tend to increase the secretion of mucus, which in turn increases the risk of choking. Some individuals may benefit from swallowing therapy, which is especially helpful if started before serious problems arise. Suction cups for plates, special tableware designed for people with disabilities, and plastic cups with tops can help prevent spilling. The individual's physician can offer additional advice about diet and about how to handle swallowing difficulties or gastrointestinal problems that might arise, such as incontinence or constipation.

Caregivers should pay attention to proper nutrition so that the individual with HD takes in enough calories to maintain his or her body weight. Sometimes people with HD, who may burn as many as 5,000 calories a day without gaining weight, require five meals a day to take in the necessary number of calories. Physicians may recommend vitamins or other nutritional supplements. In a long-term care institution, staff will need to assist with meals in order to ensure that the individual's special caloric and nutritional requirements are met. Some individuals and their families choose to use a feeding tube; others choose not to.

Individuals with HD are at special risk for dehydration and therefore require large quantities of fluids, especially during hot weather. Bendable straws can make drinking easier for the person. In some cases, water may have to be thickened with commercial additives to give it the consistency of syrup or honey.

What community resources are available?

Individuals and families affected by HD can take steps to ensure that they receive the best advice and care possible. Physicians and state and local health service agencies can provide information on community resources and family support groups that may exist. Possible types of help include:

Legal and social aid: HD affects a person's capacity to reason, make judgments, and handle responsibilities. Individuals may need help with legal affairs. Wills and other important documents should be drawn up early to avoid legal problems when the person with HD may no longer be able to represent his or her own interests. Family members should also seek out assistance if they face discrimination regarding insurance, employment, or other matters.

Home care services: Caring for a person with HD at home can be exhausting, but part-time assistance with household chores or physical care of the individual can ease this burden. Domestic help, meal programs, nursing assistance, occupational therapy, or other home services may be available from federal, state, or local health service agencies.

Recreation and work centers: Many people with HD are eager and able to participate in activities outside the home. Therapeutic work and recreation centers give individuals an opportunity to pursue hobbies and interests and to meet new people. Participation in these programs, including occupational, music, and recreational therapy, can reduce the person's dependence on family members and provides home caregivers with a temporary, much needed break.

Group housing: A few communities have group housing facilities that are supervised by a resident attendant and that provide meals, housekeeping services, social activities, and local transportation services for residents. These living arrangements are particularly suited to the needs of individuals who are alone and who, although still independent and capable, risk injury when they undertake routine chores like cooking and cleaning.

Institutional care: The individual's physical and emotional demands on the family may eventually become overwhelming. While many families may prefer to keep relatives with HD at home whenever possible, a long-term care facility may prove to be best. To hospitalize or place a family member in a care facility is a difficult decision; professional counseling can help families with this.

Finding the proper facility can itself prove difficult. Organizations such as the Huntington's Disease Society of America may be able to refer the family to facilities that have met standards set for the care of individuals with HD. Very few of these exist however, and even fewer have experience with individuals with juvenile or early-onset HD who require special care because of their age and symptoms.

What research is being done?

Although HD attracted considerable attention from scientists in the early 20th century, there was little sustained research on the disease until the late 1960s when the Committee to Combat Huntington's Disease and the Huntington's Chorea Foundation, later called the Hereditary Disease Foundation, first began to fund research and to campaign for federal funding. In 1977, Congress established the Commission for the Control of Huntington's Disease and Its Consequences, which made a series of important recommendations. Since then, Congress has provided consistent support for federal research, primarily through the National Institute of Neurological Disorders and Stroke, the government's lead agency for biomedical research on disorders of the brain and nervous system. The effort to combat HD proceeds along the following lines of inquiry, each providing important information about the disease:

- *Basic neurobiology:* Now that the HD gene has been located, investigators in the field of neurobiology—which encompasses the anatomy, physiology, and biochemistry of the nervous system— are continuing to study the HD gene with an eye toward understanding how it causes disease in the human body.

- *Clinical research:* Neurologists, psychologists, psychiatrists, and other investigators are improving our understanding of the symptoms and progression of the disease in patients while attempting to develop new therapeutics.

- *Imaging:* Scientific investigations using PET and other technologies are enabling scientists to see what the defective gene does to various structures in the brain and how it affects the body's chemistry and metabolism.

- *Animal models:* Laboratory animals, such as mice, are being bred in the hope of duplicating the clinical features of HD and can soon be expected to help scientists learn more about the symptoms and progression of the disease.

- *Fetal tissue research:* Investigators are implanting fetal tissue in rodents and nonhuman primates with the hope that success in this area will lead to understanding, restoring, or replacing functions typically lost by neuronal degeneration in individuals with HD.

These areas of research are slowly converging and, in the process, are yielding important clues about the gene's relentless destruction of mind and body. The NINDS supports much of this exciting work.

Molecular genetics: For 10 years, scientists focused on a segment of chromosome 4 and, in 1993, finally isolated the HD gene. The process of isolating the responsible gene—motivated by the desire to find a cure—was more difficult than anticipated. Scientists now believe that identifying the location of the HD gene is the first step on the road to a cure.

Finding the HD gene involved an intense molecular genetics research effort with cooperating investigators from around the globe. In early 1993, the collaborating scientists announced they had isolated the unstable triplet repeat DNA sequence that has the HD gene. Investigators relied on the NINDS-supported Research Roster for Huntington's Disease, based at Indiana University in Indianapolis, to accomplish this work. First started in 1979, the roster contains data on many American families with HD, provides statistical and demographic data to scientists, and serves as a liaison between investigators and specific families. It provided the DNA from many families affected by HD to investigators involved in the search for the gene and was an important component in the identification of HD markers.

For several years, NINDS-supported investigators involved in the search for the HD gene made yearly visits to the largest known kindred with HD—14,000 individuals—who live on Lake Maracaibo in Venezuela. The continuing trips enable scientists to study inheritance patterns of several interrelated families.

The HD gene and its product: Although scientists know that certain brain cells die in HD, the cause of their death is still unknown. Recessive diseases are usually thought to result from a gene that fails to produce adequate amounts of a substance essential to normal function. This is known as a loss-of-function gene. Some dominantly inherited disorders, such as HD, are thought to involve a gene that actively interferes with the normal function of the cell. This is known as a gain-of-function gene.

How does the defective HD gene cause harm? The HD gene encodes a protein—which has been named huntingtin—the function of which is as yet unknown. The repeated CAG sequence in the gene causes an abnormal form of huntingtin to be made, in which the amino acid glutamine is repeated. It is the presence of this abnormal form, and not the absence of the normal form, that causes harm in HD. This explains why the disease is dominant and why two copies of the defective gene—one from both the mother and the father—do not cause a more serious case than inheritance from only one parent. With the HD gene isolated, NINDS-supported investigators are now turning their attention toward discovering the normal function of huntingtin and how the altered form causes harm. Scientists hope to reproduce, study, and correct these changes in animal models of the disease.

Huntingtin is found everywhere in the body but only outside the cell's nucleus. Mice called "knockout mice" are bred in the laboratory to produce no huntingtin; they fail to develop past a very early embryo stage and quickly die. Huntingtin, scientists now know, is necessary for life. Investigators hope to learn why the abnormal version of the protein damages only certain parts of the brain. One theory is that cells in these parts of the brain may be supersensitive to this abnormal protein.

Cell death in HD: Although the precise cause of cell death in HD is not yet known, scientists are paying close attention to the process of genetically programmed cell death that occurs deep within the brains of individuals with HD. This process involves a complex series of interlinked events leading to cellular suicide. Related areas of investigation include:

- *Excitotoxicity:* Overstimulation of cells by natural chemicals found in the brain.

- *Defective energy metabolism:* A defect in the power plant of the cell, called mitochondria, where energy is produced.

- *Oxidative stress:* Normal metabolic activity in the brain that produces toxic compounds called free radicals.

- *Trophic factors:* Natural chemical substances found in the human body that may protect against cell death.

Several HD studies are aimed at understanding losses of nerve cells and receptors in HD. Neurons in the striatum are classified both by their size (large, medium, or small) and appearance (spiny or aspiny). Each type of neuron contains combinations of neurotransmitters. Scientists know that the destructive process of HD affects different subsets of neurons to varying degrees. The hallmark of HD, they are learning, is selective degeneration of medium-sized spiny neurons in the striatum. NINDS-supported studies also suggest that losses of certain types of neurons and receptors are responsible for different symptoms and stages of HD.

What do these changes look like? In spiny neurons, investigators have observed two types of changes, each affecting the nerve cells' dendrites. Dendrites, found on every nerve cell, extend out from the cell body and are responsible for receiving messages from other nerve cells.

In the intermediate stages of HD, dendrites grow out of control. New, incomplete branches form and other branches become contorted. In advanced, severe stages of HD, degenerative changes cause sections of dendrites to swell, break off, or disappear altogether. Investigators believe that these alterations may be an attempt by the cell to rebuild nerve cell contacts lost early in the disease. As the new dendrites establish connections, however, they may in fact contribute to nerve cell death. Such studies give compelling, visible evidence of the progressive nature of HD and suggest that new experimental therapies must consider the state of cellular degeneration. Scientists do not yet know exactly how these changes affect subsets of nerve cells outside the striatum.

Animal models of HD: As more is learned about cellular degeneration in HD, investigators hope to reproduce these changes in animal models and to find a way to correct or halt the process of nerve cell death. Such models serve the scientific community in general by providing a means to test the safety of new classes of drugs in nonhuman primates. NINDS-supported scientists are currently working to develop both nonhuman primate and mouse models to investigate nerve degeneration in HD and to study the effects of excitotoxicity on nerve cells in the brain.

Investigators are working to build genetic models of HD using transgenic mice. To do this, scientists transfer the altered human HD gene into mouse embryos so that the animals will develop the anatomical and biological characteristics of HD. This genetic model of mouse HD will enable in-depth study of the disease and testing of new therapeutic compounds.

Another idea is to insert into mice a section of DNA containing CAG repeats in the abnormal, disease gene range. This mouse equivalent of HD could allow scientists to explore the basis of CAG instability and its role in the disease process.

Fetal tissue research: A relatively new field in biomedical research involves the use of brain tissue grafts to study, and potentially treat, neurodegenerative disorders. In this technique, tissue that has degenerated is replaced with implants of fresh, fetal tissue, taken at the very early stages of development. Investigators are interested in applying brain tissue implants to HD research. Extensive animal studies will be required to learn if this technique could be of value in patients with HD.

Clinical studies: Scientists are pursuing clinical studies that may one day lead to the development of new drugs or other treatments to halt the disease's progression. Examples of NINDS-supported investigations, using both asymptomatic and symptomatic individuals, include:

- *Genetic studies on age of onset, inheritance patterns, and markers found within families:* These studies may shed additional light on how HD is passed from generation to generation.

- *Studies of cognition, intelligence, and movement:* Studies of abnormal eye movements, both horizontal and vertical, and tests of patients' skills in a number of learning, memory, neuropsychological, and motor tasks may serve to identify when the various symptoms of HD appear and to characterize their range and severity.

- *Clinical trials of drugs:* Testing of various drugs may lead to new treatments and at the same time improve our understanding of the disease process in HD. Classes of drugs being tested include those that control symptoms, slow the rate of progression of HD, and block effects of excitotoxins, and those that might correct or replace other metabolic defects contributing to the development and progression of HD.

Imaging: NINDS-supported scientists are using positron emission tomography (PET) to learn how the gene affects the chemical systems of the body. PET visualizes metabolic or chemical abnormalities in the body, and investigators hope to ascertain if PET scans can reveal any abnormalities that signal HD. Investigators conducting HD research are also using PET to characterize neurons that have died and chemicals that are depleted in parts of the brain affected by HD.

Like PET, a form of magnetic resonance imaging (MRI) called functional MRI can measure increases or decreases in certain brain chemicals thought to play a key role in HD. Functional MRI studies are also helping investigators understand how HD kills neurons in different regions of the brain.

Imaging technologies allow investigators to view changes in the volume and structures of the brain and to pinpoint when these changes occur in HD. Scientists know that in brains affected by HD, the basal ganglia, cortex, and ventricles all show atrophy or other alterations.

How can I help?

In order to conduct HD research, investigators require samples of tissue or blood from families with HD. Access to individuals with HD and their families may be difficult however, because families with HD are often scattered across the country or around the world. A research project may need individuals of a particular age or gender or from a certain geographic area. Some scientists need only statistical data while others may require a sample of blood, urine, or skin from family members. All of these factors complicate the task of finding volunteers. The following NINDS-supported efforts bring together families with HD, voluntary health agencies, and scientists in an effort to advance science and speed a cure.

The NINDS-sponsored HD Research Roster at the Indiana University Medical Center in Indianapolis, which was discussed earlier, makes research possible by matching scientists with patient and family volunteers. The first DNA bank was established through the roster. Although the gene has already been located, DNA from individuals who have HD is still of great interest to investigators. Of continuing interest are twins, unaffected individuals who have affected offspring, and individuals with two defective HD genes, one from each parent—a very rare occurrence. Participation in the roster and in specific research projects is voluntary and confidential. For more information about the roster and DNA bank, contact:

Indiana University Medical Center
Department of Medical and Molecular Genetics
Medical Research and Library Building
975 W. Walnut Street
Indianapolis, IN 46202-5251
Phone: 317-274-5744 (call collect)

The NINDS supports two national brain specimen banks. These banks supply research scientists around the world with nervous system tissue from patients with neurological and psychiatric disorders. They need tissue from patients with HD so that scientists can study and understand the disorder. Those who may be interested in donating should write to:

Human Brain and Spinal Fluid Resource Center
Neurology Research (127A)
W. Los Angeles Healthcare Center
11301 Wilshire Blvd. Bldg. 212
Los Angeles, CA 90073
Phone: 310-268-3536
24-hour pager: 310-636-5199
Website: http://www.loni.ucla.edu/~nnrsb/NNRSB
E-mail: RMNbbank@ucla.edu

Harvard Brain Tissue Resource Center
McLean Hospital
115 Mill Street
Belmont, Massachusetts 02478
Toll-free: 800-BRAIN-BANK (800-272-4622)
Phone: 617-855-2400
Website: http://www.ninds.nih.gov/disorders/huntington/www
.brainbank.mclean.org

What is the role of voluntary organizations?

Private organizations have been a mainstay of support and guidance for at-risk individuals, people with HD, and their families. These organizations vary in size and emphasis, but all are concerned with helping individuals and their families, educating lay and professional audiences about HD, and promoting medical research on the disorder. Some voluntary health agencies support scientific workshops and research and some have newsletters and local chapters throughout the country. These agencies enable families, health professionals, and investigators to exchange information, learn of available services and benefits, and work toward common goals.

Chapter 19

Parkinson Disease

Signs and Symptoms; Diagnoses and Dementia

Parkinsonian gait is the distinctive, unsteady walk associated with Parkinson disease. There is a tendency to lean unnaturally backward or forward, and to develop a stooped, head down, shoulder drooped stance. People with Parkinson disease tend to take small shuffling steps and arm swing is diminished or absent. (Source: Neurology Channel)

What is Parkinson disease?

Parkinson disease is a progressive disorder of the central nervous system affecting more than 1.5 million people in the United States. The disease is characterized by a decrease in spontaneous movement, gait difficulty, postural instability, rigidity, and tremor. Dr. James Parkinson discovered the disease in 1817 and identified it as shaky palsy. It was not until 1960 that changes in the brains of Parkinson patients were discovered, making it possible to develop medication for the condition.

"Parkinson's Disease: Signs and Symptoms; Diagnoses and Dementia," Gina Kemp, M.A., and John Dorsey contributed to this article, reprinted with permission from http://www.helpguide.com/elder/parkinsons_disease.htm. © 2007 Helpguide.org. All rights reserved. Helpguide provides a detailed list of related references for this article, including links to information from other websites. For a complete list of Helpguide's current resources related to Alzheimer disease and other dementias, visit www.helpguide.org.

Most people who get Parkinson disease are over 60, but there have recently been more cases in younger men and women. The cause of the disease is unknown, but genetics and environmental factors are thought to play a part in some of the cases.

What are symptoms of Parkinson disease?

There are primary levels of Parkinson disease and secondary levels. Not everyone with the disease experiences all of the symptoms and the progression of the disease is different from person to person. Most of the symptoms of the disease have to do with motor skills, but pain and lack of energy are also symptoms of the disease.

Symptoms of Parkinson Disease

Primary Symptoms

- *Bradykinesia:* Slowness in voluntary movement such as standing up, walking, and sitting down. This happens because of delayed transmission signals from the brain to the muscles.

- *Tremors:* Often occur in the hands, fingers, forearms, foot, mouth, or chin. Typically, tremors take place when the limbs are at rest as opposed to when there is movement.

- *Rigidity:* Otherwise known as stiff muscles, often produces muscle pain that is increased during movement.

- *Poor balance:* Happens because of the loss of reflexes that help posture. This causes unsteady balance which oftentimes leads to a fall.

- *Parkinson gait:* A common walk of somebody with Parkinson disease. It includes shuffling, head down, shoulders drooped, lack of arm swing, and leaning backwards or forwards unnaturally. Initiating walking is difficult and freezing mid-stride is common.

Secondary Symptoms

- Constipation

- Difficulty swallowing; saliva and food that get caught in the mouth or in the back of the throat may cause choking, coughing, or drooling

- Excessive salivation

- Excessive sweating

- Loss of bowel and/or bladder control

- Loss of intellectual capacity

- Psychosocial: anxiety, depression, isolation

- Scaling, dry skin on the face or scalp

- Slow response to questions

- Small cramped handwriting

- Soft, whispery voice

There are many secondary symptoms associated with Parkinson disease. Patients do not typically experience all the symptoms, and the intensity of each symptom varies from person to person.

How is Parkinson disease diagnosed?

There are not lab tests to definitively diagnose Parkinson disease. A systematic neurological exam will include testing your reflexes and observing things like muscle strength throughout your body, coordination, balance, and other details of movement. You may be given tests to exclude the possibility of other disorders. These tests include blood tests, urine tests, computed tomography (CT) scans, or magnetic resonance imaging (MRI) scans. Although none of these tests actually diagnose Parkinson disease, they may reveal the presence of some other conditions that could be responsible for the symptoms.

Is there a cure for Parkinson disease?

There is no cure; however, there are medications to treat the symptoms of the disease. Information about several of the medications can be found on the Parkinson's Disease Foundation website (available online at http://www.pdf.org). A surgical treatment, known as deep brain stimulation (DBS) is sometimes used to help reduce the severity of muscle rigidity and bradykinesia, and physical therapy is often recommended.

Is there a special diet or exercise program for people with Parkinson disease?

There are some things you can do to stay as healthy as possible and avoid accidents. Here are a few tips:

- Before starting an exercise regime, you should always check with your doctor.

- Cut foods into smaller portions to avoid choking and to encourage digestion.

- For upset stomachs linked to medication, try eating an oatmeal cookie when taking it.

- Exercise your face and jaw whenever possible.

- Practice bending, stretching, and breathing exercises.

- Try exercising in bed; it may be easier than on the floor.

- Build your walking skills, even if that means having to hold onto something.

- Try exercising in the water; it is easier on the joints.

There are also ways to improve your safety when living your daily life. Here are a few tips:

- Use grab bars in the tub and shower.

- Use a bath chair or stool in the shower.

- Keep your floors smooth but not slippery.

- Store supplies in easy to reach cabinets.

- Make sure stairwells are lit.

- Get nightlights for bathrooms and hallways.

- Keep walking areas free of clutter.

- Wear low heeled, comfortable shoes when walking around. Avoid walking in slippery socks and slippers.

- Make sure carpets are fully tacked to the ground.

How are Parkinson disease and dementia related?

Parkinson patients who experience hallucinations and more severe motor control problems are at risk for dementia. According to Dr. Jean Hubble of Ohio State University, dementia is a "cognitive impairment of sufficient magnitude to hinder daily activities or diminish the quality of the patient's life." Approximately 20% of people with Parkinson disease will develop dementia, usually after the age of 70. In general, there is a 10 to 15 year lag time between a Parkinson diagnosis and the onset of dementia, which typically occurs years after the motor skills begin to be affected.

Signs of dementia in Parkinson patients include:

Signs of Dementia in Parkinson Patients

- memory problems
- distractibility
- slowed thinking
- disorientation
- confusion
- moodiness
- lack of motivation

There are two types of dementia found in Parkinson patients, both involving Lewy bodies, or protein deposits in the nerve cells. The first one develops when Lewy bodies occupy the brain and the brain stem, which occurs in about 25% of the cases. The more prevalent type, accounting for the remaining 75%, is caused by Lewy bodies in the brainstem and Alzheimer changes in the brain. For both types of dementia, medication can help improve early symptoms, although some of the anticholinergic drugs may actually increase cognitive impairment (Parkinson Association of the Rockies).

Indications that the dementia may be caused by something other than Parkinson disease include agitation, delusions, language difficulties, and early onset of symptoms. If these factors are present, your physician can test for other possible causes, such as a vitamin B_{12} deficiency or an underactive thyroid gland. Depression is also common in Parkinson patients and can mimic dementia by causing similar symptoms. For this reason, antidepressant drugs often help.

Chapter 20

Down Syndrome and Dementia

Alzheimer disease, a degenerative neurological disorder character-ized by progressive memory loss, personality deterioration, and loss of functional motor capabilities, is far more common in individuals with Down syndrome than the general population. However, not all individuals with Down syndrome will develop Alzheimer disease, and even those showing Alzheimer-type symptoms may not have Alz-heimer disease since other conditions can mimic the symptoms.

How common is Alzheimer disease in individuals with Down syndrome?

Estimates vary, but a reasonable conclusion is that 25 percent or more of individuals with Down syndrome over age 35 show clinical signs and symptoms of Alzheimer-type dementia. The percentage in-creases with age. In the general population, Alzheimer disease does not usually develop before age 50, and the highest incidence (in people over age 65) is between five and 10 percent. The incidence of Alzheimer disease in the Down syndrome population is estimated to be three to five times greater than in the general population.

What are the symptoms of Alzheimer disease?

Early symptoms include loss of memory and logical thinking; per-sonality change; decline in daily living skills; new onset of seizures;

changes in coordination and gait; and loss of continence in bladder and bowel habits.

How is a final diagnosis made?

Alzheimer disease is difficult to diagnose. It is important to be certain Alzheimer-type symptoms do not arise from other conditions, namely thyroid disorders, depressive illness by psychiatric criteria, brain tumor, recurrent brain strokes, metabolic imbalances, and various neurological conditions.

The diagnosis of Alzheimer disease is made on the basis of clinical history, showing a slow, steady decrease in cognitive function, and a variety of laboratory tests which provide contributory evidence, including electroencephalogram, brain stem auditory evoked response, computerized transaxial tomography, and magnetic resonance imaging, among other tests and measurements.

Is there a baseline test that can be repeated at intervals to determine specific decrease in cognitive function?

Psychologists often use questionnaires answered by family members, companions, or caretakers that assist in the early detection of dementia. It is recommended that individuals with Down syndrome be tested at age 30 to provide a baseline reading, and periodically thereafter. If the tests show deterioration, further tests must be made to rule out conditions that present similar or overlapping symptoms.

What information has research yielded about a link between Alzheimer disease and Down syndrome?

Current research investigating how certain genes on chromosome 21 may predispose individuals with Down syndrome to Alzheimer disease. A number of centers are testing therapies in Down syndrome that appear to benefit patients with Alzheimer disease in the general population.

How can research into Alzheimer disease and Down syndrome be advanced?

As is true for Alzheimer disease in the general population, a full understanding of the disorder involves post-mortem examination of brain tissue. Contributions to a brain tissue repository for purposes of extending knowledge about the relationship between Down syndrome and Alzheimer disease will help to advance research in this area. For information for families and physicians considering such a donation, please contact the National Down Syndrome Society at 800-221-4602.

Summary

Individuals with Down syndrome are three to five times more likely than the general population to develop Alzheimer disease. Onset of Alzheimer may begin as early as age 30 in the Down syndrome population as compared to age 50 in the general population.

Symptoms of a variety of other diseases and conditions mimic the symptoms of Alzheimer disease: personality change, decline in daily living skills, memory loss, changes in coordination and gait, and other changes. Diseases and conditions such as depression, thyroid disorders, brain tumor, recurrent brain strokes, metabolic imbalances, and various neurological conditions must be ruled out prior to a diagnosis of Alzheimer disease.

It is recommended that individuals with Down syndrome take a baseline test of cognitive function at age 30, and that this test be repeated annually to determine any deterioration in this function. Some Alzheimer disease symptoms can be treated, although there is no current means of curing or arresting the disease.

Current research suggests a causative link between the extra "gene dosage" from the third chromosome 21 of Down syndrome and Alzheimer disease. To advance research, donations of brain tissue from individuals with Down syndrome and Alzheimer disease are being sought.

If you would like additional information on Alzheimer disease and Down syndrome, please refer to the National Down Syndrome Society (NDSS) Resource List on Alzheimer disease, available online at www.ndss.org or through the NDSS Helpline at 800-221-4602.

Chapter 21

Normal Pressure Hydrocephalus

What is normal pressure hydrocephalus?

Normal pressure hydrocephalus (NPH) is an abnormal increase of cerebrospinal fluid (CSF) in the brain's ventricles, or cavities. It occurs if the normal flow of CSF throughout the brain and spinal cord is blocked in some way. This causes the ventricles to enlarge, putting pressure on the brain. Normal pressure hydrocephalus can occur in people of any age, but it is most common in the elderly population. It may result from a subarachnoid hemorrhage, head trauma, infection, tumor, or complications of surgery. However, many people develop NPH even when none of these factors are present. In these cases the cause of the disorder is unknown.

Symptoms of NPH include progressive mental impairment and dementia, problems with walking, and impaired bladder control leading to urinary frequency or incontinence. The person also may have a general slowing of movements or may complain that his or her feet feel "stuck." Because these symptoms are similar to those of other disorders such as Alzheimer disease, Parkinson disease, and Creutzfeldt-Jakob disease, the disorder is often misdiagnosed. Many cases go unrecognized and are never properly treated. Doctors may use a variety of tests, including brain scans (CT or MRI), a spinal tap or lumbar catheter, intracranial pressure monitoring, and neuropsychological

"NINDS Normal Pressure Hydrocephalus Information Page," National Institute of Neurological Disorders and Stroke (NINDS), April 2007.

tests, to help them diagnose NPH and rule out other conditions. In September 2005 an international team of scientists developed clinical guidelines to help physicians diagnose NPH. The guidelines were published as a supplement to the journal *Neurosurgery* ("Diagnosing Idiopathic Normal-pressure Hydrocephalus," Vol. 57(3), Supplement: S2-4–S2-16, 2005).

Is there any treatment?

Treatment for NPH involves surgical placement of a shunt in the brain to drain excess CSF into the abdomen where it can be absorbed. This allows the brain ventricles to return to their normal size. Regular follow-up care by a physician is important in order to identify subtle changes that might indicate problems with the shunt.

What is the prognosis?

The symptoms of NPH usually get worse over time if the condition is not treated, although some people may experience temporary improvements. While the success of treatment with shunts varies from person to person, some people recover almost completely after treatment and have a good quality of life. Early diagnosis and treatment improves the chance of a good recovery.

What research is being done?

Research on disorders such as normal pressure hydrocephalus focuses on increasing knowledge and understanding of the disorder, improving diagnostic techniques, and finding improved treatments and preventions.

Chapter 22

Cerebral Atrophy

What is cerebral atrophy?

Cerebral atrophy is a common feature of many of the diseases that affect the brain. Atrophy of any tissue means loss of cells. In brain tissue, atrophy describes a loss of neurons and the connections between them. Atrophy can be generalized, which means that all of the brain has shrunk; or it can be focal, affecting only a limited area of the brain and resulting in a decrease of the functions that area of the brain controls. If the cerebral hemispheres (the two lobes of the brain that form the cerebrum) are affected, conscious thought and voluntary processes may be impaired.

Associated Diseases/Disorders: The pattern and rate of progression of cerebral atrophy depends on the disease involved. Diseases that cause cerebral atrophy include:

- stroke and traumatic brain injury

- Alzheimer disease, Pick disease, senile dementia, frontotemporal dementia, and vascular dementia

- cerebral palsy, in which lesions (damaged areas) may impair motor coordination

"NINDS Cerebral Atrophy Information Page," National Institute of Neurological Disorders and Stroke (NINDS), February 2007.

- Huntington disease, and other gene-linked, hereditary diseases that cause build-up of toxic levels of proteins in neurons

- leukodystrophies, such as Krabbe disease, which destroy the myelin sheath that protects axons

- mitochondrial encephalomyopathies, such as Kearns-Sayre syndrome, which interfere with the basic functions of neurons

- multiple sclerosis, which causes inflammation, myelin damage, and lesions in cerebral tissue

- infectious diseases, such as encephalitis, neurosyphilis, and AIDS, in which an infectious agent or the inflammatory reaction to it destroys neurons and their axons

- epilepsy, in which lesions cause abnormal electrochemical discharges that result in seizures

What are some symptoms?

Many diseases that cause cerebral atrophy are associated with dementia, seizures, and a group of language disorders called the aphasias. Dementia is characterized by a progressive impairment of memory and intellectual function that is severe enough to interfere with social and work skills. Memory, orientation, abstraction, ability to learn, visual-spatial perception, and higher executive functions such as planning, organizing and sequencing may also be impaired. Seizures can take different forms, appearing as disorientation, strange repetitive movements, loss of consciousness, or convulsions. Aphasias are a group of disorders characterized by disturbances in speaking and understanding language. Receptive aphasia causes impaired comprehension. Expressive aphasia is reflected in odd choices of words, the use of partial phrases, disjointed clauses, and incomplete sentences.

What research is being done?

The National Institute of Neurological Disorders and Stroke (NINDS) funds research looking at many of the diseases and disorders that cause cerebral atrophy. Understanding the biological mechanisms that cause neurons to die in the brain will help researchers find ways to prevent, treat, and even cure the diseases that lead to cerebral atrophy.

Chapter 23

Wernicke-Korsakoff Syndrome and Alcohol-Related Brain Damage

Wernicke-Korsakoff Syndrome

What is Wernicke-Korsakoff syndrome?

Wernicke encephalopathy is a degenerative brain disorder caused by the lack of thiamine (vitamin B_1). It may result from alcohol abuse, dietary deficiencies, prolonged vomiting, eating disorders, or the effects of chemotherapy. Symptoms include mental confusion, vision impairment, stupor, coma, hypothermia, hypotension, and ataxia. Korsakoff amnesic syndrome—a memory disorder—also results from a deficiency of thiamine and is associated with alcoholism. The heart, vascular, and nervous system are involved. Symptoms include amnesia, confabulation, attention deficit, disorientation, and vision impairment. The main features of Korsakoff amnesic syndrome are the impairments in acquiring new information or establishing new memories and in retrieving previous memories. Although Wernicke encephalopathy and Korsakoff amnesic syndrome may appear to be two different disorders, they are generally considered to be different stages of the same disorder, which is called Wernicke-Korsakoff syndrome. Wernicke encephalopathy represents the "acute" phase of the disorder, and Korsakoff amnesic syndrome represents the "chronic" phase.

This chapter includes "NINDS Wernicke-Korsakoff Syndrome Information Page," National Institute of Neurological Disorders and Stroke, 2007; and excerpts from "Alcoholism and the Brain: An Overview," by Marlene Oscar-German and Ksenija Marinkovic, *Alcohol Research and Health*, Vol. 27, No. 2, National Institute on Alcohol Abuse and Alcoholism, 2003.

Is there any treatment?

Treatment involves replacement of thiamine and providing proper nutrition and hydration. In some cases, drug therapy is also recommended.

What is the prognosis?

Most symptoms can be reversed if detected and treated promptly. However, improvement in memory function is slow and, usually, incomplete. Without treatment, these disorders can be disabling and life-threatening.

What research is being done?

The National Institute of Neurological Disorders and Stroke (NINDS) supports research on neurological disorders such as Wernicke encephalopathy, Korsakoff amnesic syndrome, and Wernicke-Korsakoff syndrome, aimed at finding ways to prevent them. The National Institute of Alcohol Abuse and Alcoholism also supports research on these disorders.

Alcoholism and the Brain

The brain, like most body organs, is vulnerable to injury from alcohol consumption. The risk of brain damage and related neuro-behavioral deficits varies from person to person. This text reviews the many factors that influence this risk, the techniques used to study the effects of alcoholism on the brain and behavior, and the implications of this research for treatment.

About half of the nearly 20 million alcoholics in the United States seem to be free of cognitive impairments. In the remaining half, however, neuropsychological difficulties can range from mild to severe. For example, up to 2 million alcoholics develop permanent and debilitating conditions that require lifetime custodial care. Examples of such conditions include alcohol-induced persisting amnesic disorder (also called Wernicke-Korsakoff syndrome) and dementia, which seriously affects many mental functions in addition to memory (for example, language, reasoning, and problem-solving abilities). Most alcoholics with neuropsychological impairments show at least some improvement in brain structure and functioning within a year of abstinence, but some people take much longer. Unfortunately, little is known about the rate and extent to which people recover specific structural and functional processes after they stop drinking. However, research has helped define the various factors that influence a person's risk for experiencing alcoholism-related brain deficits, as the following sections describe.

Risk Factors and Comorbid Conditions That Influence Alcohol-Related Brain Damage

Alcoholism's effects on the brain are diverse and are influenced by a wide range of variables. These include the amount of alcohol consumed, the age at which the person began drinking, and the duration of drinking; the patient's age, level of education, gender, genetic background, and family history of alcoholism; and neuropsychiatric risk factors such as alcohol exposure before birth and general health status. Overall physical and mental health is an important factor because comorbid medical, neurological, and psychiatric conditions can interact to aggravate alcoholism's effects on the brain and behavior. Examples of common comorbid conditions include the following:

- Medical conditions such as malnutrition and diseases of the liver and the cardiovascular system

- Neurological conditions such as head injury, inflammation of the brain (encephalopathy), and fetal alcohol syndrome (or fetal alcohol effects)

- Psychiatric conditions such as depression, anxiety, post-traumatic stress disorder, schizophrenia, and the use of other drugs

These conditions also can contribute to further drinking.

Models for Explaining Alcohol-Related Brain Damage

Some factors that are thought to influence how alcoholism affects the brain and behavior have been developed into specific models or hypotheses to explain the variability in alcoholism-related brain deficits. It should be noted that the models that focus on individual characteristics cannot be totally separated from models that emphasize affected brain systems because all of these factors are interrelated. Several of the models have been evaluated using specialized tests that enable researchers to make inferences about the type and extent of brain abnormalities.

Table 23.1. Hypotheses Proposed to Explain the Consequences of Alcoholism for the Brain

Hypotheses Emphasizing the Personal Characteristics Associated with Vulnerability

Characteristic	Hypothesis
Aging	Premature aging hypothesis: Alcoholism accelerates aging. Brains of alcoholics resemble brains of chronologically old nonalcoholics. This may occur at the onset of problem drinking ("accelerated aging") or later in life when brains are more vulnerable ("increased vulnerability" or "cumulative effects").
Gender	Alcoholism affects women more than men. Although women and men metabolize alcohol differently, it is not yet clear if women's brains are more vulnerable than men's brains to the effects of alcoholism.
Family history	Alcoholism runs in families; thus, children of alcoholics face increased risk of alcoholism and associated brain changes.
Vitamin deficiency	Thiamine deficiency can contribute to damage deep within the brain, leading to severe cognitive deficits.

Hypotheses Emphasizing the Vulnerability of Brain Regions or Systems

Region/System	Hypothesis
Entire brain	Vulnerable to cerebral atrophy.
Limbic system, thalamus,	Vulnerable to alcohol-induced persisting and hypothalamus amnesic disorder (also known as Wernicke-Korsakoff syndrome).
Frontal lobe systems	More vulnerable to the effects of alcoholism than other brain regions/systems.
Right hemisphere	More vulnerable to the effects of alcoholism than the left hemisphere.
Neurotransmitter systems (e.g., gamma-aminobutyric acid (GABA), glutamate, dopamine, acetylcholine, and serotonin systems)	Several neurotransmitter systems are vulnerable to effects of alcoholism.

Techniques for Studying Alcohol-Related Brain Damage

Researchers use multiple methods to understand the etiologies and mechanisms of brain damage across subgroups of alcoholics. Behavioral neuroscience offers excellent techniques for sensitively assessing distinct cognitive and emotional functions—for example, the measures of brain laterality (for example, spatial cognition) and frontal system integrity (for example, executive control skills) mentioned earlier. Follow-up post mortem examinations of brains of well-studied alcoholic patients offer clues about the locus and extent of pathology and about neurotransmitter abnormalities. Neuroimaging techniques provide a window on the active brain and a glimpse at regions with structural damage.

Behavioral neuroscience: Behavioral neuroscience studies the relationship between the brain and its functions—for example, how the brain controls executive functions and spatial cognition in healthy people, and how diseases like alcoholism can alter the normal course of events. This is accomplished by using specialized tests designed expressly to measure the functions of interest. Among the tests used by scientists to determine the effects of alcoholism on executive functions controlled by the frontal lobes are those that measure problem-solving abilities, reasoning, and the ability to inhibit responses that are irrelevant or inappropriate. Tests to measure spatial cognition controlled by the right hemisphere include those that measure skills important for recognizing faces, as well as those that rely on skills required for reading maps and negotiating two- and three-dimensional space (visuospatial tasks). With the advent of sophisticated neuroimaging techniques, scientists can even observe the brain while people perform many tasks sensitive to the workings of certain areas of the brain.

Neuropathology: Researchers have gained important insights into the anatomical effects of long-term alcohol use from studying the brains of deceased alcoholic patients. These studies have documented alcoholism-related atrophy throughout the brain and particularly in the frontal lobes. Post mortem studies will continue to help researchers understand the basic mechanisms of alcohol-induced brain damage and regionally specific effects of alcohol at the cellular level.

Neuroimaging: Remarkable developments in neuroimaging techniques have made it possible to study anatomical, functional, and biochemical changes in the brain that are caused by chronic alcohol use. Because of their precision and versatility, these techniques are invaluable for studying the extent and the dynamics of brain damage induced by heavy drinking. Because a patient's brain can be scanned on repeated occasions, clinicians and researchers are able to track a person's improvement with abstinence and deterioration with continued abuse. Furthermore, brain changes can be correlated with neuropsychological and behavioral measures taken at the same time. Brain imaging can aid in identifying factors unique to the individual which affect that person's susceptibility to the effects of heavy drinking and risk for developing dependence, as well as factors that contribute to treatment efficacy.

Imaging of Brain Structure: With neuroimaging techniques such as computerized tomography (CT) and magnetic resonance imaging (MRI), which allow brain structures to be viewed inside the skull, researchers can study brain anatomy in living patients. CT scans rely on x-ray beams passing through different types of tissue in the body at different angles. Pictures of the "inner structure" of the brain are based on computerized reconstruction of the paths and relative strength of the x-ray beams. CT scans of alcoholics have revealed diffuse atrophy of brain tissue, with the frontal lobes showing the earliest and most extensive shrinkage.

MRI techniques have greatly influenced the field of brain imaging because they allow noninvasive measurement of both the anatomy (using structural MRI) and the functioning (using functional magnetic resonance imaging [fMRI]) of the brain with great precision. Structural MRI scans are based on the observation that the protons derived from hydrogen atoms, which are richly represented in the body because of its high water content, can be aligned by a magnetic field like small compass needles. When pulses are emitted at a particular frequency, the protons briefly switch their alignment and "relax" back into their original state at slightly different times in different types of tissue. The signals they emit are detected by the scanner and converted into highly precise images of the tissue. MRI methods have confirmed and extended findings from post mortem and CT scan studies—namely, that chronic use of alcohol results in brain shrinkage. This shrinkage is most marked in the frontal regions and especially in older alcoholics. Other brain regions, including portions of the limbic system and the cerebellum, also are vulnerable to shrinkage.

Imaging of Brain Function: Hemodynamic Methods: Hemodynamic methods create images by tracking changes in blood flow, blood volume, blood oxygenation, and energy metabolism that occur in the brain in response to neural activity. PET and SPECT are used to map increased energy consumption by the specific brain regions that are engaged as a patient performs a task. One example of this mapping involves glucose, the main energy source for the brain. When a dose of a radioactively labeled glucose (a form of glucose that is absorbed normally but cannot be fully metabolized, thus remaining "trapped" in a cell) is injected into the bloodstream of a patient performing a memory task, those brain areas that accumulate more glucose will be implicated in memory functions. Indeed, PET and SPECT studies have confirmed and extended earlier findings that the prefrontal regions are particularly susceptible to decreased metabolism in alcoholic patients. It is important to keep in mind, however, that frontal brain systems are connected to other regions of the brain, and frontal abnormalities may therefore reflect pathology elsewhere.

Even though using low doses of radioactive substances that decay quickly minimizes the risks of radiation exposure, newer and safer methods have emerged, such as MRI methods. MRI is noninvasive, involves no radioactive risks, and provides both anatomical and functional information with high precision. The fMRI method is sensitive to metabolic changes in the parts of the brain that are activated during a particular task. A local increase in metabolic rate results in an increased delivery of blood and increased oxygenation of the region participating in a task. The blood oxygenation level–dependent (BOLD) effect is the basis of the fMRI signal. Like PET and SPECT, fMRI permits observing the brain "in action," as a person performs cognitive tasks or experiences emotions.

In addition to obtaining structural and functional information about the brain, MRI methodology has been used for other specialized investigations of the effects of alcohol on the brain. For example, structural MRI can clearly delineate gray matter from white matter but cannot detect damage to individual nerve fibers forming the white matter. By tracking the diffusion of water molecules along neuronal fibers, an MRI technique known as diffusion tensor imaging (DTI) can provide information about orientations and integrity of nerve pathways, confirming earlier findings from post mortem studies which suggested that heavy drinking disrupts the microstructure of nerve fibers. Moreover, the findings correlate with behavioral tests of attention and memory. These nerve pathways are critically important because thoughts and goal-oriented behavior depend on the concerted activity of many brain areas. Another type of MRI application, magnetic resonance spectroscopy imaging (MRSI), provides information about the neurochemistry of the living brain. MRSI can evaluate neuronal health and degeneration and can detect the presence and distribution of alcohol, certain metabolites, and neurotransmitters.

Imaging of Brain Function: Electromagnetic Methods: In spite of their excellent spatial resolution—that is, the ability to show precisely where the activation changes are occurring in the brain—hemodynamic methods such as PET, SPECT, and fMRI have limitations in showing the time sequence of these changes. Activation maps can reveal brain areas involved in a particular task, but they cannot show exactly when these areas made their respective contributions. This is because they measure hemodynamic changes (blood flow and oxygenation), indicating the neuronal activation only indirectly and with a lag of more than a second. Yet, it is important to understand the order and timing of thoughts, feelings, and behaviors, as well as the contributions of different brain areas.

The only methods capable of online detection of the electrical currents in neuronal activity are electromagnetic methods such as electroencephalography (EEG), event-related brain potentials (ERP), and magnetoencephalography (MEG). EEG reflects electrical activity measured by small electrodes attached to the scalp. Event-related potentials are obtained by averaging EEG voltage changes that are time-locked to the presentation of a stimulus such as a tone, image, or word. MEG uses sensors in a machine that resembles a large hair dryer to measure magnetic fields generated by brain electrical activity. These techniques are harmless and give us insight into the dynamic moment-to-moment changes in electrical activity of the brain. They show when the critical changes are occurring, but their spatial resolution is ambiguous and limited.

ERP and MEG have confirmed that alcohol exerts deleterious effects on multiple levels of the nervous system. These effects include impairment of the lower-level brain stem functions resulting in behavioral symptoms such as dizziness, involuntary eye movement (nystagmus), and insecure gait, as well as impairment of higher order functioning such as problem solving, memory, and emotion. ERP and MEG are remarkably sensitive to many alcohol-related phenomena and can detect changes in the brain that are associated with alcoholism, withdrawal, and abstinence. That is, these methods show different activity patterns between healthy and alcohol-dependent individuals, those in withdrawal, and those with a positive family history of alcoholism. When brain electrical activity is measured in response to target stimuli (which require the subject to respond in some way) and nontarget stimuli (to be ignored by the subject), the brains of alcoholics are less responsive than the brains of nonalcoholic control subjects. Some of the ERP abnormalities observed in alcoholics do not change with abstinence, and similar abnormalities have been reported in patients who do not drink but come from families with a history of alcoholism. The possibility that such abnormalities may be genetic markers for the predisposition for alcoholism is under intensive scrutiny in studies combining genetic and electromagnetic measures in people with or without a family history of alcoholism.

Implications for Treatment

Because alcoholism is associated with diverse changes to the brain and behavior, clinicians must consider a variety of treatment methods to promote cessation of drinking and recovery of impaired functioning. With an optimal combination of neuropsychological observations and structural and functional brain imaging results, treatment professionals may be able to develop a number of predictors of abstinence and relapse outcomes, with the purpose of tailoring treatment methods to each individual patient. Neuroimaging methods have already provided significant insight into the nature of brain damage caused by heavy alcohol use, and the integration of results from different methods of neuroimaging will spur further advances in the diagnosis and treatment of alcoholism-related damage. Clinicians also can use brain imaging techniques to monitor the course of treatment because these techniques can reveal structural, functional, and biochemical changes in living patients across time as a result of abstinence, therapeutic interventions, withdrawal, or relapse. For example, functional imaging studies might be used to evaluate the effectiveness of drugs such as naltrexone on withdrawal-induced craving. (Naltrexone is an anticraving medicine that suppresses GABA activity.) Additionally, neuroimaging research already has shown that abstinence of less than a month can result in an increase in cerebral metabolism, particularly in the frontal lobes, and that continued abstinence can lead to at least partial reversal in loss of brain tissue. Neuroimaging indicators also can be useful in prognosis, permitting identification and timely treatment of patients at high risk for relapse.

Part Three

Coping with Alzheimer Disease and Other Dementias

Chapter 24

Maintaining Cognitive Vitality as You Age

The Aging Brain

The human brain uses neurons (nerve cells) to transmit information and communicate with the environment and with the body. As the brain ages, the rate at which its neurons receive and process information slows. This, in turn, affects our fluid intelligence (ability to manipulate information) by slowing down our learning, recall, and multitasking skills.

Memory lapses and slowed retrieval of information are a normal part of the aging process and vary from person to person. Older adults are likely to have trouble recalling common items such as names, appointments, location of objects, telephone numbers, and words. Individuals experiencing normal age-related memory loss soon retrieve what they are having difficulty recalling, whereas those with cognitive impairment from disease will never remember.

From "A Practical Guide Achieving and Maintaining Cognitive Vitality With Aging," © 2005 Institute for the Study of Aging and the Alzheimer's Drug Discovery Foundation. The Alzheimer's Drug Discovery Foundation (ADDF) is a public charity established in 2004 to expand upon the programs initiated by the Institute for the Study of Aging (ISOA), a private foundation founded by the Estée Lauder family in 1998. The sole mission of the ADDF is to accelerate drug discovery research to prevent, treat, and cure Alzheimer's disease, related dementias and cognitive aging through venture philanthropy. As of spring 2007, ADDF and ISOA have awarded $28.7 million for 195 research programs and conferences worldwide. For more information about the ADDF and ISOA, visit www.alzdiscovery.org or call Howard Fillit, MD, at 212-935-2402.

Cognitive aging does have advantages. Crystallized intelligence (knowledge gained over time or by experience) increases with age, allowing older adults to reflect and ponder situations more effectively, to take a broader view, and to make decisions with less information. This is sometimes called "wisdom." Vocabulary, stored experience, and special expertise also increase with age.

Contrary to popular belief, our neurons do not die off as we age. In fact, when stimulated, the older brain is capable of neurogenesis, the process of making new brain cells.

Nine Actions That Promote Cognitive Vitality

For the brain to age successfully, its neurons must remain vital. The key to cognitive heath, then, is to protect the neurons from damage and promote their vitality. The nine strategies discussed below have a biological basis in scientific research and enable individuals of all ages to take a proactive approach to maintaining and achieving cognitive vitality with aging.

It is never too late to take concrete steps to maintain cognitive health, but the sooner you start the better. Indeed, medical and lifestyle prevention in mid-life will improve your cognitive health in late life.

1. Manage Chronic Illnesses: See Your Doctor

It is critical for middle aged and older individuals to manage medical illnesses associated with diminished cognitive function, particularly hypertension, high cholesterol and diabetes. Indeed, all the risk factors that we typically think of for heart disease are also thought to be risk factors for cognitive decline (see Table 24.1). Learn all you can about your condition in order to take responsibility for your care. Most importantly, see your doctor(s) on a regular basis and take your medications.

Older adults should also get their eyes and ears checked regularly. Sensory aids such as eyeglasses and hearing aids maximize our interaction with the environment and other people, which helps to maintain and improve cognitive vitality.

2. Physical Exercise: It's Good for Your Brain, Too

Physical activity increases blood flow to the brain, and stimulates the proteins and molecules that keep our neurons healthy and strong.

Table 24.1. Medical Risk Factors for Cognitive Decline

- Hypertension
- Heart disease
- Diabetes
- Elevated cholesterol
- Vitamin B$_{12}$ deficiency
- Transitory ischemic attacks ("mini strokes")
- Head trauma
- Environmental exposure to toxins, particularly lead
- Depression
- Sleep Disorders
- Obesity
- Sensory (vision or hearing) problems

Exercise has also been shown to reduce stress and depression and improve mood. To maintain cognitive vitality, adults should engage in moderate-intensity aerobic exercise for at least 30 minutes, three to five days per week. Physical exercise consists of aerobic, strength training, and flexibility.

The following exercises are fun and effective ways to stay active:

Aerobic Training

- Brisk Walking
- Aerobics
- Hiking
- Swimming
- Aqua aerobics
- Jogging
- Climbing stairs or hills
- Racquet sports
- Bicycling
- Skiing
- Yard work
- Dancing
- Martial arts

Flexibility / Balance Benefits

- Tai chi
- Yoga
- Pilates
- Dancing

Strength Training

- Lifting weights
- Martial arts
- Yoga
- Pilates

3. Nutrition: Eating Brain Food

Studies show that low-fat and low-calorie diets have the highest correlation with cognitive health. This may be due to their effects on preventing vascular disease in the brain, or by other mechanisms. Researchers are also investigating the role of antioxidants in preserving cognitive vitality. Antioxidants, such as vitamins C and E and beta carotene (pigment found in vegetables), act as scavengers and may protect the brain against free radicals that can damage brain cells. Free radicals are unstable molecules created by cells when burning oxygen for energy.

Dietary omega-3 fatty acids may also promote cognitive health. A component of omega-3, DHA, may enhance memory and learning by protecting and boosting our neuron's ability to communicate with each other.

Studies show that B vitamins, such as niacin and folic acid, help control inflammation and may play a role in the development of new brain cells. B vitamins are found in lean meat, fish, legumes, dairy products, whole grains, nuts and seeds, eggs, seafood, spinach, carrots, asparagus, and broccoli.

Some research suggests that drinking alcohol moderately (one to four drinks per week) may lower the risk of cognitive decline with aging. If your lifestyle includes such moderate consumption of alcohol, remember, excessive alcohol intake (more than two drinks per day), will cause cognitive impairment, and this risk increases with aging.

To promote cognitive health, a balanced, low-fat, low-calorie diet that includes five servings of antioxidant-rich fruits and vegetables is recommended. Taking a multivitamin every day is also highly recommended to insure an adequate balance of vitamins and minerals.

Examples of foods containing antioxidants and omega-3 fatty acids:

Fish Containing the Most Omega-3

- Anchovy, bluefish, herring, mackerel, sablefish, salmon, sardines, lake trout, tuna, and whitefish.

Antioxidant-Rich Vegetables

- Kale, spinach, brussels sprouts, alfalfa sprouts, beets, red bell peppers, and onions. Black and green teas are also rich in anti-oxidants.

Antioxidant-Rich Fruits

- Berries, plums, avocados, oranges, red grapes, cherries, red apples, and cranberries.

Other Omega-3 Rich Foods

- Flax seeds and flax seed oil, canola oil, walnuts, Brazilian nuts, seaweed, green leafy vegetables, tofu, and other forms of soybean. DHA is also available as a supplement.

Reduce Stress: Learn Ways to Cope

Stress affects us all differently, depending on past experiences, and coping techniques. The "stress reaction" is the body's natural response to internal and external pressures. Physically, the body reacts to stress by secreting stress hormones, tensing muscles, elevating the heart rate, and increasing blood pressure. Prolonged stress causes fatigue, disturbed sleep, poor concentration, and memory lapses. Chronically high-levels of stress hormones suppress the immune system and kill brain cells. Older adults with a high level of psychological distress have twice the risk of cognitive impairment.

The psychological reaction to stressful situations is more relevant than the stress itself because how we cope determines how stress affects our bodies—both physically and mentally. Therefore, finding ways to cope successfully with stress is critical to our physical and cognitive health. Coping takes effort, but can be learned. Effective methods for handling stress involve the following:

- Take responsibility for developing a way to cope
- Avoid rash decisions or actions
- Find a lesson in the situation
- Express your feelings privately
- Seek advice from friends, family, or counselors
- Stay confident and optimistic

- Use humor

- Regularly practice relaxation techniques such as meditation or physical exercise

5. Sleep: Snooze for Better Memory

Getting a good night's sleep is essential to cognitive health and function even with aging. The average individual needs seven to eight hours of sleep per night. Here are a few tips to improve the quality of your sleep:

- Maintain a regular bed and wake time schedule, even during the weekends

- Establish a regular bedtime routine, such as taking a hot bath, reading, or listening to soothing music

- Use the bedroom only for sleep and sex

- Eat at least two to three hours before bedtime

- Avoid exercising at least three hours before bedtime

- Avoid sleeping pills

6. Emotional Health: Depression Is Treatable

Depression is very common in older adults, yet often not diagnosed. Fortunately, today depression is very treatable with medications and psychotherapy. Depression may cause cognitive impairment, such as memory loss and difficulty paying attention. Seek help if you suffer from depression, grief, or loneliness.

Take a quick test to gage your risk for depression. Check all that apply:

_____ Persistent sad, anxious, or empty mood

_____ Feelings of hopelessness, pessimism

_____ Feelings of guilt, worthlessness, helplessness

_____ Loss of interest or pleasure in hobbies and activities that were once enjoyed, including sex

_____ Decreased energy, fatigue, being slowed down

_____ Difficulty concentrating, remembering, making decisions

_____ Insomnia, early-morning awakening, or oversleeping

_____ Changes in appetite that result in weight losses or gains unrelated to dieting

_____ Thoughts of death or suicide

_____ Restlessness, irritability

_____ Persistent physical symptoms that do not respond to treatment, such as headaches digestive disorders, and chronic pain

If you experience at least five of the symptoms listed above everyday or nearly everyday for more than two weeks, this may be a sign of depression. See your doctor. Treatment may include counseling or medication. (—Adopted from the National Institute on Mental Health)

7. Remain Engaged: Participate in Social Activities

A rich and stimulating work and social environment helps maintain cognitive function. This should be an important consideration for a person thinking about retirement. In fact, we strongly recommend planning your retirement—and we don't mean that financially. Be open to alternative ideas and ways of retiring such as volunteering, working part-time, or discovering a new career path. Retirement, after all, doesn't mean you no longer need the companionship, validation, or social connections of your peers. It simply means you're moving on to a new phase in life. So even if you are 90 years of age, ask yourself, "What am I going to do with the rest of my life?"

Adults of all ages should limit the number of hours they spend alone and socially isolated. Watching television is a mentally passive activity that has been linked with poorer performance on measures of cognitive function. Instead, engage in mentally stimulating activities associated with improving cognitive health.

Participate in group activities that provide opportunities for social interaction. Work, volunteering, and social networks, such as family and friends, are important to cognitive health, especially in old age. Playing mentally challenging, socially interactive games like bridge, and sports, such as tennis or golf, promote cognitive vitality.

Generativity is central to the mental health of older adults. Generativity is a concern for the next generation and a desire to make a difference. Generative activities include teaching, mentoring, social activism, and grandparenting. Find an activity that fulfills the desire to feel needed and connected to society and family.

8. Lifelong Learning: Stimulate the Brain

Studies demonstrate that lower education levels or low language ability in early life are associated with cognitive impairment in later years. The brain has billions of neurons, giving it a sizable reserve capacity to compensate for neurons that are damaged or destroyed. Education has been found to protect against cognitive decline, probably by providing a larger reserve in brain function.

It's never too late to acquire that extra reserve through education. Enroll in adult education courses, sign up for career development opportunities, and engage in other educational and intellectual stimulating activities. Learning to play a musical instrument, reading books, or learning a new language will all promote cognitive health.

9. Mental Exercises: Your Brain Is Like a Muscle—Use It or Lose It

Remaining socially engaged, continuing life-long learning, and engaging in activities, such as reading and writing, stimulate the brain, build cognitive reserve, and promote cognitive vitality. Mind training is another way to promote cognitive health. Even in old age the brain can rewire itself, and some areas of the brain add new cells in response to stimulation. Since the brain maintains its plasticity (adaptivity) even into very old age, activities that require repeated training, such as memory exercises, crossword puzzles, or word searches, can improve cognitive function. These "mind workouts" provide excellent training for adults of any age. Numerous books, courses, and websites are available on the subject.

Women, Menopause, and Memory

Menopause is when the ovaries stop producing the hormones estrogen and progesterone, leading to the end of women's periods. Menopause generally occurs between the ages of 45 and 55. Aside from the typical hot flashes, women going through menopause may also experience sleep disturbances and depressive symptoms such as increased irritability and anxiety. Menopausal women also complain of cognitive symptoms such as difficulty paying attention and word finding. Some women report that they became more forgetful during and after menopause. However, research studies clearly show that the menopause is not associated with any cognitive decline that impairs a woman's ability to function.

Hormone Replacement Therapy: The Role of Estrogen

Some research has shown that estrogen protects neurons from damage and may promote the production of new neurons in the brain. As a result, researchers studied whether menopausal hormone replacement therapy (HRT) would prevent or delay the onset of age-associated memory loss or cognitive impairment and dementia. However, at present, there is no conclusive clinical evidence to support this theory. Furthermore, some studies have found that HRT increases the risk of heart disease, stroke, breast cancer, and even dementia. For these reasons, long-term HRT is not recommended for women to prevent dementia or treat Alzheimer disease.

Dementia and Alzheimer Disease

Dementia is a medical condition characterized by cognitive impairment that involves multiple domains of cognitive function, including memory, language, and abstract thinking; and is severe enough to impair a person's ability to perform their usual every-day tasks. Though early dementia is sometimes difficult to distinguish from normal cognitive aging, dementia is not a normal part of aging. However, it does affect about five percent of people over age 65, and up to 25 percent of people over 75. Dementia is common and devastating for older people and their loved ones.

Alzheimer disease is the most common cause of dementia in older people. It is characterized by progressive cognitive decline caused by the degeneration of neurons and the formation of amyloid plaques and neurofibrillary tangles, both of which are abnormal in the brain. Alzheimer disease can be diagnosed, treated, and effectively managed by a doctor.

While Alzheimer disease is the most common cause of dementia, there are other causes of dementia that are preventable and treatable. These include multiple strokes, B_{12} deficiency, thyroid abnormalities, depression, and the side effects of many medications.

Since some causes of dementia are potentially reversible or preventable, and Alzheimer disease can be effectively treated and managed, getting an early diagnostic evaluation for anyone with significant memory problems in old age is very important to cognitive health.

Chapter 25

Memory Loss and Forgetfulness: When Should I Be Concerned?

Forgetfulness: It's Not Always What You Think

Many older people worry about becoming more forgetful. They think forgetfulness is the first sign of Alzheimer disease (AD). In the past, memory loss and confusion were considered a normal part of aging. However, scientists now know that most people remain both alert and able as they age, although it may take them longer to remember things.

A lot of people experience memory lapses. Some memory problems are serious, and others are not. People who have serious changes in their memory, personality, and behavior may suffer from a form of brain disease called dementia. Dementia seriously affects a person's ability to carry out daily activities. AD is one of many types of dementia.

The term dementia describes a group of symptoms that are caused by changes in brain function. Dementia symptoms may include the following:

- Asking the same questions repeatedly

- Becoming lost in familiar places

- Being unable to follow directions

This chapter includes "Forgetfulness: It's Not Always What You Think," an AgePage publication from the National Institute on Aging, August 2006. "Questions to Ask Your Doctor about Memory Changes," is from the Administration on Aging, March 2007.

- Getting disoriented about time, people, and places
- Neglecting personal safety, hygiene, and nutrition

People with dementia lose their abilities at different rates. Dementia is caused by many conditions. Some conditions that cause dementia can be reversed, and others cannot. Further, many different medical conditions may cause symptoms that seem like AD, but are not. Some of these medical conditions may be treatable. Reversible conditions can be caused by a high fever, dehydration, vitamin deficiency and poor nutrition, bad reactions to medicines, problems with the thyroid gland, or a minor head injury. Medical conditions like these can be serious and should be treated by a doctor as soon as possible.

Sometimes older people have emotional problems that can be mistaken for dementia. Feeling sad, lonely, worried, or bored may be more common for older people facing retirement or coping with the death of a spouse, relative, or friend. Adapting to these changes leaves some people feeling confused or forgetful. Emotional problems can be eased by supportive friends and family, or by professional help from a doctor or counselor.

The two most common forms of dementia in older people are AD and multi-infarct dementia (sometimes called vascular dementia). These types of dementia are irreversible, which means they cannot be cured. In AD, nerve cell changes in certain parts of the brain result in the death of a large number of cells. Symptoms of AD begin slowly and become steadily worse. As the disease progresses, symptoms range from mild forgetfulness to serious impairments in thinking, judgment, and the ability to perform daily activities. Eventually, patients may need total care.

In multi-infarct dementia, a series of strokes or changes in the brain's blood supply may result in the death of brain tissue. The location in the brain where the strokes occur and the severity of the strokes determine the seriousness of the problem and the symptoms that arise. Symptoms usually begin abruptly and progress in a stepwise fashion with repeated strokes. At this time, there is no way to reverse damage that has already been caused by a stroke. However, treatment to prevent further strokes is very important.

Diagnosis

People who are worried about memory problems should see their doctor. If the doctor believes that the problem is serious, then a thorough physical, neurological, and psychiatric evaluation may be recommended.

A complete medical examination for memory loss may include gathering information about the person's medical history, including use of prescription and over the counter medicines, diet, past medical problems, and general health. Because a correct diagnosis depends on recalling these details accurately, the doctor also may ask a family member for information about the person.

Tests of blood and urine may be done to help the doctor find any problems. There are also tests of mental abilities (tests of memory, problem solving, counting, and language). A brain computed tomography (CT) scan may assist the doctor in ruling out a curable disorder. A scan also may show signs of normal age related changes in the brain. It may be necessary to have another scan at a later date to see if there have been further changes in the brain.

Multi-infarct dementia and AD can exist together, making it hard for the doctor to diagnose either one specifically. Scientists once thought that multi-infarct dementia and other types of vascular dementia caused most cases of irreversible mental impairment. They now believe that most older people with irreversible dementia have Alzheimer disease.

Treatment

Even if the doctor diagnoses an irreversible form of dementia, much still can be done to treat the patient and help the family cope. A person with dementia should be under a doctor's care, and may see a neurologist, psychiatrist, family doctor, internist, or geriatrician. The doctor can treat the patient's physical and behavioral problems and answer the many questions that the person or family may have.

For some people in the early and middle stages of AD, the drugs tacrine (Cognex, which is still available but no longer actively marketed by the manufacturer), donepezil (Aricept), rivastigmine (Exelon), and galantamine (Razadyne, formerly known as Reminyl) are prescribed to possibly delay the worsening of some of the disease's symptoms. Another drug, memantine (Namenda), has been approved for treatment of moderate to severe AD. Doctors believe it is very important for people with multi-infarct dementia to try to prevent further strokes by controlling high blood pressure, monitoring and treating high blood cholesterol and diabetes, and not smoking.

Many people with dementia need no medication for behavioral problems. But for some people, doctors may prescribe medications to reduce agitation, anxiety, depression, or sleeping problems. These troublesome behaviors are common in people with dementia. Careful use of doctor prescribed drugs may make some people with dementia more comfortable and make caring for them easier.

A healthy diet is important. Although no special diets or nutritional supplements have been found to prevent or reverse AD or multi-infarct dementia, a balanced diet helps maintain overall good health. In cases of multi-infarct dementia, improving the diet may play a role in preventing more strokes.

Family members and friends can assist people with dementia in continuing their daily routines, physical activities, and social contacts. People with dementia should be kept up-to-date about the details of their lives, such as the time of day, where they live, and what is happening at home or in the world. Memory aids may help in the day to day living of patients in the earlier stages of dementia. Some families find that a big calendar, a list of daily plans, notes about simple safety measures, and written directions describing how to use common household items are useful aids.

Advice for Today

Scientists are working to develop new drugs that someday may slow, reverse, or prevent the damage caused by AD and multi-infarct dementia. In the meantime, people who have no dementia symptoms can try to keep their memory sharp.

Some suggestions include developing interests or hobbies and staying involved in activities that stimulate both the mind and body. Giving careful attention to physical fitness and exercise also may go a long way toward keeping a healthy state of mind. Limiting the use of alcoholic beverages is important, because heavy drinking over time can cause permanent brain damage.

Many people find it useful to plan tasks; make "things to do" lists; and use notes, calendars, and other memory aids. They also may remember things better by mentally connecting them to other meaningful things, such as a familiar name, song, or lines from a poem.

Stress, anxiety, or depression can make a person more forgetful. Forgetfulness caused by these emotions usually is temporary and goes away when the feelings fade. However, if these feelings last for a long period of time, getting help from a professional is important. Treatment may include counseling or medication, or a combination of both.

Some physical and mental changes occur with age in healthy people. However, much pain and suffering can be avoided if older people, their families, and their doctors recognize dementia as a disease, not part of normal aging.

Questions to Ask Your Doctor about Memory Changes

As we age, we experience many physical and mental changes. Many of these changes are just a part of normal aging, but sometimes, they may be an indicator of a more serious condition. One thing that people with memory problems often fear is that they have Alzheimer disease—one form of dementia. However, there are many health conditions which mimic the symptoms of Alzheimer disease but are treatable.

The following questions are designed to help you talk with your doctor about all of the possible causes of your memory loss symptoms, especially those which are treatable, before you and your doctor settle on a diagnosis of Alzheimer disease or dementia.

Ask Your Doctor

Possible medication interactions: If you take even two medications, you may be experiencing dizziness, memory loss, or other symptoms due to medication interactions. Make a list and be sure to tell your physician about all substances you are taking, including the following:

- Prescription medications
- Vitamins
- Herbal supplements
- Over the counter products (such as aspirin and cold medicine)
- Smoking cessation products
- Water and weight loss products
- Topical items (such as arthritis ointment, athlete's foot treatment, etc.)
- Other items

Be sure to be thorough, because even things that we don't think about (such as arthritis ointment) can contain substances that can cause problems for some people.

Your doctor may need to work with you over time or may need to change your prescriptions and over the counter products in order to rule out medication interactions. Of course, this may not solve your problem, but it is an important thing to rule out.

Effect of weight loss/gain and medications: If you have recently gained or lost even 10 pounds, you should ask your doctor to check your medication levels.

- Some medications are prescribed according to our weight and losing or gaining weight may mean that you have too much or too little medication in your body for your size, and you may experience a variety of symptoms that mimic dementia.

- Use the list above and share it with your physician.

- Be sure to alert your doctor to weight changes and have them adjust your medications if necessary.

Symptoms from dehydration: If you are dehydrated or malnourished, your body may not be processing your medications correctly.

- You probably know that water is an important element in our bodies. Water is also necessary for our body to digest food and to dissolve and metabolize medications properly. However, many of us do not get enough water and dehydration among older adults is common.

- In talking with your doctor about your symptoms, be sure to alert your physician of any bouts of diarrhea, vomiting, and heat exhaustion you have recently experienced.

- Ask your physician to ensure that you are not dehydrated, because if you are, the medications in your system may be more concentrated than appropriate and your body may not be metabolizing your medicines correctly.

- If you are dehydrated, your physician will work with you to ensure proper hydration and that your medication levels are appropriate.

Falls and concussions: If you have fallen or hit your head recently, you could have a concussion which can result in sudden memory loss or dizziness.

- Although you may not realize it, a recent fall or serious bump on the head may be the cause of your memory problems. Falls among older adults are common and sometimes, people fall and do not know if they hit their head or even if they were unconscious for any period of time.

- Be sure to tell your doctor about any recent falls or serious bumps on your head so that your doctor can rule out concussions and other potential problems that can arise from such events.

- Your doctor may do a series of tests to see if there is anything that needs to be done and if so, he/she will do what is necessary to address the problem.

Depression: Depression is a common problem among older adults and affects as many as one in five older people. The symptoms of depression are remarkably similar to those of dementia.

- Physicians often mistake depression for dementia, so be sure to ask for specific tests to rule out depression. Blood tests and neurological and psychological evaluations are generally necessary to rule out depression.

- Depression can have many different triggers such as loss, significant life changes, and side effects of medications. Your physician should address all possible underlying causes of depression.

- Don't be afraid to ask for a depression screening, as many older people experience the symptoms of depression but are unaware that they have a treatable condition.

- Remember that depression is treatable, so be sure that your physician checks for depression prior to providing a diagnosis of dementia.

Alcohol use: Consuming too much alcohol, or drinking alcohol while taking certain medications may result in symptoms of memory loss.

- Be sure to tell your physician if you drink alcohol on a regular basis, or if you experienced symptoms after an occasional drink.

- Advise your physician of any medications and treatments you use.

- Carefully follow your physician's advice in regards to the use of alcohol.

Hopefully, considering these will help you in speaking with your doctor about all of the possible causes of your memory problems. After considering the various treatable conditions that often mimic the symptoms of dementia, your physician may determine that a diagnosis of Alzheimer disease is correct. If you are diagnosed with Alzheimer disease or another form of dementia, you may wish to contact your State or Area Agency on Aging or the local chapter of the Alzheimer's Association for assistance in coping with Alzheimer disease.

Chapter 26

Steps to Diagnosing Alzheimer Disease

Finding the Right Doctor

The first step in following up on symptoms is finding a doctor you feel comfortable with. Alzheimer's Association clients report they are most likely to be satisfied seeing someone who is well informed about Alzheimer disease. Your local Alzheimer's Association can help you find the right doctor.

There is no single type of doctor who specializes in diagnosing and treating memory loss or Alzheimer disease. Many people contact their regular primary care physician or internist about their concerns. Primary care doctors often oversee the diagnostic process and provide treatment themselves.

In some cases, the primary care doctor may refer a patient to one of the following specialists:

- A neurologist, who specializes in diseases of the brain and nervous system

- A psychiatrist, who specializes in disorders that affect mood or the way the mind works

- A psychologist with advanced training in testing memory, concentration, problem solving, language, and other mental functions

"Steps to Diagnosis" is reprinted with permission of the Alzheimer's Association. For additional information, call the Alzheimer's Association toll-free helpline, 800-272-2900, or visit their website at www.alz.org. © 2007 Alzheimer's Association. All rights reserved.

241

Steps to Diagnosis

There is no single test that proves a person has Alzheimer disease. The medical workup is designed to evaluate overall health and identify any conditions that could affect how well the mind works.

Experts estimate a skilled physician can diagnose Alzheimer disease with more than 90 percent accuracy. Doctors can almost always determine that a person has dementia, but it may sometimes be difficult to pin down the exact cause.

Understanding the Problem

Be prepared for the doctor to ask:

- What kind of symptoms have you noticed?
- When did they begin?
- How often do they happen?
- Have they gotten worse?

Reviewing Medical History

The doctor will interview the person being examined or family members to gather information about current and past illnesses. The doctor will also obtain a history of medical conditions affecting other family members, especially whether they may have had Alzheimer disease or a related disorder.

Evaluating Mood and Mental Function

Mental status testing gives the doctor a general idea of whether a person:

- Is aware of having symptoms or feels nothing is wrong
- Knows the date, time, and where he or she is
- Can remember a short list of words, follow instructions, and do simple calculations

About the Mini-Mental State Exam (MMSE)

The mini-mental state examination (MMSE) is one of the tests most commonly used to assess mental function. In the MMSE, a health professional asks a patient a series of questions designed to test a range of everyday mental skills.

Examples of questions include:

- Remember and repeat a few minutes later the names of three common objects (for instance, horse, flower, penny)

- State the year, season, day of the week, and date

- Count backward from 100 by 7s or spell "world" backwards

- Name two familiar objects present in the office as the examiner points to them

- Identify the location of the examiner's office (state, city, street address, floor)

- Repeat a common phrase or saying after the examiner

- Copy a picture of two interlocking shapes

- Follow a three-part instruction, such as: take a piece of paper in your right hand, fold it in half, and place it on the floor

The maximum MMSE score is 30 points. A score of 20–24 suggests mild dementia, 13–20 suggests moderate dementia, and less than 12 indicates severe dementia. On average, the MMSE score of a person with Alzheimer disease declines about 2–4 points each year.

About the Mini-Cog

Another popular mental status test is the "mini-cog," which involves two tasks: (1) remembering and a few minutes later repeating the names of three common objects, and (2) drawing a face of a clock showing all 12 numbers in the right places and a time specified by the examiner.

In addition to assessing mental status, the doctor will evaluate a person's sense of well-being to detect depression or other mood disorders that can cause memory problems, loss of interest in life, and other symptoms that can overlap with dementia.

Physical Exam and Diagnostic Tests

The physician will:

- Ask about diet, nutrition, and use of alcohol.

- Review all medications. It is helpful to bring a list or the containers of all medicines currently being taken, including over-the-counter drugs and supplements.

- Check blood pressure, temperature, and pulse.
- Listen to the heart and lungs.
- Collect samples of blood and urine.

Information from these tests can help identify other disorders that may cause memory loss, confused thinking, trouble focusing attention, or other symptoms similar to dementia. Such disorders include:

- Anemia, malnutrition, or certain vitamin deficiencies
- Excess use of alcohol
- Medication side effects
- Certain infections
- Diabetes
- Kidney or liver disease
- Thyroid abnormalities
- Problems with the heart, lung, or blood vessels

Neurological Exam

The neurological examination is an important part of the physical. Its goal is to assess the function of the brain and nervous system to identify symptoms of brain disorders other than Alzheimer disease.

During the neurological exam, the physician may test:

- Reflexes
- Coordination and balance
- Muscle tone and strength
- Eye movement
- Speech
- Sensation

Brain Imaging

New imaging technologies have revolutionized our understanding of the structure and function of the living brain.

- Structural imaging provides information about the shape, position, or volume of brain tissue. Structural techniques include magnetic resonance imaging (MRI) and computed tomography (CT).

- Functional imaging reveals how well cells in various brain regions are working by showing how actively the cells use sugar or oxygen. Functional techniques include positron emission tomography (PET) and functional MRI (fMRI).

Currently, a standard medical workup for Alzheimer disease often includes structural imaging with MRI or, less frequently, CT. These images are used primarily to detect tumors, evidence of small or large strokes, damage from severe head trauma, or a buildup of fluid.

Promising Areas for Brain Imaging Research

Researchers are studying whether the use of MRI and other imaging methods may be expanded to play a more direct role in diagnosing Alzheimer disease. Many studies have shown that the brains of people with Alzheimer disease shrink significantly as the disease progresses.

Research has also shown that shrinkage in specific brain regions may be an early sign of Alzheimer disease. However, scientists have not yet agreed upon standardized values that would establish the significance of a specific amount of shrinkage for any individual person at a single point in time.

Research with PET and other functional imaging methods also suggests that those with Alzheimer disease typically have reduced brain cell activity in certain regions. However, as with the shrinkage detected by structural imaging, there is not yet enough information to translate these general patterns of reduced activity into diagnostic information about individuals.

At this time, PET is used primarily in research studies in hopes of gaining further knowledge about its potential for wider use in diagnosing Alzheimer disease and monitoring progression and response to treatment.

Today, Medicare will cover a PET scan for Alzheimer disease only to help distinguish the disease from frontotemporal dementia, a rare related disorder that may cause dramatic loss of function in the front and side regions of the brain.

Another promising area of functional imaging research focuses on developing tracer compounds that will attach to key abnormal brain deposits implicated in Alzheimer disease. For example, preliminary data suggests that one such tracer, called Pittsburgh compound B, may attach to beta-amyloid and "light up" in a PET scan.

Chapter 27

If You Have Alzheimer Disease

What is happening to me?

Alzheimer disease causes gradual, irreversible changes in the brain. These changes usually cause problems with memory, decision making, and self-care. The disease also affects the ways we communicate—both in expressing our thoughts and in understanding what others are saying.

You may be worried or anxious about the changes you've noticed so far. While there is no cure for Alzheimer disease, treatments might help you with some of your symptoms. And having information about the disease can help you cope.

It's important to know that:

- The changes you are experiencing are because of the disease.

- You will have good days and bad days.

- The disease affects each person differently, and symptoms will vary.

- Trying different ideas will help you find comfortable ways to cope.

- Some suggestions may work for you, others may not.

"If You Have Alzheimer's Disease" is reprinted with permission of the Alzheimer's Association. For additional information, call the Alzheimer's Association toll-free helpline, 800-272-2900, or visit their website at www.alz.org. © 2005 Alzheimer's Association. All rights reserved.

- You are not alone—an estimated 4.5 million Americans have Alzheimer disease.

- People who understand what you are going through can help you and your family.

What can I do?

Coping with memory loss: While you may clearly remember things that happened long ago, recent events can be quickly forgotten.

You may have trouble keeping track of time, people, and places. You may forget appointments or people's names. It might be very frustrating trying to remember where you put things.

Suggestions for coping with memory loss:

- Keep a book of important notes with you at all times that has:
  - Important telephone numbers and addresses, including emergency numbers and your own contact information;
  - People's names and their relationships to you;
  - A "To do" list of appointments;
  - A map showing where your home is;
  - Thoughts or ideas you want to hold on to.

- Label cupboards and drawers with words or pictures that describe their contents, such as dishes and silverware, or sweaters and socks.

- Get an easy-to-read, digital clock that displays the time and date, and keep it in a prominent place.

- Use an answering machine to keep track of telephone messages.

- Post phone numbers in large print next to the telephone; include emergency numbers along with your address and a description of where you live.

- Have a dependable friend call to remind you about meal times, appointments, and medication.

- Keep a set of photos of people you see regularly; label the photos with names and what each does.

- Keep track of the date by marking off each day on a calendar.

- Use pillboxes to help you organize your medication; pillboxes with sections for times of day—like morning and evening—can help remind you when you should take your pills.

Finding your way: Sometimes, things that were once familiar to you may now seem unfamiliar. A favorite place may not look the same. Or you might get lost.

Suggestions for finding your way:

- Take someone with you when you go out.

- Don't be afraid to ask for help.

- Explain to others that you have a memory problem and need assistance.

- Enroll in Alzheimer's Association Safe Return®, a 24-hour nationwide identification and support program that will reunite you with your loved ones should you ever wander. You can learn more by calling 888-572-8566 or visiting http://www.alz.org/safereturn.

Doing daily tasks: You may find familiar activities more difficult. For example, you may have trouble balancing a checkbook, following a recipe, or doing simple household repairs.

Suggestions for doing daily tasks:

- Give yourself a lot of time, and don't let others hurry you.

- Take a break if something is too difficult.

- Ask for help if you need it.

- Arrange for others to help you with difficult tasks.

- Maintain a daily routine.

Over time, certain things may become too difficult for you to do at all. This is because of the disease. Do the best you can, and accept help when it's available.

Talking to others: You may have difficulty understanding what others are saying. You may have trouble finding the right words to express your thoughts.

Suggestions for talking to others:

- Take your time.

- Tell people you have difficulty with thinking, communicating, and remembering.

- Consider with whom you will share your diagnosis—it can be helpful for family and friends to understand your condition.

- Ask the person to repeat a statement if you did not understand what was said.

- Find a quiet place to converse if loud noises or crowds are bothering you.

Is what I'm feeling normal?

Living with the changes caused by Alzheimer disease can bring about many unfamiliar emotions. These feelings are a natural response to the disease.

It is important to share these reactions with others. Tell someone with whom you are comfortable how you feel.

Also, the Alzheimer's Association can refer you to a support group where you can meet others who have Alzheimer disease.

You may find yourself saying:

"I worry more than usual." It is important to talk to your family and friends about your concerns. You may worry about what is going to happen to you in the future. Or you may wonder how quickly the disease will progress.

While there are no definite answers to these questions, most people find that doing something they enjoy—like walking or gardening—helps them take their minds off their worries.

"I sometimes think I'm going crazy." The disease can make you feel as if you are losing control. Telling those around you how you feel may give you comfort. Sharing your feelings with others who have Alzheimer disease may also help.

"I sometimes get into a bad mood." It is normal to experience mood changes. On these days, it is important to remember that tomorrow may be a better day. Try to do things that will lift your spirits.

"Sometimes I feel angry." Feeling angry is OK. Sometimes being part of a support group or talking to a counselor who knows about Alzheimer disease can help. Your doctor or your local Alzheimer's Association office can refer you.

"I sometimes feel sad." You may feel sadness when faced with the changes that the disease brings to your life. It may help to spend time with friends or family, or to do something you enjoy.

Consider consulting your doctor about medications that may help ease feelings of sadness.

"When things go wrong, I feel really embarrassed." Getting lost, forgetting a once familiar face, or not being able to find the right word can feel embarrassing. But this is a part of the disease.

Explain to people that you have memory problems to help ease any awkward feelings.

Keeping a sense of humor, whenever possible, can also be very helpful.

"I get so frustrated." Not being able to do the things you once did can be frustrating.

Talk to others about why you are feeling this way. See if there is anything that you, or those around you, can do to make things easier.

"Sometimes I feel very lonely." You may think that the people around you don't understand what you're going through.

It can be comforting to talk to others who have been diagnosed with Alzheimer disease. Your local Alzheimer's Association office can refer you to a support group.

"I feel guilty asking for help." Few of us like to ask others for help. We often resist relying on others. Over time, you will find it necessary to ask for help more often.

Try to accept the help you need. Chances are that others will be pleased to be of assistance.

How else can I take care of myself?

Two of the most important ways to maintain your well-being are to stay healthy and safe.

Health: Take good care of your body. Suggestions for your health:

- Rest when you are tired.
- Exercise regularly, with your doctor's approval.
- Eat properly.
- Cut down on alcohol—it can make your symptoms worse.
- Take your medications as prescribed, and ask for help if it is difficult to remember when medication should be taken.
- Reduce stress in your daily life.

Safety: The gradual loss of memory can bring new concerns about safety. So, too, can difficulties with decision making and communications.

Suggestions for your safety:

Consider a companion: The person you live with may worry about leaving you alone for long periods of time. While you may feel you will be fine alone, having a companion can help the time pass more pleasantly. It can also lessen worry for your loved ones.

Stop driving when it's no longer safe: Loss of memory can hinder your ability to be a safe driver. You may also become less able to make decisions and react quickly. While it is not easy to give up your license, at some point it will no longer be safe for you to drive.

Look into other ways to get around, like friends, family, taxi cabs, public transportation, or walking.

Just as people can wander while walking, they can also become lost when driving or taking a bus, train, or airplane. Some people wander hundreds of miles away from their homes. To help protect your safety, enroll in the Alzheimer's Association Safe Return® program.

Be mindful of electrical appliances: Leave written reminders to yourself like, "Turn off the stove" or "Unplug the iron." Be sure you have an automatic shut-off feature on the appliances you use most often—especially the ones that can cause harm if left unattended.

Use smoke detectors: Make sure your home has working smoke detectors. A smoke detector could save your life in a fire. Put reminders in your calendar to change the battery.

Be careful of people you don't recognize: If someone you don't recognize comes to your door, don't let them in. Instead, write down the person's name and telephone number. Later, you or a family member can call the person back.

What if I live on my own?

Many people with Alzheimer disease continue to live successfully on their own during the early stages of the disease.

Making simple adjustments, taking safety precautions, and having the support of others can make things easier.

Suggestions for living on your own:

- Talk to staff at your local Alzheimer's Association office or your doctor about where to get help for things like housekeeping, meals, or transportation.

- Inform your bank if you have difficulty with record-keeping and keeping track of your accounts; they may provide special services for people with Alzheimer disease.

- Arrange for direct deposits of checks, such as your retirement pension or Social Security benefits.

- Plan for home-delivered meals, if they are available in your community.

- Have a family member regularly sort your closet and dresser drawers to make it easier for you to get dressed.

- Leave a set of house keys with a neighbor you trust.

- Schedule family, friends, or a community service to make a daily call or visit; keep a list of things you can discuss.

At some point, it will become too difficult or dangerous for you to live alone. Make plans now for where you will live as the disease progresses.

You may want to get a helpful roommate, live with relatives, or move to a residential care setting.

What about the future?

Because Alzheimer disease is a progressive illness; the symptoms you are experiencing will gradually worsen. You will need more help.

There is no way to predict how or when this will happen. It is a good idea for you to make decisions about your future as early in the course of the disease as possible.

Suggestions for future plans:

Make Arrangements at Work

- Talk to your employer about Alzheimer disease and your symptoms, and take someone with you to help you explain and clarify your situation.

- Cut down on your hours or responsibilities if possible.

- If you own your own business, put plans in place for its future operations.

Consider Future Living Arrangements

- Talk to your family or friends about where you want to live, and with whom, to prepare for the time when you will need more care.

- Consider all of the options available, including adult day care programs, in-home care, and hospice services.

Settle Your Money and Legal Matters

- Consider naming a person to make health care decisions for you when you are unable to do so; this person should know your wishes about your health care and future living arrangements.

- Make sure your money matters are in the hands of someone you trust, like your spouse, your child, or a close friend.

- See a lawyer about naming a person to legally take care of your money matters when you can no longer do it.

- Take someone with you to the lawyer to help explain your situation and to interpret all that the lawyer says.

- Find out about any available options for long-term care insurance.

Planning ahead assures that your future will be in good hands. It also helps your loved ones make the right decisions for you in the future.

10 Quick Tips: Living with Alzheimer Disease

1. Carry a book of important notes/photos with you.

2. Enroll in Alzheimer's Association Safe Return®.

3. Be open to accepting help from others.

4. Keep doing the things you most enjoy.

5. Talk to others who have Alzheimer disease.

6. Find ways to laugh as often as you can.

7. Maintain your physical health.

8. Take steps to make your home safe.

9. Extend the time you can live safely in your home with help from your family, friends, and community.

10. Put plans in place now for your future.

Chapter 28

Living with Early-Onset Alzheimer Disease

I'm Too Young to Have Alzheimer Disease

Alzheimer disease is not just a disease of old age. Early-onset is Alzheimer disease that affects people who are under age 65. Many people with early-onset are in their 40s and 50s.

Up to 10 percent of people with Alzheimer disease have early-onset. In the United States, that's about 400,000 people.

Link to Genes

Most people with early-onset have the common type of Alzheimer disease, which is not directly linked to genes. Doctors do not know why symptoms appear at an unusually young age in these cases.

In a few hundred families worldwide, scientists have found several rare genes that directly cause Alzheimer disease. People who inherit these rare genes tend to develop symptoms in their 30s, 40s, and 50s.

Living with Early-Onset Alzheimer Disease

If you have early-onset Alzheimer disease, it's important to know that your life is not over.

You can still live a meaningful and productive life. You can still take part in activities you enjoy. You can still find comfort in your family and friends.

Living with Alzheimer disease does mean dealing with life changes sooner than you had planned.

It's important to know that:

- The disease affects each person differently, and symptoms will vary.

- You will have good days and bad days.

- You are not alone.

- People who understand what you are going through can help you and your family.

What's the Difference between Early-Onset Alzheimer Disease and Early-Stage Alzheimer Disease?

Early-onset is a diagnosis of the disease when the person is younger than 65. Early-stage is the early part of Alzheimer disease, when problems with memory and concentration may begin to appear in a doctor's interview or medical tests.

Feelings

After the diagnosis, you may be going through a range of emotions:

- **Anger:** Your life is taking a different course than the one you and your family had planned.

- **Denial:** The diagnosis seems impossible to believe.

- **Depression:** You may feel sad or hopeless about the life changes you're facing.

- **Fear:** You wonder what the future holds for you and your family, your friends, and your job.

- **Frustration:** You can't cure the disease or make yourself understood.

- **Isolation:** No one seems to understand what you're going through.

- **Sense of loss:** It's hard to accept changes in your abilities, or status in your community or job.

What you can do about your feelings:

- Find ways to express your frustrations and emotions. Don't keep your feelings to yourself.

- Join an Alzheimer's Association support group. Some are just for those with early-onset.

- Work with a well-qualified counselor.

- Share your feelings with your friends and family, and someone who can help with spiritual needs.

- Visit the message boards and chat rooms on the Alzheimer's Association website at www.alz.org and other Alzheimer-related websites.

Family

Your Spouse

Most people with Alzheimer disease continue to live in the home even as the disease progresses.

Your spouse may have to manage the household and your care. He or she may feel a sense of loss over the changes the disease brings to your relationship. You may both experience differences in how you relate to each other sexually.

What you can do to help your spouse:

- Continue to take part in all the activities that you can.

- Adapt activities to fit what you are comfortable doing.

- Talk with your spouse about how he or she can assist you.

- Work with your spouse to put together a file with information you may need later about caregiver services and their costs, including housekeeping and respite (caregiver relief) care.

- Discuss with a professional counselor any role changes in the relationship as well as sexuality issues.

- Continue to find ways for you and your spouse to fulfill the need for intimacy.

- Encourage your spouse to attend a support group for caregivers.

Your Children

Children often experience a wide range of emotions. Younger children may be afraid that they will get the disease or that they did something to cause it.

Teenagers may become resentful when they have to take on more responsibilities for helping around the home. Or they may feel embarrassed that their parent is "different."

College-bound children may be reluctant to leave home.

What you can do to help your children:

- Talk openly about the changes you are experiencing because of the disease.

- Find out what their emotional needs are. Find ways to support them, like meeting with a counselor who specializes in children who have a loved one with Alzheimer disease.

- Notify school social workers and teachers about your situation. Give them information about the disease.

- Invite children to attend support group meetings. Include them in counseling sessions.

- Record your thoughts, feelings, and wisdom in writing, audio, or video. Your children can use this counsel when they grow older. Important life stages you might want to discuss include:

  - graduation;
  - dating;
  - marriage;
  - births;
  - death.

Friends

Friends, co-workers, and neighbors may not understand what is happening to you. Some may keep their distance or resist keeping in touch.

Often they may not know what to do or say. They may be waiting for you to reach out to them.

What you can do to help your friends:

- Share your experience of living with Alzheimer disease.

- Invite them to Alzheimer's Association education programs.

- Continue social activities as much as possible.

- Let them know when you need help and support—tell them what they can do.

Job

You may find work-related tasks more difficult to perform as the disease advances. Talk to your doctor to plan when and what you'll tell your employer about the disease, and at what point you should no longer work.

Your local Alzheimer's Association office has information about the disease that you can share with your employer.

What you can do about your job:

- Continue to work as long as you and your doctor feel you are able.

- Use a daily planning calendar, memos, and other memory aids to help you organize the details of your job.

- Ask your employer if you can switch to a position that better matches your abilities and strengths—or consider reducing your work hours.

- Look into early-retirement options.

- Educate yourself, as well as your spouse or close friend or relative, about the benefits available to you and how to claim them.

Money Matters

If your earnings are the family's main source of income, you may be concerned about financially supporting your family now and in the future.

Insurance and other benefits may be more difficult to obtain. Future health care costs should be considered.

What you can do about money matters:

- Meet with a qualified financial consultant or an attorney to discuss current and future investments, insurance, and retirement options. See if long-term care insurance is still an option.

- Find out about government assistance programs such as Social Security, Medicare, and Medicaid.

- Review your employer-provided or personal disability insurance policies.

- Organize financial documents and other important information in one place. Go over them with your spouse. These include:
  - birth certificates;
  - insurance policies;
  - retirement accounts;
  - social security information;
  - wills;
  - research college scholarship and grant money for your children.

Well-Being

Two of the most important ways you can take good care of yourself are to stay healthy and safe.

Health

Take good care of your body.
What you can do about your health:

- Get regular check-ups.
- Exercise regularly, with your doctor's approval.
- Rest when you are tired.
- Eat properly.
- Take any prescribed medications according to directions.
- Cut down on alcohol—it can make your symptoms worse.
- Take care of your spiritual needs.
- Reach out for help when you need it.
- Reduce stress in your daily life, and learn new ways to relax.

Safety

Symptoms of Alzheimer disease, like loss of memory and decision-making ability, can bring about new safety needs.
What you can do about your safety:

- Keep important phone numbers nearby.
- Post reminders to lock doors and turn off electrical appliances.

- Arrange for an in-home helper to assist you when your spouse or caregiver needs to be away from home.

- Arrange for other ways to get around when it is no longer safe for you to drive.

- Enroll in Alzheimer's Association Safe Return® for services to assist you should you ever wander.

Future Plans

When you are in the early stages of Alzheimer disease, it's important to take steps right away to plan for the future.

What you can do to plan for the future:

- Work with a well-qualified attorney, accountant, and a care manager to make financial and legal plans.

- Legally appoint a person you trust to make financial and health care decisions on your behalf when you cannot. Tell the person your wishes for the future, including where you want to live and what types of treatments you want or don't want.

- Find adult day care programs and residential care settings that know how to assist people with early-onset Alzheimer disease.

- Gather all of the thoughts, memories, and family history you want to pass on to your loved ones. Work together with your family to create journals, scrapbooks, or home movies.

10 Quick Tips: Living with Early-Onset Alzheimer Disease

1. Expect to have good days and bad days.

2. Find ways to express your feelings.

3. Discuss changes in relationships with a counselor.

4. Talk openly with loved ones about the changes the disease is causing.

5. Reach out to your friends.

6. Consider adapting your job hours or duties.

7. Get professional legal and financial help.

8. Keep up your health, and reduce stress.

9. Take steps to make your home safer.

10. Record your thoughts, memories, and family history.

Chapter 29

Nutrition for People with Alzheimer Disease

While no special diet is required for people with Alzheimer disease—unless they have another condition, such as diabetes, that requires diet monitoring—eating a well-balanced, nutritious diet is extremely beneficial. With the proper diet, your body will work more efficiently, you'll have more energy, and your medications will work properly. This article addresses the basics of good nutrition. Please consult your physician before making any dietary changes.

The Basics

- Eat a variety of foods from each food category.
- Maintain your weight through a proper balance of exercise and food.
- Choose foods low in saturated fat and cholesterol.
- Try to limit sugars.
- Moderate your use of salt.
- Drink eight 8 oz. glasses of water and or other fluids per day.
- You may drink alcoholic beverages in moderation (consult your physician).

"Nutrition for Alzheimer's Disease," © 2007 The Cleveland Clinic Foundation, 9500 Euclid Avenue, Cleveland, OH 44195, www.clevelandclinic.org. Additional information is available from the Cleveland Clinic Health Information Center, 216-444-3771, toll-free 800-223-2273 extension 43771, or at http://www.clevelandclinic.org/health.

Medications

- Ask your doctor about possible food interactions with the medicines you may be taking.

Preventing Constipation

- Eat foods high in fiber. Good sources of fiber are fruits, vegetables, and whole grains. Fiber and water help the colon pass stool. Most of the fiber in fruits is found in the skins. Fruits with seeds you can eat, like strawberries, have the most fiber.
- Eat bran cereal or add bran cereal to other foods, like soup and yogurt. Bran is a great source of fiber.
- Drink 8 cups of water and other fluids a day.
- Exercise.
- Move your bowels when you feel the urge.

Tips to Relieve Constipation

- Add fruits and vegetables to your diet.
- Eat prunes and/or bran cereal.
- If needed, use a very mild stool softener or laxative. Do not use mineral oil or any other laxatives for more than two weeks without calling your health care provider.

Dining Environment

- Minimize distractions in the area where you eat.
- Stay focused on the tasks of eating and drinking.
- Do not talk with food in your mouth.

Amount and Rate

- Eat slowly.
- Cut your food into small pieces and chew it thoroughly.
- Do not try to eat more than ½ teaspoon of your food at a time.

Thirst/Dry Mouth

Often thirst diminishes with age. In addition, some medicines may dehydrate the body.

- Drink 8 or more cups of liquid each day.

- Dunk or moisten breads, toast, cookies, or crackers in milk, hot chocolate, or coffee to soften them.

- Take a drink after each bite of food to moisten your mouth and to help you swallow.

- Add sauces to foods to make them softer and moister. Try gravy, broth, sauce, or melted butter.

- Eat sour candy or fruit ice to help increase saliva and moisten your mouth.

- Don't use a commercial mouthwash. Commercial mouthwashes often contain alcohol that can dry your mouth. Ask your doctor or dentist about alternative mouthwash products.

- Ask your doctor about artificial saliva products. These products are available by prescription.

Maintaining Your Weight

Malnutrition and weight maintenance is often an issue for those with Alzheimer disease.

- Eat smaller meals more frequently. Eating five to six times a day may be more easily tolerated than eating the same amount of food in three meals.

- Take a daily vitamin/mineral supplement.

- Liquid diet supplements may be helpful.

Chapter 30

Driving and Alzheimer Disease

For most people, driving represents freedom, control, and independence. Driving enables most people to get to the places they want to go, and to see the people they want to see when they want to see them. But driving is a complex skill. Our ability to drive safely can be compromised by changes in our physical, emotional, mental, and cognitive conditions.

The goal of this chapter is to help you, your family, and your health care professional talk about how Alzheimer disease will affect your ability to drive safely.

How can having Alzheimer disease affect my driving?

There are some early and clear warning signs that Alzheimer disease is affecting your driving. For example, you might:

- Need more help than you used to with directions, or with learning a new driving route;
- Have trouble remembering where you are going, or where you left your car;
- Get lost on routes that were once familiar;
- Have trouble making turns, especially left turns;
- Feel confused when exiting a highway, or by traffic signs such as a four-way stop;

"Driving and Alzheimer's Disease," Administration on Aging, April 2007.

- Receive citations for moving violations;
- Find other drivers often honk their horns at you;
- Stop at a green light, or brake inappropriately;
- Drift out of your lane;
- Have less control over your muscles so it may be harder to push down on the pedals or turn the steering wheel;
- Find dents and scrapes on your car that you can't explain;
- Find that others are questioning your driving safety; and
- Have a hard time controlling your anger, sadness, or other emotions that can affect your driving.

What if I am experiencing these warning signs?

If you are experiencing warning signs such as those listed above, you should see your physician. If warranted, you might be referred to a driver rehabilitation specialist immediately for an evaluation.

As the disease progresses, driving will become increasingly unsafe. Your doctor can help you decide when you should stop driving.

What can I do when Alzheimer disease affects my driving?

In many communities nationwide, a driver rehabilitation specialist can give you on- and off-road tests to assess your driving. The specialist also can help you determine how your driving ability is changing and help you decide when your driving is no longer safe.

Understanding how your ability to drive is changing over time is important to keep you and others around you safe. You can call hospitals and rehabilitation facilities to find an occupational therapist with special training in driving skills assessment and remediation. Depending on where you live, you may need to travel to nearby communities to find these services.

What can I do when I have to give up driving?

You can keep your independence even when you have to stop driving. It may take some planning ahead by you and your family and friends, but that planning will get you to the places you want to go, and to the people you want to see. It may also reduce the stress of driving. Consider:

- Rides with family and friends;

- Taxi cabs;

- Shuttle buses or vans;

- Public buses, trains, and subways; and

- Walking.

If possible, ask a relative or companion to accompany you when you use public transportation or walk. That way you can avoid confusion, and be sure to get where you want to go without the risk of getting lost. To address that risk, for a modest, one-time fee you can also enroll in the Alzheimer's Association Safe Return™ program by calling 888-572-8566.

Also, senior centers, religious organizations, and other local service groups often offer transportation services for older adults in your community.

Who can I call for help with transportation?

To find transportation services in your area, call the national Elder-Care Locator at 800-677-1116 and ask for your local Office on Aging. That office will help you find transportation services in your community. You may also find your local Office on Aging by visiting their website.

Contact your regional transit authority to find out which bus or train to take. Call Easter Seals Project ACTION (Accessible Community Transportation In Our Nation) at 800-659-6428 or go to its website.

Remember, no matter who is driving or what form of transportation you decide on, always wear your safety belt. Make sure that every person who is riding with you also is buckled up. Wear your safety belt even if your car has air bags.

Chapter 31

What Medications Are Used to Treat Alzheimer Disease?

Treatment

No treatment has been proven to stop Alzheimer disease (AD). However, for some people in the early and middle stages of the disease, the drugs tacrine (Cognex®), donepezil (Aricept®), rivastigmine (Exelon®), or galantamine (Razadyne®, formerly known as Reminyl®) may help prevent some symptoms from becoming worse for a limited time in some patients. (Tacrine is no longer actively marketed by the manufacturer.) Another drug, memantine (Namenda®), has been approved to treat moderate to severe AD, although it also is limited in its effects. And the U.S. Food and Drug Administration (FDA) recently approved the use of donepezil to treat moderate to severe AD.

Also, some medicines may help control behavioral symptoms of AD such as sleeplessness, agitation, wandering, anxiety, and depression. Treating these symptoms often makes patients more comfortable and makes their care easier for caregivers.

Alzheimer Disease Medications

Five prescription drugs currently are approved by the U.S. Food and Drug Administration to treat people who have been diagnosed with Alzheimer disease. Treating the symptoms of AD can provide

---

This chapter includes text from two documents produced by the National Institute on Aging (www.nia.nih.gov): "Treatment," and "Alzheimer's Disease Medications Fact Sheet," December 2006.

patients with comfort, dignity, and independence for a longer period of time and can encourage and assist their caregivers as well.

It is important to understand that none of these medications stops the disease itself.

Treatment for Mild to Moderate AD

Four of these medications are called cholinesterase inhibitors. These drugs are prescribed for the treatment of mild to moderate AD. They may help delay or prevent symptoms from becoming worse for a limited time and may help control some behavioral symptoms. The medications are: Razadyne® (formerly known as Reminyl®) (galantamine), Exelon® (rivastigmine), Aricept® (donepezil), and Cognex® (tacrine). Scientists do not yet fully understand how cholinesterase inhibitors work to treat AD, but current research indicates that they prevent the breakdown of acetylcholine, a brain chemical believed to be important for memory and thinking. As AD progresses, the brain produces less and less acetylcholine; therefore, cholinesterase inhibitors may eventually lose their effect.

No published study directly compares these drugs. Because all four work in a similar way, it is not expected that switching from one of these drugs to another will produce significantly different results. However, an AD patient may respond better to one drug than another. Cognex® (tacrine) is no longer actively marketed by the manufacturer.

Treatment for Moderate to Severe AD

The fifth approved medication, known as Namenda® (memantine), is an N-methyl D-aspartate (NMDA) antagonist. It is prescribed for the treatment of moderate to severe AD. Studies have shown that the main effect of Namenda® is to delay progression of some of the symptoms of moderate to severe AD. The medication may allow patients to maintain certain daily functions a little longer. For example, Namenda® may help a patient in the later stages of AD maintain his or her ability to go to the bathroom independently for several more months, a benefit for both patients and caregivers.

Namenda® is believed to work by regulating glutamate, another important brain chemical that, when produced in excessive amounts, may lead to brain cell death. Because NMDA antagonists work very differently from cholinesterase inhibitors, the two types of drugs can be prescribed in combination.

The FDA has also approved Aricept® for the treatment of moderate to severe AD.

Dosage and Side Effects

Doctors usually start patients at low drug doses and gradually increase the dosage based on how well a patient tolerates the drug. There is some evidence that certain patients may benefit from higher doses of the cholinesterase inhibitor medications. However, the higher the dose, the more likely are side effects. The recommended effective dosage of Namenda® is 20 mg/day after the patient has successfully tolerated lower doses. Some additional differences among these medications exist.

Patients may be drug sensitive in other ways, and they should be monitored when a drug is started. Report any unusual symptoms to the prescribing doctor right away. It is important to follow the doctor's instructions when taking any medication, including vitamins and herbal supplements. Also, let the doctor know before adding or changing any medications.

Summary: Medications to Treat Alzheimer Disease

The following brief summary provided does not include all information important for patient use and should not be used as a substitute for professional medical advice. Consult the prescribing doctor and read the package insert before using these or any other medications or supplements. Drugs are listed in order, as approved by the U.S. Food and Drug Administration, starting with the most recent.

Namenda® (memantine): Blocks the toxic effects associated with excess glutamate and regulates glutamate activation.

- *Drug type and treatment:* N-methyl D-aspartate (NMDA) antagonist prescribed to treat symptoms of moderate to severe AD

- *Manufacturer's recommended dosage:* 5 mg, once a day, available in tablet form; increase to 10 mg/day (5 mg twice a day), 15 mg/day (5 mg and 10 mg as separate doses), and 20 mg/day (10 mg twice a day) at minimum of one week intervals if well tolerated.

Razadyne® (formerly known as Reminyl®) (galantamine): Prevents the breakdown of acetylcholine and stimulates nicotinic receptors to release more acetylcholine in the brain.

- *Drug type and treatment:* Cholinesterase inhibitor prescribed to treat symptoms of mild to moderate AD

- *Manufacturer's Recommended Dosage:* 4 mg, twice a day (8 mg/day, available in tablet or capsule form; increase by 8 mg/day after 4 weeks to 8 mg, twice a day (16 mg/day) if well tolerated; after another 4 weeks, increase to 12 mg, twice a day (24 mg/day) if well tolerated.

Exelon® (rivastigmine): Prevents the breakdown of acetylcholine and butyrylcholine (a brain chemical similar to acetylcholine) in the brain.

- *Drug type and treatment:* Cholinesterase inhibitor prescribed to treat symptoms of mild to moderate AD

- *Manufacturer's recommended dosage:* 1.5 mg, twice a day (3 mg/day, available in capsule and liquid form; increase by 3 mg/day every 2 weeks to 6 mg, twice a day (12 mg/day) if well tolerated.

Aricept® (donepezil): Prevents the breakdown of acetylcholine in the brain.

- *Drug type and treatment:* Cholinesterase inhibitor prescribed to treat symptoms of mild to moderate, and moderate to severe AD

- M*anufacturer's recommended dosage:* 5 mg, once a day, available in tablet form; increase after 4–6 weeks to 10 mg, once a day if well tolerated.

Cognex® (tacrine): Prevents the breakdown of acetylcholine in the brain. Please note that Cognex is still available but no longer actively marketed by the manufacturer.

- *Drug type and treatment:* Cholinesterase inhibitor prescribed to treat symptoms of mild to moderate AD

- *Manufacturer's recommended dosage:* 10 mg, four times a day (40 mg/day), in capsule form; increase by 40 mg/day every 4 weeks to 40 mg, four times a day (160 mg/day), if liver enzyme functions remain normal and if well tolerated

Possible Medication Side Effects and Interactions

Namenda® (memantine): Blocks the toxic effects associated with excess glutamate and regulates glutamate activation.

- *Common side effects:* Dizziness, headache, constipation, confusion

- *Possible drug interaction:* Other NMDA antagonist medications, including amantadine, an antiviral used to treat the flu, dextromethorphan, prescribed to relieve coughs due to colds or flu, and ketamine, sometimes used as an anesthetic, have not been systematically evaluated and should be used with caution in combination with this medication.

Razadyne® (formerly known as Reminyl®) (galantamine): Prevents the breakdown of acetylcholine and stimulates nicotinic receptors to release more acetylcholine in the brain.

- *Common side effects:* Nausea, vomiting, diarrhea, weight loss

- *Possible drug interactions:* Some antidepressants such as paroxetine, amitriptyline, fluoxetine, fluvoxamine, and other drugs with anticholinergic action may cause retention of excess Razadyne® (formerly known as Reminyl®) in the body, leading to complications; NSAIDs should be used with caution in combination with this medication.*

Exelon® (rivastigmine): Prevents the breakdown of acetylcholine and butyrylcholine (a brain chemical similar to acetylcholine) in the brain.

- *Common side effects:* Nausea, vomiting, weight loss, upset stomach, muscle weakness

- *Possible drug interactions:* None observed in laboratory studies; NSAIDs should be used with caution in combination with this medication.*

Aricept® (donepezil): Prevents the breakdown of acetylcholine in the brain.

- *Common side effects:* Nausea, diarrhea, vomiting

- *Possible drug interactions:* None observed in laboratory studies; NSAIDs should be used with caution in combination with this medication.*

Cognex® (tacrine): Prevents the breakdown of acetylcholine in the brain. Please note that Cognex is still available but no longer actively marketed by the manufacturer.

- *Common side effects:* Nausea, diarrhea, possible liver damage

- *Possible drug interactions:* NSAIDs should be used with caution in combination with this medication.*

* Use of cholinesterase inhibitors can increase risk of stomach ulcers, and because prolonged use of non-steroidal anti-inflammatory drugs (NSAIDs) such as aspirin or ibuprofen can also cause stomach ulcers, NSAIDs should be used with caution in combination with these medications.

Potential New Treatments

The National Institute on Aging (NIA), part of the National Institutes of Health (NIH), is the lead federal agency for AD research. NIA-supported scientists are testing a number of drugs to see if they prevent AD, slow the disease, or help reduce symptoms. Some ideas that seem promising turn out to have little or no benefit when they are carefully studied in a clinical trial. Researchers undertake clinical trials to learn whether treatments that appear promising in observational and animal studies actually are safe and effective in people.

Mild cognitive impairment: During the past several years, scientists have focused on a type of memory change called mild cognitive impairment (MCI), which is different from both AD and normal age-related memory change. People with MCI have ongoing memory problems, but they do not have other losses such as confusion, attention problems, and difficulty with language. The NIA-funded Memory Impairment Study compared donepezil (Aricept), vitamin E, or placebo in participants with MCI to see whether the drugs might delay or prevent progression to AD. The study found that the group with MCI taking the drug donepezil were at reduced risk of progressing to AD for the first 18 months of a 3-year study when compared with their counterparts on placebo. The reduced risk of progressing from MCI to a diagnosis of AD among participants on donepezil disappeared after 18 months, and by the end of the study, the probability of progressing to AD was the same in the two groups. Vitamin E had no effect at any time point in the study when compared with placebo.

Neuroimaging: Scientists are finding that damage to parts of the brain involved in memory, such as the hippocampus, can sometimes be seen on brain scans before symptoms of the disease occur. An NIA public-private partnership—the AD Neuroimaging Initiative (ADNI)—is a large study that will determine whether magnetic resonance imaging (MRI) and positron emission tomography (PET) scans, or other imaging or biological markers, can see early AD changes or measure disease progression. The project is designed to help speed clinical trials and find new ways to determine the effectiveness of treatments.

AD genetics: The NIA is sponsoring the AD Genetics Study to learn more about risk factor genes for late onset AD. To participate in this study, families with two or more living siblings diagnosed with AD should contact the National Cell Repository for AD (NCRAD) toll-free at 800-526-2839. Information may also be requested through the study's website: http://ncrad.iu.edu.

Inflammation: There is evidence that inflammation in the brain may contribute to AD damage. Some studies have suggested that drugs such as nonsteroidal anti-inflammatory drugs (NSAIDs) might help slow the progression of AD, but clinical trials thus far have not demonstrated a benefit from these drugs. A clinical trial studying two of these drugs, rofecoxib (Vioxx) and naproxen (Aleve), showed that they did not delay the progression of AD in people who already have the disease. Another trial, testing whether the NSAIDs celecoxib (Celebrex) and naproxen could prevent AD in healthy older people at risk of the disease, has been suspended. However, investigators are continuing to follow the participants and are examining data regarding possible cardiovascular risk. Researchers are continuing to look for ways to test how other anti-inflammatory drugs might affect the development or progression of AD.

Antioxidants: Several years ago, a clinical trial showed that vitamin E slowed the progress of some consequences of AD by about seven months. Additional studies are investigating whether antioxidants—vitamins E and C—can slow AD. Another clinical trial is examining whether vitamin E and/or selenium supplements can prevent AD or cognitive decline, and additional studies on other antioxidants are ongoing or being planned.

Ginkgo biloba: Early studies suggested that extracts from the leaves of the ginkgo biloba tree may be of some help in treating AD symptoms. There is no evidence yet that ginkgo biloba will cure or prevent AD, but scientists now are trying to find out in a clinical trial whether ginkgo biloba can delay cognitive decline or prevent dementia in older people.

Estrogen: Some studies have suggested that estrogen used by women to treat the symptoms of menopause also protects the brain. Experts also wondered whether using estrogen could reduce the risk of AD or slow the disease. Clinical trials to test estrogen, however, have not shown that estrogen can slow the progression of already diagnosed AD. And one study found that women over the age of 65 who used estrogen with a progestin were at greater risk of dementia, including AD, and that older women using only estrogen could also increase their chance of developing dementia.

Scientists believe that more research is needed to find out if estrogen may play some role in AD. They would like to know whether starting estrogen therapy around the time of menopause, rather than at age 65 or older, will protect memory or prevent AD.

Chapter 32

Alternative Treatments and Therapies for Alzheimer Disease

Alternative Treatments

Several herbal remedies and other dietary supplements are promoted as effective treatments for Alzheimer disease and related diseases. Claims about the safety and effectiveness of these products, however, are based largely on testimonials, tradition, and a rather small body of scientific research. The rigorous scientific research required by the U.S. Food and Drug Administration for the approval of a prescription drug is not required by law for the marketing of dietary supplements.

Concerns about Alternative Therapies

Although many of these remedies may be valid candidates for treatments, there are legitimate concerns about using these drugs as an alternative or in addition to physician-prescribed therapy:

- Effectiveness and safety are unknown. The maker of a dietary supplement is not required to provide the U.S. Food and Drug Administration (FDA) with the evidence on which it bases its claims for safety and effectiveness.

This chapter includes "Alternative Treatments" and "Music, Art, and Other Therapies," reprinted with permission of the Alzheimer's Association. For additional information, call the Alzheimer's Association toll-free helpline, 800-272-2900, or visit their website at www.alz.org. © Alzheimer's Association. All rights reserved.

- Purity is unknown. The FDA has no authority over supplement production. It is a manufacturer's responsibility to develop and enforce its own guidelines for ensuring that its products are safe and contain the ingredients listed on the label in the specified amounts.

- Bad reactions are not routinely monitored. Manufacturers are not required to report to the FDA any problems that consumers experience after taking their products. The agency does provide voluntary reporting channels for manufacturers, health care professionals, and consumers, and will issue warnings about products when there is cause for concern.

- Dietary supplements can have serious interactions with prescribed medications. No supplement should be taken without first consulting a physician.

Coenzyme Q10

Coenzyme Q10, or ubiquinone, is an antioxidant that occurs naturally in the body and is needed for normal cell reactions to occur. This compound has not been studied for its effectiveness in treating Alzheimer disease.

A synthetic version of this compound, called idebenone, was tested for Alzheimer disease but did not show favorable results. Little is known about what dosage of coenzyme Q10 is considered safe, and there could be harmful effects if too much is taken.

Ginkgo Biloba

Ginkgo biloba is a plant extract containing several compounds that may have positive effects on cells within the brain and the body. Ginkgo biloba is thought to have both antioxidant and anti-inflammatory properties, to protect cell membranes, and to regulate neurotransmitter function. Ginkgo has been used for centuries in traditional Chinese medicine and currently is being used in Europe to alleviate cognitive symptoms associated with a number of neurological conditions.

In a study published in the *Journal of the American Medical Association* (October 22/29, 1997), Pierre L. Le Bars, MD, PhD, of the New York Institute for Medical Research, and his colleagues observed in some participants a modest improvement in cognition, activities of daily living (such as eating and dressing), and social behavior. The researchers found no measurable difference in overall impairment.

Results from this study show that ginkgo may help some individuals with Alzheimer disease, but further research is needed to determine the exact mechanisms by which Ginkgo works in the body. Also, results from this study are considered preliminary because of the low number of participants, about 200 people.

Few side effects are associated with the use of Ginkgo, but it is known to reduce the ability of blood to clot, potentially leading to more serious conditions, such as internal bleeding. This risk may increase if Ginkgo biloba is taken in combination with other blood-thinning drugs, such as aspirin and warfarin.

Currently, multicenter trial with about 3,000 participants is investigating whether Ginkgo may help prevent or delay the onset of Alzheimer disease or vascular dementia.

Huperzine A

Huperzine A is a moss extract that has been used in traditional Chinese medicine for centuries. Because it has properties similar to those of FDA-approved Alzheimer medications, it is promoted as a treatment for Alzheimer disease.

Evidence from small studies shows that the effectiveness of huperzine A may be comparable to that of the approved drugs. Large-scale trials are needed to better understand the effectiveness of this supplement.

In Spring 2004, the National Institute on Aging (NIA) launched the first U.S. clinical trial of huperzine A as a treatment for mild to moderate Alzheimer disease.

Because huperzine A is a dietary supplement, it is unregulated and manufactured with no uniform standards. If used in combination with FDA-approved Alzheimer drugs, an individual could increase the risks of serious side effects.

Omega-3 Fatty Acids

Omega-3s are a type of polyunsaturated fatty acid (PUFA). Research has linked certain types of omega-3s to a reduced risk of heart disease and stroke.

The U.S. Food and Drug Administration (FDA) permits supplements and foods to display labels with "a qualified health claim" for two omega-3s called docosahexaenoic acid (DHA) and eicosapentaenoic acid (EPA). The labels may state, "Supportive but not conclusive research shows that consumption of EPA and DHA omega-3 fatty acids may reduce the risk of coronary heart disease," and then list the amount of DHA or EPA in the product. The FDA recommends taking no more than a combined total of 3 grams of DHA or EPA a day, with no more than 2 grams from supplements.

Research has also linked high intake of omega-3s to a possible reduction in risk of dementia or cognitive decline. The chief omega-3 in the brain is DHA, which is found in the fatty membranes that surround nerve cells, especially at the microscopic junctions where cells connect to one another.

A January 25, 2006, literature review by the Cochrane Collaboration found that published research does not currently include any clinical trials large enough to recommend omega-3 supplements to prevent cognitive decline or dementia. But the reviewers found enough laboratory and epidemiological studies to conclude this should be a priority area for further research.

According to the review, results of at least two larger clinical trials are expected in 2008. The Cochrane Collaboration is an independent, nonprofit organization that makes objective assessments of available evidence on a variety of issues in treatment and health care.

Theories about why omega-3s might influence dementia risk include their benefit for the heart and blood vessels; anti-inflammatory effects; and support and protection of nerve cell membranes. There is also preliminary evidence that omega-3s may also be of some benefit in depression and bipolar disorder (manic depression).

A report in the April 2006 *Nature* described the first direct evidence for how omega-3s might have a helpful effect on nerve cells (neurons). Working with laboratory cell cultures, the researchers found that omega-3s stimulate growth of the branches that connect one cell to another. Rich branching creates a dense "neuron forest," which provides the basis of the brain's capacity to process, store and retrieve information.

In 2004 the U.S. Food and Drug Administration (FDA) announced an extension of the qualified health claim for omega-3s and coronary heart disease from supplements to foods. You can read a press release regarding this announcement outline at http://www.fda.gov/bbs/topics/news/2004/NEW01115.html.

Phosphatidylserine

Phosphatidylserine is a kind of lipid, or fat, that is the primary component of cell membranes of neurons. In Alzheimer disease and similar disorders, neurons degenerate for reasons that are not yet understood. The strategy behind the possible treatment with phosphatidylserine is to shore up the cell membrane and possibly protect cells from degenerating.

The first clinical trials with phosphatidylserine were conducted with a form derived from the brain cells of cows. Some of these trials had promising results. However, most trials were with small samples of participants.

This line of investigation came to an end in the 1990s over concerns about mad cow disease. There have been some animals studies since then to see whether phosphatidylserine derived from soy may be a potential treatment. A report was published in 2000 about a clinical trial with 18 participants with age-associated memory impairment who were treated with phosphatidylserine. The authors concluded that the results were encouraging but that there would need to be large carefully controlled trials to determine if this could be a viable treatment.

Coral Calcium

"Coral" calcium supplements have been heavily marketed as a cure for Alzheimer disease, cancer, and other serious illnesses. Coral calcium is a form of calcium carbonate claimed to be derived from the shells of formerly living organisms that once made up coral reefs.

In June 2003, the Federal Trade Commission (FTC) and the Food and Drug Administration (FDA) filed a formal complaint against the promoters and distributors of coral calcium. The agencies state that they are aware of no competent and reliable scientific evidence supporting the exaggerated health claims and that such unsupported claims are unlawful.

Coral calcium differs from ordinary calcium supplements only in that it contains traces of some additional minerals incorporated into the shells by the metabolic processes of the animals that formed them. It offers no extraordinary health benefits. Most experts recommend that individuals who need to take a calcium supplement for bone health take a purified preparation marketed by a reputable manufacturer.

You can read a copy of the FDA/FTC press release on the coral calcium complaint online at http://www.ftc.gov/opa/2003/06/trudeau.shtm.

Music, Art, and Other Therapies

Music, art, pet, and other types of therapies can help enrich the lives of people with Alzheimer disease. Pets, for instance, have been shown to reduce depression and boost self-esteem. Art provides an outlet for expression. Music stirs memories, emotions, and, when accompanied by singing, encourages group activity.

Music Therapy

- Identify music that's familiar and enjoyable to the listeners.

- Use live music, tapes or CDs; radio programs, interrupted by too many commercials, can cause confusion.

- Use music to create the mood you want.

- Link music with other reminiscence activities; use photographs to help stir memories.

- Encourage movement (clapping, dancing) to add to the enjoyment.

- Avoid sensory overload; eliminate competing noises by shutting windows and doors and by turning off the television.

Art Therapy

- Keep the project on an adult level. Avoid anything that might be demeaning or seem child-like.

- Build conversation into the project. Provide encouragement; discuss what the person is creating, and try to initiate a bit of creative storytelling or reminiscence.

- Help the person begin the activity. If the person is painting, you may need to start the brush movement. Most other projects should only require basic instruction and assistance.

- Use safe materials. Avoid toxic substances and sharp tools.

- Allow plenty of time to complete the art project.

- The person doesn't have to finish the project in one sitting.

- And remember: The artwork is complete when the person says it is.

Pet Therapy Guidelines

- Not everyone will react positively to animals. Those who owned pets previously tend to be more responsive.

- Match the animal's activity and energy level with that of the individual. For example, a lively dog might be appropriate for someone who can go out for a walk; a cat may be more appropriate for a person who is less mobile.

For more information about alternative therapies, contact your local Alzheimer's Association or refer to the resource list provided by the Alzheimer's Association's Green-Field Library [e-mail greenfield @alz.org for more information].

Chapter 33

Planning Guide for Long-Term Care

This chapter is designed to help you learn how to own your future by maintaining the lifestyle you have worked for all your life. It will get you started planning for your future needs.

Long-term care is a variety of services that help people with health or personal needs and activities of daily living over a period of time. The fact is, 60 percent of people over 65 will need some type of long-term care. Long-term care does not mean a complete loss of independence or control over your life. The keys to owning your future are planning early and wisely, knowing your options, and taking action. It is about living well.

Focus on Your Finances

Long-term care can be very expensive. Many Americans are surprised to learn that Medicare and most health insurance plans, including Medigap policies (Medicare supplemental insurance), do not cover long-term care. State Medicaid programs cover some long-term care services only for people who have a low income and few resources.

While costs for nursing home care vary widely, they average about $4,500 a month. This can cost approximately $50,000 to $60,000 a

---

"Own Your Future," Centers for Medicare and Medicaid Services, December 2002. Text under the heading "How to Compare Long-Term Care Insurance Policies," is from *A Shopper's Guide to Long Term Care Insurance*, © 2006 National Association of Insurance Commissioners. Reprinted with permission.

year. People who receive long-term care services at home spend an average of $1,500 a month.

You can plan to cover the cost of long-term care you may need in the future with long-term care insurance, savings plan annuities, certain life insurance policies, and reverse mortgages. The best way to pay for long-term care depends on your personal finances and family circumstances.

Putting a financial plan in place now can help to preserve both your savings and your peace of mind.

Steps You Can Take Now

• Think about how much of the cost of long-term care you could afford from your own resources.

• Talk with an independent financial planner for more information.

• Ask your current or former employer if you are eligible for group long-term care insurance, savings plan annuities, or similar long-term care benefits.

• Learn about long-term care insurance, trusts, annuities, reverse mortgages, or other options and whether they might be right for you.

Call your local Area Agency on Aging to find out about other programs that might help pay for long-term care. Look under "Aging" or "Human Services" in the local government blue pages of the phone book for the number. The Eldercare Locator (800-677-1116), a toll-free information line, can also give you this number.

If your income is low, you may qualify for Medicaid. Call your State Medical Assistance Office for more information about Medicaid eligibility and coverage. Look under "Medicaid" in the county government blue pages of the phone book for the number.

Understand Long-Term Care Insurance

Deciding to buy a long-term care insurance policy is an important decision. These policies can help pay for many types of long-term care, but they are not for everyone. Compare the costs and benefits of policies from different insurance companies when shopping. If you decide to buy, make sure you buy from a reliable company that is licensed by your state to sell long-term care insurance.

What does it cover?

Long-term care insurance policies may cover nursing home stays, community services such as adult day care, in-home care, or a combination of these services. Some policies may cover costs for an assisted living facility. You can choose the type of coverage that is appropriate for you.

You can also choose how much coverage you want from the long-term care policy. Policies pay for a maximum amount of costs for each day of care. You can also decide how long you will want the coverage. For example, your policy may cover $50 of in-home nursing care per day for a period of three years. To help you determine the daily benefit amount that is right for you, find out the costs of long-term care in your local area.

A policy covering three to five years is the most cost-effective option for most people. However, if you are concerned about care for Alzheimer disease or other types of dementia, you may want to consider more comprehensive coverage.

How does it work?

Generally, you can start receiving benefits from a long-term care policy when a licensed health practitioner declares that you are eligible. You may qualify for benefits if you need long-term assistance with activities of daily living, such as bathing, dressing, toileting, eating, and moving in and out of a bed or chair. A cognitive impairment, such as Alzheimer disease, may also qualify you. Once it is determined that you are eligible for benefits, there is generally a waiting period before the policy begins paying for your care. You may have to pay for the services received during this waiting period.

Is it right for me?

Generally, financial planners recommend considering long-term care insurance if you own assets of at least $75,000 (this does not include your home or car); have annual retirement income of at least $25,000 to $35,000 for an individual or $35,000 to $50,000 for a couple; or are able to pay premiums without financial difficulty, even if premiums increase over time.

Long-term care insurance is probably not for you if these factors do not apply to you. Long-term care insurance can be expensive, depending on your age and health status when you buy the policy and how much coverage you want. Policy costs also vary according to the benefits you choose. It is better to buy long-term care insurance at a younger age when premiums are lower. As an example, in 2002, America's Health Insurance Plans (AHIP) states that a comprehensive policy with a $150 daily benefit, four years of coverage, and 5% compounded inflation protection costs about $1,134 per year when purchased for a 50-year-old. The same policy costs about $2,346 per year for a 65-year-old and $7,572 per year for a 79-year-old.

Where do I shop?

Compare the costs and benefits of policies from different insurance companies when shopping. If you decide to buy, make sure you buy from a reliable company that is licensed by your state to sell long-term care insurance. You may also be able to purchase a long-term care insurance policy through your employer.

What else should I consider?

- Is there a waiting period? Some companies require you to receive care for a certain period before the policy will begin to cover the services. Find out if there is more than one waiting period in your lifetime.

- Does the policy include a nonforfeiture benefit? If you stop paying premiums, this option can either provide you with limited benefits or return some of the premium amount that you already paid.

- Does the policy have inflation protection? This feature automatically increases your benefits by a small percentage each year so that your policy will continue to be able to cover costs as service prices increase. If you buy a policy before age 75, you may need this protection.

- Is the policy "tax-qualified" or "non-tax-qualified?" Be sure to ask if you are eligible for long-term care insurance tax incentives.

- Does the policy have a benefit that your spouse can use if you die first?

- Can you choose your own care manager?

Steps You Can Take Now

- Consider long-term care policies from at least three different companies that are licensed in your state.

- Read the outline of coverage for each policy that must come with the application or enrollment form.

Contact your State Health Insurance Assistance Program (SHIP) for free one-on-one counseling and assistance regarding long-term care insurance.

Contact your State Insurance Department to find out where to buy long-term care insurance in your area.

Establish Clear Legal Directions

Putting your legal affairs in order will give you peace of mind and make sure your wishes are followed.

Think about what you want while you have the time to think through the options clearly. You should put your wishes in writing, just in case you cannot speak for yourself or lose the ability to make decisions for yourself.

Steps You Can Take Now

- Review all legal documents that are more than five years old to make sure they still express your wishes and meet your needs. These papers should be kept in one convenient place.

- Make sure you have a living will, and a durable power-of-attorney for health care or health care proxy.

- Find a lawyer in your area who can help you. Ask about the fees for a consultation and preparation of the documents that you need.

- If you live in a community with a law school, find out if there is a free legal clinic for seniors or contact your local community legal aid.

Visit www.aoa.gov. Select "Area Agencies on Aging."

Call your local Area Agency on Aging to find out if your state has any legal services to help you. Look under "Aging" or "Human Services" in the local government blue pages of the phone book for the number. The Eldercare Locator (800-677-1116), a toll-free information line, can also give you this number.

Decide Who You Can Count on for Help

The first step in planning ahead is to pick someone who can help you make decisions about long-term care planning. Talk to them before you need services. Family members and friends can sometimes help you with personal activities. Other people prefer to hire caregivers or get help from volunteers or agencies. One of the advantages of getting help from your family for long-term care needs is that it may lower the cost.

Steps You Can Take Now

- Talk to your family members about long-term care. Share your concerns and preferences, where you may want to live and any medical history which may be important in making decisions.

- Think about sharing your home with someone or a group of people in the future.

Contact the American Health Care Association for more information on how to talk with your family and friends about long-term care at 800-628-8140 or www.ahca.org.

Learn What Your Community Has to Offer

There are many local organizations with services and programs that can help with personal activities. They can help you plan for long-term care by explaining their different services and programs. For example, most communities have adult daycare, senior centers, meal programs and help with shopping and transportation. Others offer tips on how to stay healthy as you age or where to go for support. Some of these services are free. Other community services are available for a cost.

Steps You Can Take Now

- Learn about community services, programs, and whether they are available at no or low cost. Explore resources in your local community to find out what is available for you.

- Contact your faith community to find out if they can help with future long-term care needs, such as transportation or in-home services.

- Check with your doctor, local social service agency or hospital to help you locate different kinds of long-term care services available to meet your needs now and in the future.

Call your local AARP (formerly known as American Association of Retired Persons) for tips on how to stay healthy as you age. Check under "Associations" in the yellow pages of the phone book for the number.

Call your local Area Agency on Aging to get information on all the community services available for older people where you live. Look under "Aging" or "Human Services" in the local government blue pages of the phone book for the number.

Make Sure Your Home Remains a Good Fit

Most people would prefer to stay in their own homes for as long as possible. However, homes that are easy to live in at age 50 can present problems later in life.

Some improvements can be inexpensive, like removing scatter rugs, making sure that smoke detectors are in working order, or replacing doorknobs. Bigger changes may include adding railings to outside steps, replacing floor coverings with slip-resistant carpet, or adding a bathroom to the ground floor of your home. Most home modifications will actually increase the value of your home.

Steps You Can Take Now

- Start thinking about small changes to your home to keep it safe in the years ahead.

Visit www.aarp.org to get a home modification checklist.

For help in locating a local contractor trained in counseling seniors about home modification, call the National Association of Home Builders at 800-368-5242.

Call your local Area Agency on Aging to ask about subsidized senior housing and home repair in your area. Look under "Aging" or "Human Services" in the local government blue pages of the phone book for the number.

Contact the U.S. Department of Housing & Urban Development (HUD) for local contacts who can tell you about the FHA 203K program for home repairs for low income families at 888-466-3487 or www.hud.gov.

If you live in a rural area, call the local office of the U.S. Department of Agriculture about their Farmer's Home Administration loans to low income borrowers for home improvements. The telephone number is in the government blue pages of the phone book.

How to Compare Long-Term Care Insurance Policies

Text under this heading is from *A Shopper's Guide to Long Term Care Insurance,* © 2006 National Association of Insurance Commissioners. Reprinted with permission.

Answer the questions below so that you can compare long-term care insurance policies. Most of the information you need is in the outline of coverage provided in the policies you are comparing. Even so, you will need to calculate some information and talk to the agent or a company representative to get the rest.

Insurance Company Information

1. Name of the insurance company's agent.

2. Is the company licensed in your state?

3. Insurance rating service and rating.

What levels of care are covered by this policy?

4. Does the policy provide benefits for these levels of care?

    - Skilled nursing care?

    - Personal / Custodial Care? (In many states, both levels of care are required)

5. Does the policy pay for any nursing home stay, no matter what level of care you receive?

    - If not, what levels aren't covered?

Where can you receive care covered under the policy?

6. Does the policy pay for care in any licensed facility?

    - If not, what doesn't it pay for?

7. Does the policy provide home care benefits for:

    - skilled nursing care?

    - personal care given by home health aides?

    - homemaker services?

    - other _____?

8. Does the policy pay for care received in:

   - adult day care centers?

   - assisted living facilities?

   - other settings?

How long are benefits paid and what amounts are covered?

You may be considering a policy that pays benefits on a different basis, so you may have to do some calculations to determine comparable amounts.

9. How much will the policy pay per day for:

   - nursing home care?

   - assisted living facility care?

   - home care?

10. Are there limits on the number of days or visits per year for which benefits will be paid? If yes, what are the limits for:

    - nursing home care?

    - assisted living facility care?

    - home care? (days or visits?)

11. What is the length of the benefit period that you are considering?

12. Are there limits on the amounts the policy will pay during your lifetime? If yes, what are the limits for:

    - nursing home care?

    - assisted living facility care?

    - home care? (days or visits?)

    - total lifetime limit

How does the policy decide when you are eligible for benefits?

13. Which of the "benefit triggers" does the policy use to decide your eligibility for benefits? (It may have more than one)

    - unable to do activities of daily living (ADLs)

- cognitive impairment (older policies may discriminate against Alzheimer disease; newer ones don't)
- doctor certification of medical necessity
- prior hospital stay
- bathing is one of the ADLs

When do benefits start?

14. How long is the waiting period before benefits begin for:
    - nursing home care?
    - assisted living care?
    - home health care?
    - waiting period: service days or calendar days?

15. Are the waiting periods for home care cumulative or consecutive?

16. How long will it be before you are covered for a pre-existing condition? (Usually 6 months)

17. How long will the company look back on your medical history to determine a pre-existing condition? (Usually 6 months)

Does the policy have inflation protection?

18. Are the benefits adjusted for inflation?

19. Are you allowed to buy more coverage? If yes,
    - When can you buy more coverage?
    - How much can you buy?
    - When can you no longer buy more coverage?

20. Do the benefits increase automatically? If yes,
    - What is the rate of increase?
    - Is it a simple or compound increase?
    - When do automatic increases stop?

21. If you buy inflation coverage, what daily benefit would you receive for nursing home care:
    - 5 years from now?
    - 10 years from now?

Assisted living facility care:

- 5 years from now?
- 10 years from now?

Home health care:

- 5 years from now?
- 10 years from now?

22. If you buy inflation coverage, what will your premium be:

- 5 years from now?
- 10 years from now?
- 15 years from now?

What other benefits are covered under the policy?

23. Is there a waiver of premium benefit? If yes,

- How long do you have to be in a nursing home before it begins?
- Does the waiver apply when you receive home care?

24. Does the policy have a nonforfeiture benefit? If yes, what kind?

25. Does the policy have a return of premium benefit?

26. Does the policy have a death benefit? If yes, are there any restrictions before the benefit is paid?

27. Will the policy cover one person or two?

Tax-qualified status

28. Is the policy tax-qualified?

What does the policy cost?

29. What is the premium excluding all riders?

- monthly
- yearly

30. What is the premium if home care is covered?

- monthly
- yearly

31. What is the premium if assisted living is covered?
    - monthly
    - yearly

32. What is the premium if you include an inflation rider?
    - monthly
    - yearly

33. What is the premium if you include a nonforfeiture benefit?
    - monthly
    - yearly

34. Is there any discount if you and your spouse both buy policies?
    - If yes, what is the amount of the discount?
    - Do you lose the discount when one spouse dies?

35. What is the total annual premium including all riders and discounts?
    - total monthly premium
    - total annual premium

36. When looking at the results of Questions 29 through 35, how much do you think you are willing to pay in premiums?

Finding Phone Numbers for Your Local State Health Insurance Programs

You can find the most up-to-date phone numbers by looking at www.medicare.gov on the internet. Or call 866-PLANLTC (866-752-6582). TTY users should call 877-486-2048.

Chapter 34

Legal Issues in Planning for Incapacity

When a family member has been diagnosed with Alzheimer disease or another disabling health condition, it's easy to feel overwhelmed by the many legal and financial questions that can arise as a result of the diagnosis. Determining how to pay for long-term care is often confusing for families. It is important to find an attorney with whom you feel comfortable and who has the expertise to advise you on these matters.

What legal matters should be discussed when a family member has a health condition that affects his ability to function independently?

There are several legal issues to consider when a person is (or may become) incapacitated:

- The management of the person's financial affairs during his or her lifetime

- The management of the person's personal care: medical decisions, residence, placement in a nursing facility, etc.

- Arranging for payment of long-term health care: use of private insurance, Medicare, Medicaid (Medi-Cal in California), and Supplemental Security Income (SSI) when applicable

---

- Preserving the family assets: ensuring that the patient's spouse and any disabled family members are adequately protected

- The distribution of the person's assets on his or her death (If the person has a disabled spouse, child, or other family member that they wish to provide for, special arrangements need to be made.)

In addition to issues that are clearly "legal," other important issues should be discussed in the course of legal planning. For example, a full discussion of housing options is critical in making certain legal and financial decisions; that is, is the person planning to stay in his home? Is this feasible, both physically and financially? Is he thinking of moving to a retirement facility? What level of care is provided? Is it a rental or a "buy-in" arrangement? Is a move to a nursing home probable?

When should an attorney be consulted?

Consult an attorney as early as possible. The maximum number of planning options will be available while the patient still has the legal capacity to make his or her own decisions. The question of capacity is a gray area, and must be determined on a case-by-case basis.

What are the options for managing assets?

Options for managing assets include:

- Durable Powers of Attorney;
- Revocable living trusts;
- Designation of a representative payee; and
- Conservatorship (or Guardianship) of the estate and of the person.

Each of these has advantages and disadvantages, which should be discussed thoroughly with an attorney. Further, for making medical decisions, you should discuss the use of a durable power of attorney for health care, directive to physicians, and conservatorship (or guardianship) of the person.

What are the options for paying for long-term care?

Investigate first the availability of private insurance to cover long-term care, whether at home or at an assisted living or skilled nursing facility. Also, examine the government benefit programs that may help pay for care:

- Medicare
- Medicaid or Medi-Cal
- Supplemental Security Income (SSI)
- In-Home Supportive Services (IHSS)

If the person served in the United States Military, federal, or state veteran assistance may be available.

Can any assets be protected—for a well spouse, for example—if a patient needs long-term custodial care in a skilled nursing facility?

Various planning options may be available to finance long-term care. Much depends on the individual's circumstances; that is, marital status, mental capacity, age and health of the care recipient, and, most importantly, the applicable law in the state where the individual resides. Medicaid, a federal program administered by the states, may pay for care in a facility. The rules regarding planning vary from state to state. Planning options can include:

- Converting non-exempt assets into exempt assets;
- Transfer of the family residence to a spouse;
- Transfer of the principal residence with the retention of a life estate;
- Use of court orders to increase the amount of resources and/or income the spouse of a nursing home resident can retain;
- Trusts;
- Gifting of assets.

Each of these options has significant implications and should be thoroughly discussed with an attorney knowledgeable in Medicaid law.

How can an individual provide for the distribution of his or her property upon death?

The options for distributing assets on death include:

- Will;
- Revocable Living Trust;
- Joint Tenancy Accounts;

299

- Payable on Death Accounts;
- Transfer with a Retained Life Estate.

Each of these has significant legal ramifications and should be discussed with a knowledgeable advisor. Also, some financial products, such as life insurance, IRAs, and annuities, provide for the distribution on death to a designated beneficiary.

How do you find an attorney to assist with legal planning?

One of the best ways to find an attorney specializing in elder law is through a personal recommendation from a friend, relative, or co-worker, or from another attorney whom you know and trust. Another way to get a personal recommendation is to attend a caregiver support group. Someone there may already have had experience with a knowledgeable attorney and be able to share his or her experience. Referrals, and advice for individuals aged 60 or over also may be obtained from senior legal services provided by your local Area Agency on Aging. Independent community legal aid agencies also may offer assistance to people of all ages.

Another way to locate an attorney is through an attorney referral service. The local bar association in your community may have a panel which refers callers to lawyers in various specializations. After describing your needs, you will be referred to the most appropriate specialist. Initial consultations generally include a nominal fee.

Caution should be exercised if such a referral service is used. Panel-referred attorneys need meet only minimum requirements and may have little experience. It is important to check the qualifications of an attorney and to make calls to compare fees and experience. Keep in mind that laws vary from state to state. The National Academy of Elder Law Attorneys may also be able to help you.

What kind of attorney should be consulted?

Most attorneys concentrate on one or two areas of law. It is especially important for caregivers to find an attorney who has the appropriate expertise. Attorneys advising caregivers on planning for long-term care should have knowledge of the following areas of law:

- Medicaid (Medi-Cal) laws and regulations
- Social Security
- Trusts (special needs trusts)

- Conservatorships
- Durable power of attorney for health care and asset management
- Tax (income, estate and gift) planning
- Housing and health care contracts

Some attorneys are certified specialists. For example, an attorney can be a certified specialist in elder law, taxation, or estate planning. In the case of an accident, a personal injury attorney is needed. In that case, it is advisable to select someone who has had jury trial experience.

Attorneys often do not know about all of the above-mentioned areas. In the case of a personal injury, two attorneys may be needed—one to litigate an accident settlement and another to help plan for long-term financial or health care needs.

What should you do to prepare for a legal consultation?

It's helpful to have a clear idea of what you would like as the outcome of a legal consultation—that is, what you would like to gain from the appointment. Learning as much as possible ahead of time will help ensure a productive consultation.

More specifically, individuals who are interested in a health care directive may wish to think about the type of life-sustaining procedures they would want used in the case of a serious illness. In addition, it may be helpful to identify a first, second, and third choice of family member or trusted friend to make personal health care and financial decisions in the event you are unable to do this for yourself.

Items to Bring to the Consultation

- List of major assets (real estate, stocks, cash, jewelry, insurance, etc.)
- Any documents of title (for example, copies of deeds, stock certificates, loan papers, etc.) which show who the asset owners are and how title is held
- Contracts or other legally binding documents
- Lists of all major debts
- Existing wills or Durable Powers of Attorney
- Bank statements, passbooks, CDs—again showing who the owners are and how title is held

Glossary

Advance Health Care Directive: An Advance Health Care Directive is a document in which you can: 1) instruct your physician as to the kinds of medical treatment you might want or not want in the future (in many states, this is called a Living Will); and 2) choose someone to make medical decisions for you in the event you are unable to make those decisions yourself (in many states, this is called a Durable Power of Attorney for Health Care, or just a Power of Attorney for Health Care).

Attorney-in-Fact: The person named in a Durable Power of Attorney to act as an agent. This person need not be an attorney.

Beneficiary: An individual who receives the benefit of a transaction, for example, a beneficiary of a life insurance policy, a beneficiary of a trust, beneficiary under a will.

Conservatee or Ward: The incapacitated person for whom a conservatorship or guardianship has been established.

Conservator or Guardian: An individual who is appointed by the court to act on behalf of an incapacitated person.

Conservatorship or Guardianship: A court proceeding in which the court supervises the management of an incapacitated person's affairs or personal care.

Directive to Physicians: A written document in which an individual states his or her desire to have life-sustaining procedures withheld or withdrawn under certain circumstances. This document must meet certain requirements under the law to be valid.

Durable Power of Attorney for Health Care: A type of Advance Health Care Directive, this is a document in which an individual nominates a person as his or her agent to make health care decisions for him or her if he or she is not able to give medical consent. This document can give the agent the power to withdraw or continue life-sustaining procedures.

Durable Power of Attorney for Asset Management: A document in which an individual (the "principal") nominates a person as his or her agent (attorney-in-fact) to conduct financial transactions on his or her behalf. This document can be either "springing," which means that it is effective only upon the principal's incapacity, or "fixed," which means that the document becomes effective when it is signed.

Executor: The individual named in a will who is responsible for administering an estate during probate. The Executor is the person responsible for making sure all taxes and other expenses are paid and distributing the property of the deceased person in accordance with the will.

Federal Estate Taxes: A tax is due at death if the estate exceeds $1,500,000 (as of 2004), and is calculated on the value of the deceased person's estate at the time of death.

Health Insurance Portability and Accountability Act of 1996 (aka HIPAA): Federal legislation which limits the informal communication of information from doctors and other health care providers.

In-Home Supportive Services (IHSS): A program in California that pays for non-medical services for persons who meet certain financial criteria and who could not remain safely at home without such services.

Irrevocable Trust: A trust that has terms and provisions which cannot be changed.

Joint Tenancy: A form of property ownership by two or more persons designated as "joint tenants." When a joint tenant dies, his or her interest in the property automatically passes to the surviving joint tenant and is not controlled by the will of the deceased joint tenant and is not subject to probate.

Life Estate: An interest in property that lasts for the life of the person retaining the life estate. When a person who has a life estate interest dies, the property passes to the person holding the remainder interest, without the need for probate.

Living Will: A written document in which an individual conveys his or her desire to die a natural death and not be kept alive by artificial means. Unlike a Durable Power of Attorney for Health Care, the wishes in this document are not legally enforceable in California.

Long-Term Care Insurance: Private insurance which, depending on the terms of the policy, can pay for home care, or care in an assisted living facility or skilled nursing facility.

Medicaid: A state and federally financed program that provides medical care to low income persons. In California it's called Medi-Cal.

Medicare: A federal medical coverage program for persons who are over 65 years old or who are disabled. It is funded by Social Security deductions and has no income or resource restrictions. It does not pay for long-term custodial care.

Probate: The court proceeding which oversees the administration of a deceased person's estate. Wills are subject to probate; living trusts (if properly funded) are not.

Revocable Living Trust: A device that describes certain property, names a trustee (who manages the property), and names a beneficiary who receives benefit from the trust. A living trust is an effective means of avoiding probate and providing for management of assets. It can be revoked by the person who created it during that person's lifetime.

Social Security Retirement Benefits: Benefits, which eligible workers and their families receive when the worker retires. The worker must work for a specified period at a job that is covered by Social Security in order to be eligible for benefits. A worker must be at least 62 years old to receive retirement benefits.

Social Security Disability Benefits: Social Security benefits payable to disabled workers and their families.

Special Needs Trust: A specially drafted trust that provides a fund to supplement the governmental benefits of a beneficiary while not affecting that beneficiary's eligibility for public benefits.

Supplemental Security Income (SSI): A federal program which provides cash assistance to the aged, blind, and disabled who have limited income and resources.

Testator: The person who executes a will.

Trustor (Settlor): A person who creates a trust.

Trustee: The individual who is responsible for managing the property in the trust for the benefit of the beneficiary.

Will: The document a person signs which tells how he or she wants his or her estate administered and distributed upon death. It must conform to certain legal requirements in order to be valid. The terms of a will become operational only upon the testator's death.

Resources

Family Caregiver Alliance
180 Montgomery Street
Suite 1100
San Francisco, CA 94104
Toll-Free: 800-445-8106
Phone: 415-434-3388
Fax: 415-434-3508
Website: http://www.caregiver.org
E-mail: info @caregiver.org

Family Caregiver Alliance (FCA) seeks to improve the quality of life for caregivers through education, services, research, and advocacy.

FCA's National Center on Caregiving offers information on current social, public policy, and caregiving issues and provides assistance in the development of public and private programs for caregivers.

For residents of the greater San Francisco Bay Area, FCA provides direct family support services for caregivers of those with Alzheimer disease, stroke, ALS, head injury, Parkinson's disease, and other debilitating health conditions that strike adults.

American Bar Association (ABA)
Commission on Legal Problems of the Elderly
740 Fifteenth Street, NW
Washington, DC 20005-1022
Phone: 202-662-8690
Fax: 202-662-8698
Website: www.abanet.org/elderly

The general public may contact the ABA to obtain information on county bar associations. County bar associations provide attorney referrals through local attorney referral offices throughout the U.S.

National Academy of Elder Law Attorneys
1604 N. Country Club Rd.
Tucson, AZ 85716
Phone: 520-881-4005
Website: www.naela.com

Provides information on how to choose an elder law attorney and referrals to elder law attorneys.

National Association of Area Agencies on Aging
1730 Rhode Island Ave., NW, Suite 1200
Washington, DC 20036
Phone: 202-872-0888
Website: www.n4a.org

Provides information on local Area Agencies on Aging which coordinate a variety of community-based services for senior citizens, including legal services.

National Senior Citizens Law Center
1101 14th Street, NW, Suite 400
Washington, DC 20005
Phone: 202-289-6976
Fax: 202-289-7224
Website: http://www.nsclc.org
E-mail: nsclc@nsclc.org

NSCLC closely monitors court rulings, legislation, and regulatory changes which affect older persons. They also publish a weekly newsletter.

Part Four

Caregiver Concerns

Chapter 35

Alzheimer Disease: A Guide for Caregivers

Tips for Caregivers

Caring for a person with Alzheimer disease (AD) at home is a difficult task and can become overwhelming at times. Each day brings new challenges as the caregiver copes with changing levels of ability and new patterns of behavior. Research has shown that caregivers themselves often are at increased risk for depression and illness, especially if they do not receive adequate support from family, friends, and the community.

One of the biggest struggles caregivers face is dealing with the difficult behaviors of the person they are caring for. Dressing, bathing, eating—basic activities of daily living—often become difficult to manage for both the person with AD and the caregiver. Having a plan for getting through the day can help caregivers cope. Many caregivers have found it helpful to use strategies for dealing with difficult behaviors and stressful situations. Through trial and error you will find that some of the following tips work, while others do not. Each person with AD is unique and will respond differently, and each person changes over the course of the disease. Do the best you can, and remind yourself to take breaks.

"Caregiver Guide," National Institute on Aging (http://www.nia.nih.gov), March 2007. You can download a copy of this guide online at http://www.nia.nih .gov/Alzheimers/Publications/caregiverguide.htm, or you can order a copy from the Alzheimer's Disease Education and Referral (ADEAR) Center; call toll-free at 800-438-4380.

Dealing with the Diagnosis

Finding out that a loved one has Alzheimer disease can be stressful, frightening, and overwhelming. As you begin to take stock of the situation, here are some tips that may help:

- Ask the doctor any questions you have about AD. Find out what treatments might work best to alleviate symptoms or address behavior problems.

- Contact organizations such as the Alzheimer's Association and the Alzheimer's Disease Education and Referral (ADEAR) Center for more information about the disease, treatment options, and caregiving resources. Some community groups may offer classes to teach caregiving, problem-solving, and management skills.

- Find a support group where you can share your feelings and concerns. Members of support groups often have helpful ideas or know of useful resources based on their own experiences. Online support groups make it possible for caregivers to receive support without having to leave home.

- Study your day to see if you can develop a routine that makes things go more smoothly. If there are times of day when the person with AD is less confused or more cooperative, plan your routine to make the most of those moments. Keep in mind that the way the person functions may change from day to day, so try to be flexible and adapt your routine as needed.

- Consider using adult day care or respite services to ease the day-to-day demands of caregiving. These services allow you to have a break while knowing that the person with AD is being well cared for.

- Begin to plan for the future. This may include getting financial and legal documents in order, investigating long-term care options, and determining what services are covered by health insurance and Medicare.

Communication

Trying to communicate with a person who has AD can be a challenge. Both understanding and being understood may be difficult.

- Choose simple words and short sentences and use a gentle, calm tone of voice.

- Avoid talking to the person with AD like a baby or talking about the person as if he or she weren't there.

- Minimize distractions and noise—such as the television or radio—to help the person focus on what you are saying.

- Call the person by name, making sure you have his or her attention before speaking.

- Allow enough time for a response. Be careful not to interrupt.

- If the person with AD is struggling to find a word or communicate a thought, gently try to provide the word he or she is looking for.

- Try to frame questions and instructions in a positive way.

Bathing

While some people with AD don't mind bathing, for others it is a frightening, confusing experience. Advance planning can help make bath time better for both of you.

- Plan the bath or shower for the time of day when the person is most calm and agreeable. Be consistent. Try to develop a routine.

- Respect the fact that bathing is scary and uncomfortable for some people with AD. Be gentle and respectful. Be patient and calm.

- Tell the person what you are going to do, step by step, and allow him or her to do as much as possible.

- Prepare in advance. Make sure you have everything you need ready and in the bathroom before beginning. Draw the bath ahead of time.

- Be sensitive to the temperature. Warm up the room beforehand if necessary and keep extra towels and a robe nearby. Test the water temperature before beginning the bath or shower.

- Minimize safety risks by using a handheld showerhead, shower bench, grab bars, and nonskid bath mats. Never leave the person alone in the bath or shower.

- Try a sponge bath. Bathing may not be necessary every day. A sponge bath can be effective between showers or baths.

Dressing

For someone who has AD, getting dressed presents a series of challenges: choosing what to wear, getting some clothes off and other clothes on, and struggling with buttons and zippers. Minimizing the challenges may make a difference.

- Try to have the person get dressed at the same time each day so he or she will come to expect it as part of the daily routine.

- Encourage the person to dress himself or herself to whatever degree possible. Plan to allow extra time so there is no pressure or rush.

- Allow the person to choose from a limited selection of outfits. If he or she has a favorite outfit, consider buying several identical sets.

- Arrange the clothes in the order they are to be put on to help the person move through the process.

- Provide clear, step-by-step instructions if the person needs prompting.

- Choose clothing that is comfortable, easy to get on and off, and easy to care for. Elastic waists and Velcro enclosures minimize struggles with buttons and zippers.

Eating

Eating can be a challenge. Some people with AD want to eat all the time, while others have to be encouraged to maintain a good diet.

- View mealtimes as opportunities for social interaction and success for the person with AD. Try to be patient and avoid rushing, and be sensitive to confusion and anxiety.

- Aim for a quiet, calm, reassuring mealtime atmosphere by limiting noise and other distractions.

- Maintain familiar mealtime routines, but adapt to the person's changing needs.

- Give the person food choices, but limit the number of choices. Try to offer appealing foods that have familiar flavors, varied textures, and different colors.

- Serve small portions or several small meals throughout the day. Make healthy snacks, finger foods, and shakes available. In the earlier stages of dementia, be aware of the possibility of overeating.

- Choose dishes and eating tools that promote independence. If the person has trouble using utensils, use a bowl instead of a plate, or offer utensils with large or built-up handles. Use straws or cups with lids to make drinking easier.

- Encourage the person to drink plenty of fluids throughout the day to avoid dehydration.

- As the disease progresses, be aware of the increased risk of choking because of chewing and swallowing problems.

- Maintain routine dental checkups and daily oral health care to keep the mouth and teeth healthy.

Activities

What to do all day? Finding activities that the person with AD can do and is interested in can be a challenge. Building on current skills generally works better than trying to teach something new.

- Don't expect too much. Simple activities often are best, especially when they use current abilities.

- Help the person get started on an activity. Break the activity down into small steps and praise the person for each step he or she completes.

- Watch for signs of agitation or frustration with an activity. Gently help or distract the person to something else.

- Incorporate activities the person seems to enjoy into your daily routine and try to do them at a similar time each day.

- Try to include the person with AD in the entire activity process. For instance, at mealtimes, encourage the person to help prepare the food, set the table, pull out the chairs, or put away the dishes. This can help maintain functional skills, enhance feelings of personal control, and make good use of time.

- Take advantage of adult day services, which provide various activities for the person with AD, as well as an opportunity for caregivers to gain temporary relief from tasks associated with caregiving. Transportation and meals often are provided.

Exercise

Incorporating exercise into the daily routine has benefits for both the person with AD and the caregiver. Not only can it improve health, but it also can provide a meaningful activity for both of you to share.

313

- Think about what kind of physical activities you both enjoy, perhaps walking, swimming, tennis, dancing, or gardening. Determine the time of day and place where this type of activity would work best.

- Be realistic in your expectations. Build slowly, perhaps just starting with a short walk around the yard, for example, before progressing to a walk around the block.

- Be aware of any discomfort or signs of overexertion. Talk to the person's doctor if this happens.

- Allow as much independence as possible, even if it means a less-than-perfect garden or a scoreless tennis match.

- See what kinds of exercise programs are available in your area. Senior centers may have group programs for people who enjoy exercising with others. Local malls often have walking clubs and provide a place to exercise when the weather is bad.

- Encourage physical activities. Spend time outside when the weather permits. Exercise often helps everyone sleep better.

Incontinence

As the disease progresses, many people with AD begin to experience incontinence, or the inability to control their bladder or bowels. Incontinence can be upsetting to the person and difficult for the caregiver. Sometimes incontinence is due to physical illness, so be sure to discuss it with the person's doctor.

- Have a routine for taking the person to the bathroom and stick to it as closely as possible. For example, take the person to the bathroom every 3 hours or so during the day. Don't wait for the person to ask.

- Watch for signs that the person may have to go to the bathroom, such as restlessness or pulling at clothes. Respond quickly.

- Be understanding when accidents occur. Stay calm and reassure the person if he or she is upset. Try to keep track of when accidents happen to help plan ways to avoid them.

- To help prevent nighttime accidents, limit certain types of fluids—such as those with caffeine—in the evening.

- If you are going to be out with the person, plan ahead. Know where restrooms are located, and have the person wear simple, easy-to-remove clothing. Take an extra set of clothing along in case of an accident.

Sleep Problems

For the exhausted caregiver, sleep can't come too soon. For many people with AD, however, the approach of nighttime may be a difficult time. Many people with AD become restless, agitated, and irritable around dinnertime, often referred to as "sundowning" syndrome. Getting the person to go to bed and stay there may require some advance planning.

- Encourage exercise during the day and limit daytime napping, but make sure that the person gets adequate rest during the day because fatigue can increase the likelihood of late afternoon restlessness.

- Try to schedule more physically demanding activities earlier in the day. For example, bathing could be earlier in the morning, or large family meals could be at midday.

- Set a quiet, peaceful tone in the evening to encourage sleep. Keep the lights dim, eliminate loud noises, even play soothing music if the person seems to enjoy it.

- Try to keep bedtime at a similar time each evening. Developing a bedtime routine may help.

- Restrict access to caffeine late in the day.

- Use night lights in the bedroom, hall, and bathroom if the darkness is frightening or disorienting.

Hallucinations and Delusions

As the disease progresses, a person with AD may experience hallucinations or delusions. Hallucinations are when the person sees, hears, smells, tastes, or feels something that is not there. Delusions are false beliefs from which the person cannot be dissuaded.

- Sometimes hallucinations and delusions are a sign of a physical illness. Keep track of what the person is experiencing and discuss it with the doctor.

315

- Avoid arguing with the person about what he or she sees or hears. Try to respond to the feelings he or she is expressing, and provide reassurance and comfort.

- Try to distract the person to another topic or activity. Sometimes moving to another room or going outside for a walk may help.

- Turn off the television set when violent or disturbing programs are on. The person with AD may not be able to distinguish television programming from reality.

- Make sure the person is safe and does not have access to anything he or she could use to harm anyone.

Wandering

Keeping the person safe is one of the most important aspects of caregiving. Some people with AD have a tendency to wander away from their home or their caregiver. Knowing what to do to limit wandering can protect a person from becoming lost.

- Make sure that the person carries some kind of identification or wears a medical bracelet. Consider enrolling the person in the Alzheimer's Association Safe Return program if the program is available in your area. If the person gets lost and is unable to communicate adequately, identification will alert others to the person's medical condition. Notify neighbors and local authorities in advance that the person has a tendency to wander.

- Keep a recent photograph or videotape of the person with AD to assist police if the person becomes lost.

- Keep doors locked. Consider a keyed deadbolt or an additional lock up high or down low on the door. If the person can open a lock because it is familiar, a new latch or lock may help.

- Be sure to secure or put away anything that could cause danger, both inside and outside the house.

Home Safety

Caregivers of people with AD often have to look at their homes through new eyes to identify and correct safety risks. Creating a safe environment can prevent many stressful and dangerous situations.

- Install secure locks on all outside windows and doors, especially if the person is prone to wandering. Remove the locks on bathroom doors to prevent the person from accidentally locking himself or herself in.

- Use childproof latches on kitchen cabinets and anyplace where cleaning supplies or other chemicals are kept.

- Label medications and keep them locked up. Also make sure knives, lighters and matches, and guns are secured and out of reach.

- Keep the house free from clutter. Remove scatter rugs and anything else that might contribute to a fall. Make sure lighting is good both inside and out.

- Be alert to and address kitchen-safety issues, such as the person forgetting to turn off the stove after cooking. Consider installing an automatic shut-off switch on the stove to prevent burns or fire.

Driving

Making the decision that a person with AD is no longer safe to drive is difficult, and it needs to be communicated carefully and sensitively. Even though the person may be upset by the loss of independence, safety must be the priority.

- Look for clues that safe driving is no longer possible, including getting lost in familiar places, driving too fast or too slow, disregarding traffic signs, or getting angry or confused.

- Be sensitive to the person's feelings about losing the ability to drive, but be firm in your request that he or she no longer do so. Be consistent—don't allow the person to drive on "good days" but forbid it on "bad days."

- Ask the doctor to help. The person may view the doctor as an "authority" and be willing to stop driving. The doctor also can contact the Department of Motor Vehicles and request that the person be reevaluated.

- If necessary, take the car keys. If just having keys is important to the person, substitute a different set of keys.

- If all else fails, disable the car or move it to a location where the person cannot see it or gain access to it.

Visiting the Doctor

It is important that the person with AD receive regular medical care. Advance planning can help the trip to the doctor's office go more smoothly.

- Try to schedule the appointment for the person's best time of day. Also, ask the office staff what time of day the office is least crowded.

- Let the office staff know in advance that this person is confused. If there is something they might be able to do to make the visit go more smoothly, ask.

- Don't tell the person about the appointment until the day of the visit or even shortly before it is time to go. Be positive and matter-of-fact.

- Bring along something for the person to eat and drink and any activity that he or she may enjoy.

- Have a friend or another family member go with you on the trip, so that one of you can be with the person while the other speaks with the doctor.

Coping with Holidays

Holidays are bittersweet for many AD caregivers. The happy memories of the past contrast with the difficulties of the present, and extra demands on time and energy can seem overwhelming. Finding a balance between rest and activity can help.

- Keep or adapt family traditions that are important to you. Include the person with AD as much as possible.

- Recognize that things will be different, and have realistic expectations about what you can do.

- Encourage friends and family to visit. Limit the number of visitors at one time, and try to schedule visits during the time of day when the person is at his or her best.

- Avoid crowds, changes in routine, and strange surroundings that may cause confusion or agitation.

- Do your best to enjoy yourself. Try to find time for the holiday things you like to do, even if it means asking a friend or family member to spend time with the person while you are out.

- At larger gatherings such as weddings or family reunions, try to have a space available where the person can rest, be by themselves, or spend some time with a smaller number of people, if needed.

Visiting a Person with AD

Visitors are important to people with AD. They may not always remember who the visitors are, but just the human connection has value. Here are some ideas to share with someone who is planning to visit a person with AD.

- Plan the visit at the time of the day when the person is at his or her best. Consider bringing along some kind of activity, such as something familiar to read or photo albums to look at, but be prepared to skip it if necessary.

- Be calm and quiet. Avoid using a loud tone of voice or talking to the person as if he or she were a child. Respect the person's personal space and don't get too close.

- Try to establish eye contact and call the person by name to get his or her attention. Remind the person who you are if he or she doesn't seem to recognize you.

- If the person is confused, don't argue. Respond to the feelings you hear being communicated, and distract the person to a different topic if necessary.

- If the person doesn't recognize you, is unkind, or responds angrily, remember not to take it personally. He or she is reacting out of confusion.

Choosing a Nursing Home

For many caregivers, there comes a point when they are no longer able to take care of their loved one at home. Choosing a residential care facility—a nursing home or an assisted living facility—is a big decision, and it can be hard to know where to start.

- It's helpful to gather information about services and options before the need actually arises. This gives you time to explore fully all the possibilities before making a decision.

- Determine what facilities are in your area. Doctors, friends and relatives, hospital social workers, and religious organizations may be able to help you identify specific facilities.

- Make a list of questions you would like to ask the staff. Think about what is important to you, such as activity programs, transportation, or special units for people with AD.

- Contact the places that interest you and make an appointment to visit. Talk to the administration, nursing staff, and residents.

- Observe the way the facility runs and how residents are treated. You may want to drop by again unannounced to see if your impressions are the same.

- Find out what kinds of programs and services are offered for people with AD and their families. Ask about staff training in dementia care, and check to see what the policy is about family participation in planning patient care.

- Check on room availability, cost and method of payment, and participation in Medicare or Medicaid. You may want to place your name on a waiting list even if you are not ready to make an immediate decision about long-term care.

- Once you have made a decision, be sure you understand the terms of the contract and financial agreement. You may want to have a lawyer review the documents with you before signing.

- Moving is a big change for both the person with AD and the caregiver. A social worker may be able to help you plan for and adjust to the move. It is important to have support during this difficult transition.

Chapter 36

Answers for Long-Distance Caregivers

What is long-distance caregiving?

Long-distance caregiving takes many forms—from helping manage the money to arranging for in-home care; from providing respite care for a primary caregiver to helping a parent move to a new home or facility. Many long-distance caregivers act as information coordinators, helping aging parents understand the confusing maze of home health aides, insurance benefits, and durable medical equipment.

Caregiving is often a long-term task. What may start out as an occasional social phone call to share family news can eventually turn into regular phone calls about managing health insurance claims, getting medical information, and arranging for respite services. What begins as a monthly trip to check on Mom may turn into a larger project to move her to a nursing facility close to your home.

If you are a long-distance caregiver, you are not alone. Approximately 7 million adults are long-distance caregivers, mostly caring for aging parents who live an hour or more away. Historically, caregivers have been primarily mid-life, working women who have other family responsibilities. That's changing. More and more men are becoming caregivers; in fact, men now represent over 40 percent of caregivers. Clearly, anyone, anywhere can be a long-distance caregiver.

Excerpted from "So Far Away: Twenty Questions for Long-Distance Caregivers," National Institute on Aging (http://www.nia.nih.gov), NIH Pub. No. 06-5496, January 2006.

Gender, income, age, social status, employment—none of these prevent you from taking on caregiving responsibilities.

How will I know if help is needed?

In some cases, the sudden start of a severe illness will make it clear that help is needed. In other cases, your relative may ask for help. When you live far away, you have to think carefully about possible signs that support or help is needed. You might want to use holiday trips home to take stock.

Some questions to answer during your visit include:

- Are the stairs manageable or is a ramp needed?

- Are there any tripping hazards at exterior entrances or inside the house (throw rugs, for instance)?

- If a walker or wheelchair is needed, can the house be modified?

- Is there food in the fridge? Are there staple foods in the cupboards?

- Are bills being paid? Is mail piling up?

- Is the house clean?

- If your parents are still driving, can you assess their road skills?

- How is their health? Are they taking several medications? If so, are they able to manage their medications?

- What about mood: Does either parent seem depressed or anxious?

What can I really do from far away?

Many long-distance caregivers provide emotional support and occasional respite to a primary caregiver who is in the home. Long-distance caregivers can play a part in arranging for professional caregivers, hiring home health and nursing aides, or locating assisted living and nursing home care. Some long-distance caregivers help a parent pay for care, while others step in to manage finances.

Caregiving is not easy for anyone, not for the caregiver and not for the care recipient. From a distance, it may be especially hard to feel that what you are doing is enough, or that what you are doing is important. It usually is.

Some Good Ideas

- Know what you need to know. Experienced caregivers recommend that you learn as much as you can about your parent's illness and treatment. Information can help you understand what is going on, anticipate the course of an illness, prevent crises, and assist in disease management. It can also make talking with the doctor easier. Learn as much as you can about the resources available. Make sure at least one family member has written permission to receive medical and financial information. Try putting together a notebook, or something similar, that includes all the vital information about health care, social services, contact numbers, financial issues, and so on. Make copies for other caregivers.

- Plan your visits. When visiting your parent, you may feel that there is just too much to do in the time that you have. You can get more done and feel less stressed by talking to your parent ahead of time and finding out what he or she would like to do. This may help you set clear-cut and realistic goals for the visit. For instance, does your mother need to go to the mall or to visit another family member? Could your father use help fixing things around the house? Would you like to talk to your mother's physician? Decide on the priorities and leave other tasks to another visit.

- Remember to actually spend time visiting with your family member. Try to make time to do things unrelated to being a caregiver. Maybe you could rent a movie to watch with your parents, or visit with old friends or other family members. Perhaps your aunt or uncle would like to attend worship services. Offer to play a game of cards or a board game. Take a drive, or go to the library together. Finding a little bit of time to do something simple and relaxing can help everyone.

- Get in touch and stay in touch. Many families schedule conference calls with doctors, the assisted living facility team, or nursing home staff to get up-to-date information about a parent's health and progress. If your parent is in a nursing home, you can request occasional teleconferences with the facility's staff. Some families schedule conference calls so several relatives can participate in one conversation. Sometimes a social worker is good to talk to for updates as well as for help in making decisions. The human touch is important too. Try to find people in your parent's community who can be your eyes and ears and provide a realistic view of what is going on. In some cases, this will be your other parent.

- Help your parent stay in contact. For one family, having a private phone line installed in their father's nursing home room allowed him to stay in touch. For another family, giving the grandmother a cell phone (and then teaching her to use it) gave everyone some peace of mind. You can program telephone numbers (such as doctors', neighbors', and your own) into your parent's phone so that he or she can speed-dial contacts. Such simple strategies can be a lifeline for you and your parent. But be prepared—you may find you are inundated with calls from your parent. It's good to think in advance about a workable approach for coping with numerous calls.

- Get a phone book, either hardcopy or online, that lists resources in your parent's neighborhood. Having a copy of the phone book for your parent's city or town can be really helpful. The "Blue Pages" can provide an easy guide to State and local services available in your parent's hometown.

How can my family decide who does what?

Be sure to talk with other family members and decide who will be responsible for which tasks. Think about your schedules and how to adapt them to give respite to a primary caregiver or to coordinate holiday and vacation times. One family found that it worked to have the long-distance caregiver come to town while the primary caregiver was on a family vacation. And remember, if you aren't the primary caregiver, offering appreciation, reassurance, and positive feedback is also a contribution.

Are there things I can do that will help me feel less frustrated?

Feeling frustrated and angry with everyone, from your parent to his or her doctors, is a common caregiving experience. It can be hard to acknowledge that you feel this way, but try not to criticize yourself even more. Caregiving, especially from a distance, is likely to bring out a full range of human emotions, both positive and negative. If you feel angry, it could be a sign that you are overwhelmed or that you are trying to do too much. If you can, give yourself a break: Take a walk, talk with your friends, get some sleep, join a support group—try to do something for yourself.

Consider joining a caregiver support group, either in your own community or online. Meeting other caregivers can relieve your sense of isolation and will give you a chance to exchange stories and ideas. By focusing on what you can do, you may be able to free yourself from some of the worry and focus on being supportive and loving.

What is a geriatric care manager and how can I find one?

Professional care managers are usually licensed nursing or social work professionals who specialize in geriatrics. Some families hire a geriatric care manager to evaluate and assess a parent's needs and to coordinate care through community resources. The cost of an initial evaluation varies and may be expensive, but geriatric care managers can offer a useful service. They are a sort of "professional relative" to help you and your family to identify needs and how to meet them. These professionals can also be helpful in leading family discussions about sensitive subjects.

When interviewing a geriatric care manager, you might want to ask:

- Are you a licensed geriatric care manager?
- Are you a member of the National Association of Professional Geriatric Care Managers?
- How long have you been providing care management services?
- Are you available for emergencies?
- Does your company also provide home care services?
- How will you communicate information to me?
- What are your fees? Will you provide them in writing prior to starting services?
- Can you provide references?

The National Association of Professional Geriatric Care Managers can help you find a care manager near your family member's community. You can also call or write the Eldercare Locator for recommendations. In some cases, local chapters of the Alzheimer's Association may be able to recommend geriatric care managers who have assisted other families.

How can I keep up with my parents' medical care?

Health care experts recommend that you start by learning as much as you can about your parent's illness, current treatments, and its likely course. This information will be essential as you help your parent and the primary caregiver cope with day-to-day concerns, make decisions, and plan for the future.

When you visit your parent, consider going along on a doctor's appointment (check that your parent does not mind having you there). Some long-distance caregivers say that making a separate appointment with a doctor allows them to seek more detailed information and answers to questions. These appointments must be paid for out-of-pocket.

You must have permission to have any conversation with your parent's doctor. Ask your parent to complete a release form that allows the doctor to discuss his or her health care with you. Be sure the release is up-to-date and that there's a copy in your parent's records in addition to keeping a back-up copy for your files.

How can I make the most of a visit with my parent's doctor? I don't want to waste the doctor's time.

If you go with your parent to see the doctor, here are a few tips that will help you be an ally and advocate:

- Bring a prioritized list of questions and take notes on what the doctor recommends. Both can be helpful later, either to give information to the primary caregiver, or to remind your parent what the doctor said.

- Before the appointment, ask your parent, the primary caregiver, and your siblings if they have any questions or concerns they would like you to bring up.

- Bring a list of ALL medications your parent is taking, both prescription and over-the-counter, and include dosage and schedule (if your parent sees several different doctors one may not necessarily know what another has prescribed).

- When the doctor asks a question, do not answer for your parent unless you have been asked to do so. Always talk to the doctor and to your parent.

- Respect your parent's privacy, and leave the room when necessary.

- Ask the doctor if she or he can recommend community resources that might be helpful.

- Larger medical practices and hospitals may have a social worker on staff. Ask to speak with the social worker. She or he may have valuable information about community resources.

How on earth can my parents afford everything they need?

You are not alone in worrying about how much everything costs. Health care expenses can be crushing, even for middle-class families who thought they had saved enough. Your parents may be eligible for some health care benefits. People on fixed incomes who have limited resources may qualify for Medicaid, a program of the Centers for Medicare and Medicaid Services (CMS), a Federal agency. CMS covers the costs of health care for people of all ages who meet income requirements and who are disabled. Because the guidelines change often, you should check with CMS regularly.

Medicare offers insurance for prescription drugs. For information about this coverage, visit www.medicare.gov or call 800-MEDICARE (800-633-4227).

The State Health Insurance Assistance Program (SHIP) is a national program offering one-on-one counseling and assistance to people and their families on Medicare. SHIP provides free counseling and assistance to Medicare beneficiaries on a wide range of Medicare, Medicaid, and Medigap matters. To find your State program, visit www.shipusa.org.

If prescription medications cost too much, talk to the doctor about the possibility of prescribing a less expensive medication. The Partnership for Prescription Assistance can provide a list of patient assistance programs supported by pharmaceutical companies.

What kinds of documents do we need? It sounds like caregiving requires a lot of paperwork.

Effective caregiving depends on keeping a great deal of information in order and up-to-date. Often, long-distance caregivers will need to have information about a parent's personal, health, financial, and legal records. If you have ever tried to gather and organize your own personal information, you know what a chore it can be. Gathering and organizing this information from far away can seem even more challenging. Maintaining up-to-date information about your parent's health and medical care, as well as finances, home ownership, and other legal issues, lets you get a handle on what is going on and allows you to respond quickly if there is a crisis.

If you do not see your parent often, one visit may not be enough time for you to get all the paperwork organized. Instead, try to focus on gathering the essentials first; you can fill in the blanks as you go along. You might begin by talking to your parent and his or her primary caregiver about the kinds of records that need to be pulled together. If a primary caregiver is already on the scene, chances are that some of the information has already been assembled. Talk about any missing information or documentation and how you might help to organize the records.

Your parents may be reluctant to share personal information with you. Explain that you are not trying to invade their privacy or take over their personal lives—you are only trying to assemble what they (and you) will need in the event of an emergency. Assure them that you will respect their privacy and keep your promise. If your parents are still uncomfortable, ask if they would be willing to work with an attorney (some lawyers specialize in elder affairs) or perhaps with another trusted family member or friend.

Should I encourage my parents to get more help?

If you do not see your parent often, changes in his or her health may seem dramatic. In contrast, the primary caregiver might not notice such changes, or realize that more help, medical treatment, or supervision is needed. Sometimes a geriatric care manager or other professional is the first to notice changes. For families dealing with Alzheimer disease and other dementias, it can be easier to "cover" for the patient—doing things for him or her, filling in information in conversations, and so on—than to acknowledge what is happening.

A few good conversation starters are:

- If you thought there might be a change in Aunt Joan's condition, whose opinion would you seek?

- I didn't notice Dad repeating himself so much the last time I was here. Do you remember when it started?

Some changes may not be what you think. Occasional forgetfulness does not necessarily indicate Alzheimer disease. Before you raise the issue of what needs to be done, talk to your parent and the primary caregiver about your concerns. Try not to sound critical when you raise the subject. Instead, mention your particular worry, for example, "Mom, it looks like you don't have much food in the house—are you having trouble getting to the store?" and explain why you are concerned. Listen to what the primary caregiver says about the situation, and whether he or she feels there are problems.

Discuss what you think needs to be done: "Do we need to get a second opinion about the diagnosis? Can you follow the medication schedule? Would you like some help with housework?" Try to follow up your suggestions with practical help, and give specific examples of what you can do. For example, you might arrange to have a personal or home health aide come in once a week. You might schedule doctors' appointments or arrange for transportation.

In some cases you may have to be forceful, especially if you feel that the situation is unhealthy or unsafe. Do not leave a frail adult at risk. If you have to act against the wishes of your parent or the primary caregiver, be direct and explain what you are going to do. Discuss your plan and say why you are taking action.

How can we make the house safer for my parent who has Alzheimer disease?

You can take many precautions that will make the house safer, more accessible, and comfortable. Because you are not present, you may want to evaluate the safety of your parent's home during one of your visits (with the understanding that you must quickly correct any real dangers). On future visits, you should be alert for hazards and aware of things you can do to make the house safer.

If you are worried about your parent's safety, don't wait until the next visit. If you feel that your parent is unsafe alone, make note of which behaviors have become most worrisome and discuss these with the primary caregiver and the doctor. Behavior that is unsafe or unhealthy may have become familiar to the primary caregiver. The kitchen in particular presents many opportunities for accidents, especially when a parent misuses appliances or forgets that something is cooking. Discuss your concerns and offer to help adapt the environment to meet your parent's changing safety needs.

Consider these principles about home safety for older people:

Think prevention: It is hard to predict or anticipate every problem, but you can go through the house room-by-room and evaluate safety problems. Checking the safety of your parent's home may prevent a hazardous situation. Some easy steps to take:

- Remind the primary caregiver to lock all doors and windows on the inside and outside to prevent wandering.

- Make sure all potentially harmful items, such as medications, weapons, machinery, or electrical cords are put away in a safe, preferably locked, place when they're not in use.

- Use child-resistant caps on medicine bottles and childproof door latches on storage units as well.

Adapt the environment: Because it is easier to change a place than to change a person, consider the following:

- Install at least one stairway handrail that extends beyond the first and last steps.

- Place carpet or safety grip strips on stairs.

- Avoid clutter, which can cause disorientation and confusion.

- Keep all walk areas free of furniture, and extension and electrical cords.

- Cover unused outlets with childproof plugs.

- Make sure all rooms have adequate lighting.

How can I help my folks decide if it's time for them to move?

The decision about whether your parents should move is often tricky and emotional. Each family will have its own reasons for wanting (or not wanting) to take such a step. One family may decide a move is right because the parents no longer need so much space or cannot manage the home. For another family the need for hands-on care in a long-term care facility motivates a change. In some cases, a move frees up cash so that the parent can afford a more suitable situation.

In the case of long-distance caregivers, the notion of moving can seem like a solution to the problem of not being close enough to help. For some caregivers, moving a sick or aging parent to their own home or community can be a viable alternative. In some cases, an adult child moves back to the parent's home to become the primary caregiver. Keep in mind that leaving a home, community, and familiar medical care can be very disruptive and difficult.

Older adults and their families have some choices when it comes to deciding where to live, but these choices can be limited by factors such as illness, financial resources, and personal preferences. Making a decision that is best for your parent—and making that decision with your parent—can be difficult. Try to learn as much as you can about possible housing options.

Older adults, or those with serious illness, can:

- stay in their own home, or move to a smaller one,

- move to an assisted living facility or retirement community,

- move to a long-term care facility, or

- move in with another family member.

Experts advise families to think carefully before moving an aging adult into an adult child's home. The Family Caregiver Alliance suggests considering the following issues before deciding whether or not to move your parent to your home:

- Evaluate whether your parent needs constant supervision or assistance throughout the day, and consider how this will be provided.

- Identify which activities of daily living (eating, bathing, toileting) your parent can perform independently.

- Determine your comfort level for providing personal care such as bathing or changing an adult diaper.

- Take an honest look at your health and physical abilities, and decide if you are able to provide care for your parent.

- Expect changes in your parent's medical or cognitive condition.

- Explore the availability of services such as a friendly visitor, in-home care, or adult day services.

- Investigate back-up options if living with your parent does not work or is not your choice.

- Consider the type of medical care your parent needs and find out if appropriate doctors and services are available in your community.

What happens if my parents ask me to promise that I won't "put" them in a nursing home?

This request usually reflects what most of us want: to stay in our own homes, to maintain independence, to turn to family and friends for help. Sometimes, however, parents really do want their adult children to make a promise. Think carefully before doing so. According to the Centers for Medicare and Medicaid Services, "Quality of care means doing the right thing, at the right time, in the right way, for the right person, and having the best possible results." Agreeing that you will not "put someone" in a nursing home may close the door to the right care option for your family. It requires you to know that no matter what happens you will be able to care for your parent. The fact is that for some illnesses, and for some people, professional health care in a long-term care facility is the only reasonable choice.

When faced with a parent who is truly ill or frail, long-distance caregivers may find that some promises hamper their ability to do what is necessary, either for their own health, or for their parent's. Many people discover too late that the promises they made ("Of course you will be able to die at home.") cannot be kept.

Try to focus your commitments on what you know here and now. If asked to make a promise, you could say something like, "Dad, I will make sure you have the best care we can arrange. You can count on me to try and do what's best for everyone. I can't think of a situation where I'd walk out on you." Base your promises and decisions on a realistic assessment of the current situation or diagnosis, and realize that you may need to revisit your agreement. Your father's situation might change. Your situation might change. You truly do not know what will happen in the future—disease and illness can lead to enormous changes. And, of course, it's not only your parent's health that changes—your own health may alter over time, too.

If you've already made a promise to a parent, remember you can bring the subject up again; you can change your answer to something more specific, something you feel you can undertake. As hard as that conversation might be, it may be better than risking the guilt of a promise not kept.

How is it that long-distance caregiving makes me feel so guilty all the time?

You might think that being far away gives you some immunity from feeling overwhelmed by what is happening to your parent—but long-distance caregivers report that this is not so. Although you may not feel as physically exhausted and drained as the primary, hands-on caregiver, you may still feel worried and anxious. Many long-distance caregivers describe feeling terribly guilty about not being there, about not being able to do enough or spend enough time with the parent. Remind yourself that you are doing the best you can given the circumstances, and you can only do what you can do.

If you are like most long-distance caregivers, you already have many people who rely on you: Your spouse, children, perhaps even grandchildren, as well as friends, coworkers, and colleagues. Adding one more "to-do" to your list may seem impossible.

You may find some consolation or comfort in knowing that you are not alone. Many people find that support groups are a great resource and a way to learn caregiving tips and techniques that work—even from a distance. Others find the camaraderie and companionship helpful. Some enjoy meeting monthly or weekly, while others find what they need in online support groups. The Eldercare Locator may be able to help you find a local group.

How can I be sure that my parent's caregiver isn't mistreating him?

From a distance, it can be hard to assess the quality of your parent's caregivers. Ideally, if there is a primary caregiver on the scene, he or she can keep tabs on how things are going. Sometimes a geriatric care manager can help. You can stay in touch by phone and take note of any concerns that might indicate neglect or mistreatment. These can happen in any setting, at any socioeconomic level. They can take many forms, including domestic violence, emotional abuse, financial abuse, and basic neglect.

The stress that may happen when adult children care for their aging parents can take a toll on everyone. In some families, abuse continues a long-standing family pattern. In others, the older adult's need for constant care can cause a caregiver to lash out verbally or physically. In some cases, especially in the mid-to-late stages of Alzheimer disease, the older adult may become physically aggressive and difficult to manage. This might cause a caregiver to respond angrily. But no matter what the cause or who is the perpetrator, abuse and neglect are never acceptable responses.

If you feel that your parent is in physical danger, contact the authorities right away. If you suspect abuse, but do not feel there is an immediate risk, contact someone who can act on your behalf: your parent's doctor, for instance, or your contact at a home health agency. Suspected abuse must be reported to adult protective services.

How can I help my parents think about their future health care preferences?

Making advance care plans is a key step for your parent to take to be sure that his or her health care preferences are known. Health care providers can only respect those wishes that have been made known and are documented in the medical record. Advance care planning can help your family avoid some of the conflicts that can occur when family members disagree over treatment decisions.

It may be easier to make certain decisions after discussing them with family, clergy members, or health care providers. Decisions about forgoing treatment, for instance, or ending life support, involve complex emotional issues and are hard for many people to make alone. Try to make peace with yourself and your family, whatever the decision. When thinking about the future consider:

- Naming a surrogate decision maker (a surrogate has the authority to make decisions on behalf of someone who is too ill to do so),

- Stating which treatment results are desirable and which ones are unacceptable,

- Discussing what to do in an emergency,

- Noting preferences regarding any possible treatments, and whether or not a time-limited trial would be acceptable (for instance, five days on a ventilator to recover some strength; a week with a feeding tube, and so on),

- Talking to the doctor and surrogate about preferences and including written instructions in the medical record.

Advance care planning is an ongoing process. As an illness progresses and circumstances change, your parent may want to revisit his or her preferences. If so, be sure to update all written instructions and share the changes with health care providers and anyone who assists with care.

Try to approach decision-making tasks by recognizing that you are working with a parent, not for a parent (unless you are healthcare proxy or agent, in which case, you will be implementing a family member's decisions). How will you know when the advance care plans are complete and that you have covered all the bases? A complete plan will:

- Be very specific and detailed and cover what is to be done in a variety of medical situations,

- Name a healthcare proxy,

- Be recorded in the medical record,

- Be readily available to any caregiver in the home, nursing home, or hospital.

What if I'm told my parent only has a few months to live?

The news that a family member is dying is difficult to bear—and yet, it is a basic part of life. When you hear that a parent has a terminal illness, you may be flooded with emotions: Sorrow, disbelief, anger, anxiety. It can be hard to know what to do or what to say. Fortunately, many organizations are working to improve the lives of dying people and their families. Try to locate a hospice program. Hospice provides special care for people who are near the end of life. Check with Medicare for information on hospice benefits.

Talk to your own friends, clergy, or colleagues. Just about everyone has experienced the serious illness and death of a beloved friend or family member. Exchanging stories can help you as you cope with your own loss and with trying to decide what you can do.

Contact your parent's doctor and talk to your own doctor as well to find out what will need to be done, the kinds of care that your mother or father is likely to need, and how you can arrange for it to happen.

Some people find that it is very hard to talk about death and dying, and will go to great lengths to avoid the subject. Difficult as it is, talk to your parents about what is going on, but if you can't have that conversation, don't let that add to your worry. There is no single "right" way to approach the death of a loved one.

Chapter 37

Caregiver Stress

What is a caregiver?

Caregivers are people who take care of other adults, most often parents or spouses, who are ill or disabled. The people who receive care usually need help with basic daily tasks. Caregivers help with many things such as the following:

- Grocery shopping
- Cooking
- Paying bills
- Toileting
- Dressing

- House cleaning
- Shopping
- Giving medicine
- Bathing
- Eating

Usually caregivers take care of elderly people. Less often, caregivers are grandparents who are raising their grandchildren. The terms informal caregiver and family caregiver refer to people who are not paid to provide care. As the American population ages, the number of caregivers and the demands placed on them will grow.

"Caregiver Stress," National Women's Health Information Center (http://www.womenshealth.gov), January 2006. This document is available online at http://www.womenshealth.gov/faq/caregiver.htm. Additional information can also be obtained frm the National Women's Health Information Center by calling toll-free, 800-994-9662.

Who are our nation's caregivers?

About one in four American families or 22.4 million households care for someone over the age of 50. The number of American households involved in caregiving may reach 39 million by 2007.

- About 75% of caregivers are women.

- Two-thirds of caregivers in the United States have jobs in addition to caring for another person.

- Most caregivers are middle-aged: 35–64 years old.

What is caregiver stress?

Caregiver stress is the emotional strain of caregiving. Studies show that caregiving takes a toll on physical and emotional health. Caregivers are more likely to suffer from depression than their peers. Limited research suggests that caregivers may also be more likely to have health problems like diabetes and heart disease than non-caregivers.

Caring for another person takes a lot of time, effort, and work. Plus, most caregivers juggle caregiving with full-time jobs and parenting. In the process, caregivers put their own needs aside. Caregivers often report that it is difficult to look after their own health in terms of exercise, nutrition, and doctor's visits. So, caregivers often end up feeling angry, anxious, isolated, and sad.

Caregivers for people with Alzheimer disease (AD) or other kinds of dementia are particularly vulnerable to burnout. Research shows that most dementia caregivers suffer from depression and stress. Also, studies show that the more hours spent on caregiving, the greater the risk of anxiety and depression.

Women caregivers are particularly prone to feeling stress and overwhelmed. Studies show that female caregivers have more emotional and physical health problems, employment-related problems, and financial strain than male caregivers. Other research shows that people who care for their spouses are more prone to caregiving-related stress than those who care for other family members.

It is important to note that caring for another person can also create positive emotional change. Aside from feeling stress, many caregivers say their role has had many positive effects on their lives. For example, caregivers report that caregiving has given them a sense of purpose. They say that their role makes them feel useful, capable and that they are making a difference in the life of a loved one.

How can I tell if caregiving is putting too much stress on me?

If you have any of the following symptoms, caregiving may be putting too much strain on you:

- Sleeping problems—sleeping too much or too little

- Change in eating habits—resulting in weight gain or loss

- Feeling tired or without energy most of the time

- Loss of interest in activities you used to enjoy such as going out with friends, walking, or reading

- Easily irritated, angered, or saddened

- Frequent headaches, stomach aches, or other physical problems

What can I do to prevent or relieve stress?

Take care of yourself. In the process, you'll become a better caregiver. Take the following steps to make your health a priority:

- Find out about community caregiving resources.

- Ask for and accept help.

- Stay in touch with friends and family. Social activities can help you feel connected and may reduce stress.

- Find time for exercise most days of the week.

- Prioritize, make lists and establish a daily routine.

- Look to faith-based groups for support and help.

- Join a support group for caregivers in your situation (like caring for a person with dementia). Many support groups can be found in the community or on the internet.

- See your doctor for a checkup. Talk to her about symptoms of depression or sickness you may be having.

- Try to get enough sleep and rest.

- Eat a healthy diet rich in fruits, vegetables, and whole grains and low in saturated fat.

- Ask your doctor about taking a multivitamin.

- Take one day at a time.

Caregivers who work outside the home should consider taking some time off. If you are feeling overwhelmed, taking a break from your job may help you get back on track. Employees covered under the federal Family and Medical Leave Act may be able to take up to 12 weeks of unpaid leave per year to care for relatives. Ask your human resources office about options for unpaid leave.

What is respite care?

The term respite care means care that gives the regular caregiver some time off. Respite care gives family caregivers a much-needed break. In the process, respite care reduces caregiver stress.

Respite care may be provided by resources such as the following:

* Home health care workers

* Adult day-care centers

* Short-term nursing homes

* Assisted living homes

Respite care is essential to family caregivers. Studies show that respite care helps caregivers keep their loved ones at home for longer periods of time.

What is the National Family Caregiver Support Program (NFCSP)?

The National Family Caregiver Support Program (NFCSP) is a federally-funded program through the Older Americans Act. The NFCSP helps states provide services that assist family caregivers. To be eligible for the NFCSP, caregivers must meet these criteria:

* Care for adults aged 60 years and older, or

* Be grandparents or relatives caring for a child under the age of 18.

Each state offers different amounts and types of services. These include the following:

* Information about available services

* Help accessing support services

* Individual counseling and organization of support groups

- Caregiver training

- Respite care

- Limited supplemental services to complement the care provided by caregivers

How can I find out about caregiving resources in my community?

A number of resources can help direct you to the caregiver services you need. These agencies will be able to tell you facts such as these:

- What kind of services are available in your community

- If these services are right for you

- If you are eligible for these services

- Whom to contact and hours of operation

People who need help caring for an older person should contact their local Area Agency on Aging (AAA). AAAs are usually listed in the government sections of the telephone directory under "Aging" or "Social Services." A listing of state and area agencies on aging is also available online at: http://www.aoa.gov/eldfam/How_To_Find/ Agencies/Agencies.asp

The National Eldercare Locator, a toll-free service of the Administration on Aging, is another good resource. They can be reached by telephone at 800-677-1116 or online at http://www.eldercare.gov/ Eldercare/Public/Home.asp. The Eldercare Locator can help find your local or state AAA. Operators are available Monday through Friday, 9:00 a.m. to 8:00 p.m., Eastern Time. When contacting the Eldercare Locator, callers should have the address, zip code, and county of residence for the person needing assistance.

What kind of caregiver services can I find in my community?

There are many kinds of community care services, including the following:

- Transportation

- Meals

- Adult day care

- Home care

- Cleaning and yard work services

- Home modification

- Senior centers

- Hospice care

- Support groups

- Legal and financial counseling

What kind of home care help is available?

There are two kinds of home care: home health care and non-medical home care services. Both types help sick and disabled people live independently in their homes for as long as possible. Caregivers and doctors decide what services are necessary and most helpful. Home health care includes health-related services such as medicine assistance, nursing services, and physical therapy. Non-medical home care services include housekeeping, cooking, and companionship.

How will I pay for home health care?

Medicare, Medicaid and some private insurance companies will cover the cost of limited home care. Coverage varies from state to state. Other times, you will have to pay out of pocket for these services.

The cost of home care depends on what types of services are used. Non-medical workers like housekeepers are much less expensive than nurses or physical therapists. Also, some home care agencies are cheaper than others.

Who is eligible for Medicare home health care services?

To get Medicare home health care, a person must meet all of the following four conditions:

- A doctor must decide that the person needs medical care in the home and make a plan for home care.

- The person must need at least one of the following: sporadic (and not full time) skilled nursing care, physical therapy, speech language pathology services, or continue to need occupational therapy.

- The person must be homebound. This means that he or she is normally unable to leave home. When the person leaves home, it must be infrequent, for a short time, or to get medical care, or to attend religious services.

- The home health agency caring for the person must be approved by the Medicare program.

To find out if a person is eligible for Medicare home health care services, call the Regional Home Health Intermediary at 800-MEDICARE or visit the Medicare website at: http://www.medicare.gov and select "Helpful Contacts."

Will Medicaid help pay for home health care?

To qualify for Medicaid, a person must have a low income and few other assets. Medicaid coverage differs from state to state. In all states, Medicaid pays for basic home health care and medical equipment. In some cases, Medicaid will pay for a homemaker, personal care, and other services not covered by Medicare.

For more information on Medicaid coverage of home health care in your state, call your state medical assistance office. For state telephone numbers, call 800-MEDICARE.

Chapter 38

Home Safety for People with Alzheimer Disease

Caring for a person with Alzheimer disease (AD) is a challenge that calls upon the patience, creativity, knowledge, and skills of each caregiver. Hopefully this information will help you cope with some of these challenges and develop creative solutions to increase the security and freedom of the person with AD in your home, as well as your own peace of mind.

This chapter is for those who provide in-home care for people with AD or related disorders. The goal is to improve home safety by identifying potential problems in the home and offering possible solutions to help prevent accidents.

First, there is a checklist to help you make each room in your home a safer environment for the person with AD. Next, hopefully this information will increase your awareness of the ways specific impairments associated with the disease can create particular safety hazards in the home. Specific home safety tips are listed to help you cope with some of the more hazardous behaviors that may occur as the disease advances. Also included are tips for managing driving and planning for natural disaster safety.

General Safety Concerns

People with AD become increasingly unable to take care of themselves. However, individuals will move through the disease in their

From "Home Safety for People with Alzheimer's Disease," National Institute on Aging (http://www.nia.nih.gov), March 2007.

own unique manner. As a caregiver, you face the ongoing challenge of adapting to each change in the person's behavior and functioning. The following general principles may be helpful.

- **Think prevention:** It is very difficult to predict what a person with AD might do. Just because something has not yet occurred, does not mean it should not be cause for concern. Even with the best-laid plans, accidents can happen. Therefore, checking the safety of your home will help you take control of some of the potential problems that may create hazardous situations.

- **Adapt the environment:** It is more effective to change the environment than to change most behaviors. While some AD behaviors can be managed with special medications prescribed by a doctor, many cannot. You can make changes in an environment to decrease the hazards and stressors that accompany these behavioral and functional changes.

- **Minimize danger:** By minimizing danger, you can maximize independence. A safe environment can be a less restrictive environment where the person with AD can experience increased security and more mobility.

Is It Safe to Leave the Person with AD Alone?

This issue needs careful evaluation and is certainly a safety concern. The following points may help you decide. Does the person with AD:

- become confused or unpredictable under stress?

- recognize a dangerous situation; for example, fire?

- know how to use the telephone in an emergency?

- know how to get help?

- stay content within the home?

- wander and become disoriented?

- show signs of agitation, depression, or withdrawal when left alone for any period of time?

- attempt to pursue former interests or hobbies that might now warrant supervision such as cooking, appliance repair, or woodworking?

You may want to seek input and advice from a health care professional to assist you in these considerations. As Alzheimer disease progresses, these questions will need ongoing evaluation.

Home Safety Room-by-Room

Prevention begins with a safety check of every room in your home. Use the following room-by-room checklist to alert you to potential hazards and to record any changes you need to make. You can buy products or gadgets necessary for home safety at stores carrying hardware, electronics, medical supplies, and children's items.

Keep in mind that it may not be necessary to make all of the suggested changes. This chapter covers a wide range of safety concerns that may arise, and some modifications may never be needed. It is important, however, to re-evaluate home safety periodically as behavior and abilities change.

Your home is a personal and precious environment. As you go through this checklist, some of the changes you make may impact your surroundings positively, and some may affect you in ways that may be inconvenient or undesirable. It is possible, however, to strike a balance. Caregivers can make adaptations that modify and simplify without severely disrupting the home. You may want to consider setting aside a special area for yourself, a space off-limits to anyone else and arranged exactly as you like. Everyone needs private, quiet time, and as a caregiver, this becomes especially crucial.

A safe home can be a less stressful home for the person with AD, the caregiver, and family members. You don't have to make these changes alone. You may want to enlist the help of a friend, professional, or community service such as the Alzheimer's Association.

Throughout the Home

- Display emergency numbers and your home address near all telephones.

- Use an answering machine when you cannot answer phone calls, and set it to turn on after the fewest number of rings possible. A person with AD often may be unable to take messages or could become a victim of telephone exploitation. Turn ringers on low to avoid distraction and confusion. Put all portable and cell phones and equipment in a safe place so that they will not be easily lost.

- Install smoke alarms near all bedrooms and carbon monoxide detectors in appropriate places; check their functioning and batteries frequently.

- Avoid the use of flammable and volatile compounds near gas water heaters. Do not store these materials in an area where a gas pilot light is used.

- Install secure locks on all outside doors and windows.

- Hide a spare house key outside in case the person with AD locks you out of the house.

- Avoid the use of extension cords if possible by placing lamps and appliances close to electrical outlets. Tack extension cords to the baseboards of a room to avoid tripping.

- Cover unused outlets with childproof plugs.

- Place red tape around floor vents, radiators, and other heating devices to deter the person with AD from standing on or touching a hot grid.

- Check all rooms for adequate lighting.

- Place light switches at the top and the bottom of stairs.

- Stairways should have at least one handrail that extends beyond the first and last steps. If possible, stairways should be carpeted or have safety grip strips.

- Keep all medications (prescription and over-the-counter) locked. Each bottle of prescription medicine should be clearly labeled with the patient's name, name of the drug, drug strength, dosage frequency, and expiration date. Child-resistant caps are available if needed.

- Keep all alcohol in a locked cabinet or out of reach of the person with AD. Drinking alcohol can increase confusion.

- If smoking is permitted, monitor the person with AD while he or she is smoking. Remove matches, lighters, ashtrays, cigarettes, and other means of smoking from view. This reduces potential fire hazards, and with these reminders out of sight, the person may forget the desire to smoke.

- Avoid clutter, which can create confusion and danger. Throw out or recycle newspapers and magazines regularly. Keep all walk areas free of furniture.

- Keep plastic bags out of reach. A person with AD may choke or suffocate.

- Remove all guns or other weapons from the home, or safety proof them by installing safety locks or by removing ammunition and firing pins.

- Lock all power tools and machinery in the garage, workroom, or basement.

- Remove all poisonous plants from the home. Check with local nurseries or poison control centers for a list of poisonous plants.

- Make sure all computer equipment and accessories, including electrical cords, are kept out of the way. If valuable documents or materials are stored on a home computer, protect the files with passwords. Password protect access to the internet also, and restrict the amount of online time without supervision. Consider monitoring the person with AD's computer use, and installing software that screens for objectionable or offensive material on the internet.

- Keep fish tanks out of reach. The combination of glass, water, electrical pumps, and potentially poisonous aquatic life could be harmful to a curious person with AD.

Outside Approaches to the House

- Keep steps sturdy and textured to prevent falls in wet or icy weather.

- Mark the edges of steps with bright or reflective tape.

- Consider a ramp with handrails into the home rather than steps.

- Eliminate uneven surfaces or walkways, hoses, or other objects that may cause a person to trip.

- Restrict access to a swimming pool by fencing it off with a locked gate, covering it, and keeping it closely supervised when in use.

- In the patio area, remove the fuel source and fire starters from any grills when not in use, and supervise use when the person with AD is present.

- Place a small bench or table by the entry door to hold parcels while unlocking the door.

- Make sure outside lighting is adequate. Light sensors that turn on lights automatically as you approach the house are available and may be useful. They also may be used in other parts of the home.

- Prune bushes and foliage well away from walkways and doorways.

- Consider a NO SOLICITING sign for the front gate or door.

Entryway

- Remove scatter rugs and throw rugs.

- Use textured strips or nonskid wax on hardwood floors to prevent slipping.

Kitchen

- Install childproof door latches on storage cabinets and drawers designated for breakable or dangerous items. Lock away all household cleaning products, matches, knives, scissors, blades, small appliances, and anything valuable.

- If prescription or nonprescription drugs are kept in the kitchen, store them in a locked cabinet.

- Remove scatter rugs and foam pads from the floor.

- Remove knobs from the stove, or install an automatic shut-off switch.

- Do not use or store flammable liquids in the kitchen. Lock them in the garage or in an outside storage unit.

- Keep a night-light in the kitchen.

- Remove or secure the family "junk drawer." A person with AD may eat small items such as matches, hardware, erasers, plastics, etc.

- Remove artificial fruits and vegetables or food-shaped kitchen magnets, which might appear to be edible.

- Insert a drain trap in the kitchen sink to catch anything that may otherwise become lost or clog the plumbing.

- Consider dismantling the garbage disposal. People with AD may place objects or their own hands in the disposal.

Bedroom

- Anticipate the reasons a person with AD might get out of bed, such as hunger, thirst, going to the bathroom, restlessness, and pain, and try to meet these needs by offering food and fluids, and scheduling ample toileting.

- Use a night-light.

- Use an intercom device (often used for infants) to alert you to any noises indicating falls or a need for help. This also is an effective device for bathrooms.

- Remove scatter rugs.

- Remove portable space heaters. If you use portable fans, be sure that objects cannot be placed in the blades.

- Be cautious when using electric mattress pads, electric blankets, electric sheets, and heating pads, all of which can cause burns. Keep controls out of reach.

- When the person with AD is at risk of falling out of bed, place mats next to the bed, as long as this does not create a greater risk of accident.

- Use transfer or mobility aids.

- If you are considering using a hospital-type bed with rails or wheels, understand that many people can sleep safely without bed rails, and reassess the need for using bed rails on a regular basis:

  - Use beds that can be raised and lowered close to the floor to accommodate both the person with AD and your needs.

  - Keep the bed in the lowest position with wheels locked.

  - Use a proper size mattress or mattress with raised foam edges to prevent the person from being trapped between the mattress and rail.

  - Reduce the gaps between the mattress and side rails.

  - Monitor the person with AD frequently.

Bathroom

- Do not leave a severely impaired person with AD alone in the bathroom.

351

- Remove the lock from the bathroom door to prevent the person with AD from getting locked inside.

- Place nonskid adhesive strips, decals, or mats in the tub and shower. If the bathroom is uncarpeted, consider placing these strips next to the tub, toilet, and sink.

- Use washable wall-to-wall bathroom carpeting to prevent slipping on wet tile floors.

- Use an extended toilet seat with handrails, or install grab bars beside the toilet.

- Install grab bars in the tub/shower. A grab bar in contrasting color to the wall is easier to see.

- Use a foam rubber faucet cover (often used for small children) in the tub to prevent serious injury should the person with AD fall.

- Use plastic shower stools and a hand-held showerhead to make bathing easier.

- In the shower, tub, and sink, use a single faucet that mixes hot and cold water to avoid burns.

- Adjust the water heater to 120 degrees to avoid scalding tap water.

- Insert drain traps in sinks to catch small items that may be lost or flushed down the drain.

- Store medications (prescription and nonprescription) in a locked cabinet. Check medication dates and throw away outdated medications.

- Remove cleaning products from under the sink, or lock them away.

- Use a night-light.

- Remove small electrical appliances from the bathroom. Cover electrical outlets. If men use electric razors, have them use a mirror outside the bathroom to avoid water contact.

Living Room

- Clear all walk areas of electrical cords.

- Remove scatter rugs or throw rugs. Repair or replace torn carpet.

- Place decals at eye level on sliding glass doors, picture windows, or furniture with large glass panels to identify the glass pane.

- Do not leave the person with AD alone with an open fire in the fireplace. Consider alternative heating sources. Remove matches and cigarette lighters.

- Keep the controls for cable or satellite TV, VCR, and stereo system out of sight.

Laundry Room

- Keep the door to the laundry room locked if possible.

- Lock all laundry products in a cabinet.

- Remove large knobs from the washer and dryer if the person with AD tampers with machinery.

- Close and latch the doors and lids to the washer and dryer to prevent objects from being placed in the machines.

Garage/Shed/Basement

- Lock access to all garages, sheds, and basements if possible.

- Inside a garage or shed, keep all potentially dangerous items, such as tools, tackle, machines, and sporting equipment either locked away in cabinets or in appropriate boxes/cases.

- Secure and lock all motor vehicles and keep them out of sight if possible. Consider covering those vehicles, including bikes, which are not frequently used. This may reduce an AD person's thoughts of leaving.

- Keep all toxic materials, such as paint, fertilizers, gasoline, or cleaning supplies out of view. Put them either in a high, dry place, or lock them in a cabinet.

- If a person with AD is permitted in a garage, shed, or basement, preferably with supervision, make sure the area is well lit and that stairs have a handrail and are safe to walk up and down. Keep walkways clear of debris and clutter, and place overhanging items out of reach.

Home Safety Behavior-by-Behavior

Although a number of behavior and sensory problems may accompany Alzheimer disease, not every person will experience the disease in exactly the same way. As the disease progresses, particular behavioral changes can create safety problems. The person with AD may or may not have these symptoms. However, should these behaviors occur, the following safety recommendations may help reduce risks.

Wandering

- Remove clutter and clear the pathways from room to room to allow the person with AD to move about more freely.

- Make sure floors provide good traction for walking or pacing. Use nonskid floor wax or leave floors unpolished. Secure all rug edges, eliminate throw rugs, or install nonskid strips. The person with AD should wear nonskid shoes or sneakers.

- Place locks on exit doors high or low on the door out of direct sight. Consider double locks that require a key. Keep a key for yourself and hide one near the door for emergency exit purposes.

- Use loosely fitting doorknob covers so that the cover turns instead of the actual knob. Due to the potential hazard they could cause if an emergency exit is needed, locked doors and doorknob covers should be used only when a caregiver is present.

- Install safety devices found in hardware stores to limit the distance that windows can be opened.

- If possible, secure the yard with fencing and a locked gate. Use door alarms such as loose bells above the door or devices that ring when the doorknob is touched or the door is opened.

- Divert the attention of the person with AD away from using the door by placing small scenic posters on the door; placing removable gates, curtains, or brightly colored streamers across the door; or wallpapering the door to match any adjoining walls.

- Place STOP, DO NOT ENTER, or CLOSED signs in strategic areas on doors.

- Reduce clues that symbolize departure such as shoes, keys, suitcases, coats, or hats.

- Obtain a medical identification bracelet for the person with AD with the words "memory loss" inscribed along with an emergency telephone number. Place the bracelet on the person's dominant hand to limit the possibility of removal, or solder the bracelet closed. Check with the local Alzheimer's Association about the Safe Return program.

- Place labels in garments to aid in identification.

- Keep an article of the person's worn, unwashed clothing in a plastic bag to aid in finding someone with the use of dogs.

- Notify neighbors of the person's potential to wander or become lost. Alert them to contact you or the police immediately if the individual is seen alone and on the move.

- Give local police, neighbors, and relatives a recent picture, along with the name and pertinent information about the person with AD, as a precaution should he or she become lost. Keep extra pictures on hand.

- Consider making an up-to-date home video of the person with AD.

- Do not leave a person with AD who has a history of wandering unattended.

Rummaging/Hiding Things

- Lock up all dangerous or toxic products, or place them out of the person's reach.

- Remove all old or spoiled food from the refrigerator and cupboards. A person with AD may rummage for snacks but may lack the judgment or taste to rule out spoiled foods.

- Simplify the environment by removing clutter or valuable items that could be misplaced, lost, or hidden by the person with AD. These include important papers, checkbooks, charge cards, and jewelry.

- If your yard has a fence with a locked gate, place the mailbox outside the gate. People with AD often hide, lose, or throw away mail. If this is a serious problem, consider obtaining a post office box.

- Create a special place for the person with AD to rummage freely or sort (for example, a chest of drawers, a bag of selected objects, or a basket of clothing to fold or unfold). Often, safety problems occur when the person with AD becomes bored or does not know what to do.

- Provide the person with AD a safe box, treasure chest, or cupboard to store special objects.

- Close access to unused rooms, thereby limiting the opportunity for rummaging and hiding things.

- Search the house periodically to discover hiding places. Once found, these hiding places can be discreetly and frequently checked.

- Keep all trashcans covered or out of sight. The person with AD may not remember the purpose of the container or may rummage through it.

- Check trash containers before emptying them in case something has been hidden there or accidentally thrown away.

Hallucinations, Illusions, and Delusions

Due to the complex changes occurring in the brain, people with AD may see or hear things that have no basis in reality. Hallucinations come from within the brain and involve hearing, seeing, or feeling things that are not really there. For example, a person with AD may see children playing in the living room when no children exist. Illusions differ from hallucinations because the person with AD is misinterpreting something that actually does exist. Shadows on the wall may look like people, for example. Delusions are persistent thoughts that the person with AD believes are true but in reality, are not. Often, stealing is suspected, for example, but cannot be verified.

It is important to seek medical evaluation if a person with AD has ongoing disturbing hallucinations, illusions, or delusions. Often, these symptoms can be treated with medication or behavior management techniques. With all of the above symptoms, the following environmental adaptations also may be helpful.

- Paint walls a light color to reflect more light. Use solid colors, which are less confusing to an impaired person than a patterned wall. Large, bold prints (for example, floral wallpaper or drapes) may cause confusing illusions.

- Make sure there is adequate lighting, and keep extra bulbs handy in a secured place. Dimly lit areas may produce confusing shadows or difficulty with interpreting everyday objects.

- Reduce glare by using soft light or frosted bulbs, partially closing blinds or curtains, and maintaining adequate globes or shades on light fixtures.

- Remove or cover mirrors if they cause the person with AD to become confused or frightened.

- Ask if the person can point to a specific area that is producing confusion. Perhaps one particular aspect of the environment is being misinterpreted.

- Vary the home environment as little as possible to minimize the potential for visual confusion. Keep furniture in the same place.

- Avoid violent or disturbing television programs. The person with AD may believe the story is real.

- Do not confront the person with AD who becomes aggressive. Withdraw and make sure you have access to an exit as needed.

Special Occasions/Gatherings/Holidays

When celebrations, special events, or holidays include large numbers of people, remember that it is possible that large groups may cause a person with AD some confusion and anxiety. The person with AD may find some situations easier and more pleasurable than others.

- Large gatherings, weddings, family reunions, or picnics may be cause for anxiety. Consider having a more intimate gathering with only a few people in your home. Think about having friends and family visit in small groups rather than all at once. If you are hosting a large group, remember to prepare the person with AD ahead of time. Try to have a space available where they can rest, be by themselves, or spend some time with a smaller number of people, if needed.

- Consider simplifying your holidays around the home and remember that you already may have more responsibilities than in previous years. For example, rather than cooking an elaborate dinner at Thanksgiving or Christmas, invite family and friends for a potluck dinner. Instead of elaborate decorations, consider choosing a few select items to celebrate holidays. Make sure holiday decorations do not significantly alter the environment, which might confuse the person with AD.

- Holiday decorations, such as Christmas trees, lights, or menorahs, should be secured so that they do not fall or catch on fire. Anything flammable should be monitored at all times, and extra precautions should be taken so that lights or anything breakable are fixed firmly, correctly, and out of the way of those with AD.

- As suggested by most manufacturers, candles of any size should never be lit without supervision. When not in use, they should be put away.

- Try to avoid clutter in general, especially in walkways, during the holidays.

Impairment of the Senses

Alzheimer disease can cause changes in the ability to interpret what a person can see, hear, taste, feel, or smell, even though his or her sense organs may still be intact. The person with AD should be evaluated periodically by a physician for any such changes that may be correctable with glasses, dentures, hearing aids, or other treatments.

Vision: People with AD may experience a number of changes in visual abilities. For example, they may lose their ability to comprehend visual images. Although there is nothing physically wrong with their eyes, people with AD may no longer be able to interpret accurately what they see due to changes in their brain. Also, their sense of perception and depth may be altered. These changes can cause safety concerns.

- Create color contrast between floors and walls to help the person see depth. Floor coverings are less visually confusing if they are a solid color.

- Use dishes and placemats in contrasting colors for easier identification.

- Mark the edges of steps with brightly colored strips of tape to outline changes in elevation.

- Place brightly colored signs or simple pictures on important rooms (the bathroom, for example) for easier identification.

- Be aware that a small pet that blends in with the floor or lies in walkways may be a hazard. The person with AD may trip over a small pet.

Smell: A loss or decrease in smell often accompanies Alzheimer disease.

- Install good quality smoke detectors and check them frequently. The person with AD may not smell smoke or may not associate it with danger.

- Keep refrigerators clear of spoiled foods.

Touch: People with AD may experience loss of sensation or may no longer be able to interpret feelings of heat, cold, or discomfort.

- Adjust water heaters to 120 degrees to avoid scalding tap water. Most hot water heaters are set at 150 degrees, which can cause burns.

- Color code separate water faucet handles, with red for hot and blue for cold.

- Place a sign on the oven, coffee maker, toaster, crock-pot, iron, or other potentially hot appliances that says DO NOT TOUCH or STOP! VERY HOT. The person with AD should not use appliances without supervision. Unplug appliances when not in use.

- Use a thermometer to tell you whether the water in the bathtub is too hot or too cold.

- Remove furniture or other objects with sharp corners or pad them to reduce potential for injury.

Taste: People with AD may lose taste sensitivity. As their judgment declines, they also may place dangerous or inappropriate things in their mouth.

- If possible, keep a spare set of dentures. If the person keeps removing dentures, check for correct fit.

- Keep all condiments such as salt, sugar, or spices away from easy access if you see the person with AD using excess amounts. Too much salt, sugar, or spice can be irritating to the stomach or cause other health problems.

- Remove or lock up medicine cabinet items such as toothpaste, perfume, lotions, shampoos, rubbing alcohol, or soap, which may look and smell like edible items to the person with AD.

- Consider a childproof latch on the refrigerator, if necessary.

- Keep the poison control number by the telephone. Keep a bottle of Ipecac (vomit inducing) available, but use only with instructions from poison control or 911.

- Keep pet litter boxes inaccessible to the person with AD. Do not store pet food in the refrigerator.

- Learn the Heimlich maneuver or other techniques to use in case of choking. Check with your local Red Cross chapter for more information and instruction.

Hearing: People with AD may have normal hearing, but they may lose their ability to interpret what they hear accurately. This may result in confusion or over-stimulation.

- Avoid excessive noise in the home such as having the stereo and the TV on at the same time.

- Be sensitive to the amount of noise going on outside, and close windows or doors, if necessary.

- Avoid large gatherings of people in the home if the person with AD shows signs of agitation or distress in crowds.

- Check hearing aid batteries and functioning frequently.

Driving

Driving is a complex activity that demands quick reactions, alert senses, and split-second decision-making. For a person with AD, driving becomes increasingly more difficult. Memory loss, impaired judgment, disorientation, impaired visual and spatial perception, slow reaction time, certain medications, diminished attention span, inability to recognize cues such as stop signs and traffic lights can make driving particularly hazardous.

People with AD who continue to drive can be a danger to themselves, their passengers, and the community at large. As the disease progresses, they lose driving skills and must stop driving. Unfortunately, people with AD often cannot recognize when they should no longer drive. This is a tremendous safety concern. It is extremely important to have the impaired person's driving abilities carefully evaluated.

Warning Signs of Unsafe Driving: Often, it is the caregiver, a family member, neighbor, or friend who becomes aware of the safety hazards. If a person with AD experiences one of more of the following problems, it may be time to limit or stop driving.

Does the person with AD:

- get lost while driving in a familiar location?
- fail to observe traffic signals?
- drive at an inappropriate speed?
- become angry, frustrated, or confused while driving?
- make slow or poor decisions?

Please do not wait for an accident to happen. Take action immediately!

Explaining to the person with AD that he or she can no longer drive can be extremely difficult. Loss of driving privileges may represent a tremendous loss of independence, freedom, and identity. It is a significant concern for the person with AD and the caregiver. The issue of not driving may produce anger, denial, and grief in the person with AD, as well as guilt and anxiety in the caregiver. Family and concerned professionals need to be both sensitive and firm. Above all, they should be persistent and consistent.

The doctor of a person with AD can assist the family with the task of restricting driving. Talk with the doctor about your concerns. Most people will listen to their doctor. Ask the doctor to advise the person with AD to reduce his or her driving, go for a driving evaluation or test, or stop driving altogether. An increasing number of States have laws requiring physicians to report AD and related disorders to the Department of Motor Vehicles. The Department of Motor Vehicles then is responsible for retesting the at-risk driver. Testing should occur regularly, at least yearly.

When dementia impairs driving and the person with AD continues to insist on driving, a number of different approaches may be necessary.

- Work as a team with family, friends, and professionals, and use a single, simple explanation for the loss of driving ability such as: "You have a memory problem, and it is no longer safe to drive." "You cannot drive because you are on medication." or "The doctor has prescribed that you no longer drive." Ask the doctor to write on a prescription pad DO NOT DRIVE. Ask the doctor to write to the Department of Motor Vehicles or Department of Public Safety saying this person should no longer drive. Show the letter to the person with AD as evidence.

- Offer to drive.

- Walk when possible, and make these outings special events.

- Use public transportation or any special transportation provided by community organizations. Ask about senior discounts or transportation coupons. The person with AD should not take public transportation unsupervised.

- Park the car at a friend's home.

- Hide the car keys.

- Exchange car keys with a set of unusable keys. Some people with AD are in the habit of carrying keys.

- Place a large note under the car hood requesting that any mechanic call you before doing work requested by the person with AD.

- Have a mechanic install a "kill switch" or alarm system that disengages the fuel line to prevent the car from starting.

- Consider selling the car and putting aside the money saved from insurance, repairs, and gasoline for taxi funds.

- Do not leave a person with AD alone in a parked car.

Natural Disaster Safety

Natural disasters come in many forms and degrees of severity. They seldom give warning, and they call upon good judgment and ability to follow through with crisis plans. People with AD are at a serious disadvantage. Their impairments in memory and reasoning severely limit their ability to act appropriately in crises.

It is always important to have a plan of action in case of fire, earthquake, flood, tornado, or other disasters. Specific home safety precautions may apply and environmental changes may be needed. The American Red Cross is an excellent resource for general safety information and preparedness guides for comprehensive planning. If there is a person with AD in the home, the following precautions apply:

- Get to know your neighbors, and identify specific individuals who would be willing to help in a crisis. Formulate a plan of action with them should the person with AD be unattended during a crisis.

- Give neighbors a list of emergency numbers of caregivers, family members, and primary medical resources.

- Educate neighbors beforehand about the person's specific disabilities, including inability to follow complex instructions, memory loss, impaired judgment, and probable disorientation and confusion. Give examples of some of the simple one-step instructions that the person may be able to follow.

- Have regular emergency drills so that each member of the household has a specific task. Realize that the person with AD cannot be expected to hold any responsibility in the crisis plan and that someone will need to take primary responsibility for supervising the individual.

- Always have at least an extra week's supply of any medical or personal hygiene items critical to the person's welfare, such as food and water, medications, incontinence undergarments, hearing aid batteries, and glasses.

- Be sure that the person with AD wears an identification bracelet stating "memory loss" should he or she become lost or disoriented during the crisis. Contact your local Alzheimer's Association chapter and enroll the person in the Safe Return program.

- Under no circumstances should a person with AD be left alone following a natural disaster. Do not count on the individual to stay in one place while you go to get help. Provide plenty of reassurance.

Who Would Take Care of the Person with AD If Something Happened to You?

It is important to have a plan in case of your own illness, disability, or death.

- Consult a lawyer regarding a living trust, durable power of attorney for health care and finances, and other estate planning tools.

- Consult with family and close friends to decide who will take responsibility for the person with AD. You also may want to seek information about your local public guardian's office, mental health conservator's office, adult protective services, or other case management services. These organizations may have programs to assist the person with AD in your absence.

- Maintain a notebook for the responsible person who will be assuming caregiving. Such a notebook should contain the following information:
  - emergency numbers
  - current problem behaviors and possible solutions
  - ways to calm the person with AD
  - assistance needed with toileting, feeding, or grooming
  - favorite activities or food

363

Preview board and care or long-term care facilities in your community and select a few as possibilities. If the person with AD is no longer able to live at home, the responsible person will be better able to carry out your wishes for long-term care.

Conclusion

Home safety takes many forms. This information focuses on the physical environment and specific safety concerns. But the home environment also involves the needs, feelings, and lifestyles of the occupants, of you the caregiver, your family, and the person with AD. Disability affects all family members, and it is crucial to maintain your emotional and physical welfare in addition to a safe environment.

We encourage you to make sure you have quiet time, time out, time to take part in something you enjoy. Protect your own emotional and physical health. Your local Alzheimer's Association chapter can help you with the support and information you may need as you address this very significant checkpoint in your home safety list. You are extremely valuable and as you take on a commitment to care for a person with AD, please take on the equally important commitment to care for yourself.

Chapter 39

Depression and Alzheimer Disease

Do people who have Alzheimer disease become depressed?

Yes. Depression is very common among people who have Alzheimer disease. In many cases, they become depressed when they realize that their memory and ability to function are getting worse.

Unfortunately, depression may make it even harder for a person who has Alzheimer disease to function, to remember things and to enjoy life.

How can I tell if my family member who has Alzheimer disease is depressed?

It may be difficult for you to know if your family member is depressed. You can look for some of the typical signs of depression, which include the following:

- Not wanting to move or do things (called apathy)

- Expressing feelings of worthlessness and sadness

- Refusing to eat and losing weight

- Sleeping too much or too little

Other signs of depression include crying and being unusually emotional, being angry or agitated, and being confused. Your family member who has Alzheimer disease may refuse to help with his or her own personal care (for example, getting dressed or taking medicines). He or she may wander away from home more often.

Alzheimer disease and depression have many symptoms that are alike. It can be hard to tell the difference between them. If you think that depression is a problem for your relative who has Alzheimer disease, talk to his or her family doctor.

How can the doctor help?

The doctor will talk with your relative. The doctor will also ask you and other family members and caregivers whether the person has any new or changed behaviors. The doctor will check your relative and may wish to do some tests to rule out other medical problems. He or she may suggest medicines to help your family member feel better. The doctor may also have some advice for you and other family members and caregivers on how to cope. He or she may recommend support groups that can help you.

What medicines can help reduce depression?

Antidepressant medicines can be very helpful for people who have Alzheimer disease and depression. These medicines can improve the symptoms of sadness and apathy, and they may also improve appetite and sleep problems. Don't worry—these medicines are not habit-forming. The doctor may also suggest other medicines that can help reduce upsetting problems, such as hallucinations or anxiety.

What can I do to help my family member?

Try to keep a daily routine for your family member who has Alzheimer disease. Avoid loud noises and over stimulation. A pleasant environment with familiar faces and mementos helps soothe fear and anxiety. Have a realistic expectation of what your family member can do. Expecting too much can make you both feel frustrated and upset. Let your family member help with simple, enjoyable tasks, such as preparing meals, gardening, doing crafts, and sorting photos. Most of all, be positive. Frequent praise for your family member will help him or her feel better—and it will help you as well.

As the caregiver of a person who has Alzheimer disease, you must also take care of yourself. If you become too tired and frustrated, you will be less able to help your family member. Ask for help from relatives, friends, and local community organizations. Respite care (short-term care that is given to the patient who has Alzheimer disease in order to provide relief for the caregiver) may be available from your local senior citizens' group or a social services agency. Look for caregiver support groups. Other people who are dealing with the same problems may have some good ideas on how you can cope better and on how to make caregiving easier. Adult day care centers may be helpful. They can give your family member a consistent environment and a chance to socialize.

Chapter 40

Activities at Home: Planning the Day for the Person with Dementia

Activities are the "things that we do," like getting dressed, doing chores, playing cards—even paying bills. They can be active or passive, done alone or with others. Activities represent who we are and what we're about.

A person with dementia needs assistance from a caregiver to organize the day. These planned activities can enhance the person's sense of dignity and self-esteem by giving more purpose and meaning to his or her life.

Activities structure time. They can make the best of a person's abilities. Activities can also reduce behavior like wandering or agitation.

Both the person with dementia and the caregiver can enjoy the sense of security and togetherness that activities can provide.

Types of Activities

Daily Routines

Chores: Dusting, sweeping, doing laundry

Mealtime: Preparing food, cooking, eating

Personal care: Bathing, shaving, getting dressed

Other Activities

Creative: Painting, playing the piano

Intellectual: Reading a book, doing crossword puzzles

Physical: Taking a walk, playing catch

Social: Having coffee, talking, playing cards

Spiritual: Praying, singing a hymn

Spontaneous: Going out to dinner, visiting friends

Work-related: Making notes, typing, fixing something

Planning Activities

Person

Planning activities for the person with dementia is best when you continually explore, experiment, and adjust. Consider the person's likes and dislikes; strengths and abilities; and interests. As the disease progresses, keep activities flexible, and be ready to make adjustments.

Keep the person's skills and abilities in mind: He or she may be able to play simple songs learned on the piano years ago. Bring these types of skills into daily activities.

Pay special attention to what the person enjoys: Take note when the person seems happy, anxious, distracted, or irritable. Some people enjoy watching sports, while others may be frightened by the fast pace or noise.

Consider if the person begins activities without direction: Does he or she set the table before dinner or begin sweeping the kitchen floor mid-morning? If so, you may wish to plan these activities as part of the daily routine.

Be aware of physical problems: Does he or she get tired quickly, have difficulty seeing, hearing, or performing simple movements? If so, you may want to avoid certain activities.

Activity

Focus on enjoyment, not achievement: Find activities that build on remaining skills and talents. A professional artist might become frustrated over the declining quality of work, but an amateur might enjoy a new opportunity for self-expression.

Encourage involvement in daily life: Activities that help the individual feel like a valued part of the household—like setting the table, wiping counter tops or emptying wastebaskets—provide a sense of success and accomplishment.

Relate activity to work life: A former office worker might enjoy activities that involve organizing, like putting coins in a holder, helping to assemble a mailing, or making a "to do" list. A farmer or gardener will probably take pleasure in working in the yard.

Look for favorites: The person who always enjoyed drinking coffee and reading the newspaper may still find these activities enjoyable, even if he or she is no longer able to completely understand what the newspaper says.

Change activities as needed: Try to be flexible and acknowledge the person's changing interests and abilities.

Consider time of day: Caregivers may find they have more success with certain activities at specific times of day, such as bathing and dressing in the morning. Whatever the case, your typical daily routine may need to change somewhat.

Adjust activities to stages of the disease: As the disease progresses, you may want to introduce more repetitive tasks. Be prepared for the person to eventually take a less-active role in activities.

Approach

Offer support and supervision: You may need to show the person how to perform the activity and provide simple, step-by-step directions.

Concentrate on the process, not the result: Does it really matter if the towels are folded properly? Not really. What matters is that you were able to spend time together, and the person feels as if he or she has helped do something useful.

Be flexible: When the person insists that he or she doesn't want to do something, it may be because he or she can't do it or fears doing it. Or if the person insists on doing it a different way, let it happen, and fix it later.

Be realistic and relaxed: Don't be concerned about filling every minute of the day with an activity. The person with Alzheimer disease needs a balance of activity and rest, and may need more frequent breaks and varied tasks.

Help get the activity started: Most people with dementia still have the energy and desire to do things but lack the ability to organize, plan, initiate, and successfully complete the task.

Break activities into simple, easy-to-follow steps: Too many directions at once often overwhelm a person with dementia. Focus on one task at a time.

Assist with difficult parts of the task: If you're cooking, and the person can't measure the ingredients, finish the measuring and say, "Would you please stir this for me?"

Let the individual know he or she is needed: Ask, "Could you please help me?" Be careful, however, not to place too many demands upon the person.

Stress a sense of purpose: If you ask the person to make a card, he or she may not respond. But, if you say that you're sending a special get-well card to a friend, the person may enjoy working on this task with you.

Don't criticize or correct the person: If the person enjoys a harmless activity, even if it may seem insignificant or meaningless to you, you should encourage the person to continue.

Encourage self-expression: Include activities that allow the person a chance for expression. These types of activities could include painting, drawing, music, or conversation.

Involve the person through the use of conversation: While you're polishing shoes, washing the car, or cooking dinner, talk to the person about what you're doing. Even if the person cannot respond, he or she is likely to benefit from your communication.

Substitute an activity for a behavior: If a person with dementia rubs his or her hand on a table, put a cloth in his or her hand, and encourage the person to wipe the table. Or, if the person is moving his or her feet on the floor, play some music so the person can tap them to the beat.

Try again later: If something isn't working, it may just be the wrong time of day or the activity may be too complicated. Try again later, or adapt the activity.

Place

Make activities safe: Modify a workshop by removing toxic materials and dangerous tools so an activity such as sanding a piece of wood can be safe and pleasurable.

Change your surroundings: to encourage activities Place in key locations scrapbooks, photo albums, or old magazines that help the person reminisce.

Minimize distractions that can frighten or confuse: A person with dementia may not be able to recall familiar sounds and places or may feel uncomfortable in certain settings.

Creating a Daily Plan

Consider how you organize your own day when planning the day for the person with dementia. There are times when you want variety and other times when you welcome routine. The challenge for caregivers is to find activities that provide meaning and purpose, as well as pleasure.

Begin by thinking about the past week. Try keeping a daily journal, and make notes about:

- Which activities worked best and which didn't? Why?

- Were there times when there was too much going on or too little to do?

- Were spontaneous activities enjoyable and easily completed?

Use what you've learned to set up a written daily plan. A planned day allows you to spend less time and energy trying to figure out what to do from moment to moment. Allow yourself and the person with dementia some flexibility for spontaneous activities.

Effective activities:

- Bring meaning, purpose, joy, and hope to the person's life;
- Use the person's skills and abilities;

- Give the person a sense of being normal;

- Involve family and friends;

- Are dignified and appropriate for adults;

- Are enjoyable.

Example of a Daily Plan

Morning

- Wash, brush teeth, get dressed

- Prepare and eat breakfast

- Have coffee and make conversation

- Discuss the newspaper, try a craft project, reminisce about old photos

- Take a break, have some quiet time

- Do some chores together

- Take a walk, play an active game

Afternoon

- Prepare and eat lunch, read mail, wash dishes

- Listen to music, do crossword puzzles, watch TV

- Do some gardening, take a walk, visit a friend

- Take a short break or nap

Evening

- Prepare and eat dinner, clean up the kitchen

- Reminisce over coffee and dessert

- Play cards, watch a movie, give a massage

- Take a bath, get ready for bed, read a book

Measuring the Plan's Success

To decide how the daily plan is working, look at each activity. Think about how the person responds and how well the activity meets your needs.

The success of an activity can vary from day to day. In general, if the person seems bored, distracted, or irritable, it may be time to introduce another activity or to take time out for rest.

Oftentimes, structured and pleasant activities reduce agitation and improve mood. The type of activity and how well it's completed are not as important as the joy and sense of accomplishment the person gets from doing it.

10 Quick Tips: Activities at Home

1. Be flexible and patient.

2. Encourage involvement in daily life.

3. Avoid correcting the person.

4. Help the person remain as independent as possible.

5. Offer opportunities for choice.

6. Simplify instructions.

7. Establish a familiar routine.

8. Respond to the person's feelings.

9. Simplify, structure and supervise.

10. Provide encouragement and praise.

Chapter 41

Tips for Traveling with a Person with Dementia

If someone you love has Alzheimer disease, there are many things to consider when planning a trip. A few simple measures will help to ensure that your traveling companion remains safe and comfortable. It is also essential that you contact your doctor and develop a realistic travel plan. That way, you can both enjoy your vacation to its fullest.

Bring along an identification tag that your companion can wear around his or her neck. In addition, register him or her with the safe return program in your area. Information about the safe return program in your area can be found at your local Alzheimer's Association chapter.

Keep things as familiar as possible. For example, keep bedtimes and eating times as close to normal as possible, and bring the person's favorite pajamas or pillow. If the person has never traveled on an airplane before, this is not the best time to introduce something new.

Be prepared. Get plenty of rest before the trip. Pack for the patient, allowing extra time for everything. Bathe and dress him or her without rushing, and make sure you both wear comfortable clothing during the trip. Research in advance what medical services are offered at your destination, in case you need them. Bring a brief medical history with you, including a current medication list, doctor's telephone numbers, and a list of any allergies.

Plan your itinerary well in advance. If staying with friends or family, make them aware of what Alzheimer disease is and what the symptoms can look like. Minimize time spent with large groups, noisy places, or energetic children. Avoid busy, chaotic locations. Check in with family members daily during the trip.

Be realistic. Carefully assess what the person's limitations and strengths are and shape the vacation accordingly. Also be realistic about your own and other caregivers' limitations and strengths—can you handle the person if he or she becomes agitated or wanders or is unable to sleep? Get your doctor's feedback on what is realistic and whether he or she recommends prescribing medication for the trip.

Limit the length of plane or car rides. If a trip is over four hours, two caregivers should be present. Bring along toys, photos, hobbies, or other distractions in case the person with Alzheimer disease becomes agitated. Carry moist wipes for any spills. Avoid caffeine.

If you are driving and the person with Alzheimer disease becomes agitated, pull over. Do not try to calm him or her and drive at the same time. He or she may become more disoriented and try to leave a moving car.

If you are traveling by air, avoid layovers, and try to fly on direct flights only. Carry all boarding passes, passports, and other important papers yourself, rather than giving them to the person with Alzheimer disease. Request a middle seat for your companion and an aisle seat for yourself so that he or she cannot wander away without your noticing. Pre-board the aircraft. Pack all medications in a carry-on bag—do not put it in checked luggage, which can get lost.

If you are staying in a hotel, request a large and quiet room. To protect against wandering order a door alarm or a childproof door-knob cover. Avoid rooms with sliding glass doors.

Have a back up plan. That way you can react to mishaps without become overly anxious yourself. Recognize when the patient is becoming upset or agitated, and stop any activities when necessary in order to get some rest.

In short, planning is the key to having a vacation that is enjoyable and safe. It is realistic to assume that the confusion of dementia will increase on a trip, leading to discomfort, fear, or agitation. Being prepared can help mediate any mishaps and make for a safe and enjoyable trip.

Chapter 42

Understanding and Handling Dementia-Related Behaviors

Caring for a loved one with dementia poses many challenges for families and caregivers. People with dementia from conditions such as Alzheimer disease and related diseases have a progressive brain disorder that makes it more and more difficult for them to remember things, think clearly, communicate with others, or take care of themselves. In addition, dementia can cause mood swings and even change a person's personality and behavior. This chapter provides some practical strategies for dealing with the troubling behavior problems and communication difficulties often encountered when caring for a person with dementia.

Ten Tips for Communicating with a Person with Dementia

We aren't born knowing how to communicate with a person with dementia—but we can learn. Improving your communication skills will help make caregiving less stressful and will likely improve the quality of your relationship with your loved one. Good communication skills will also enhance your ability to handle the difficult behavior you may encounter as you care for a person with a dementing illness.

---

1. Set a positive mood for interaction. Your attitude and body language communicate your feelings and thoughts stronger than your words. Set a positive mood by speaking to your loved one in a pleasant and respectful manner. Use facial expressions, tone of voice and physical touch to help convey your message and show your feelings of affection.

2. Get the person's attention. Limit distractions and noise—turn off the radio or TV, close the curtains or shut the door, or move to quieter surroundings. Before speaking, make sure you have her attention; address her by name, identify yourself by name and relation, and use nonverbal cues and touch to help keep her focused. If she is seated, get down to her level and maintain eye contact.

3. State your message clearly. Use simple words and sentences. Speak slowly, distinctly and in a reassuring tone. Refrain from raising your voice higher or louder; instead, pitch your voice lower. If she doesn't understand the first time, use the same wording to repeat your message or question. If she still doesn't understand, wait a few minutes and rephrase the question. Use the names of people and places instead of pronouns or abbreviations.

4. Ask simple, answerable questions. Ask one question at a time; those with yes or no answers work best. Refrain from asking open-ended questions or giving too many choices. For example, ask, "Would you like to wear your white shirt or your blue shirt?" Better still, show her the choices—visual prompts and cues also help clarify your question and can guide her response.

5. Listen with your ears, eyes, and heart. Be patient in waiting for your loved one's reply. If she is struggling for an answer, it's okay to suggest words. Watch for nonverbal cues and body language, and respond appropriately. Always strive to listen for the meaning and feelings that underlie the words.

6. Break down activities into a series of steps. This makes many tasks much more manageable. You can encourage your loved one to do what he can, gently remind him of steps he tends to forget, and assist with steps he's no longer able to accomplish on his own. Using visual cues, such as showing him with your hand where to place the dinner plate, can be very helpful.

7. When the going gets tough, distract and redirect. When your loved one becomes upset, try changing the subject or the environment. For example, ask him for help or suggest going for a walk. It is important to connect with the person on a feeling level, before you redirect. You might say, "I see you're feeling sad—I'm sorry you're upset. Let's go get something to eat."

8. Respond with affection and reassurance. People with dementia often feel confused, anxious, and unsure of themselves. Further, they often get reality confused and may recall things that never really occurred. Avoid trying to convince them they are wrong. Stay focused on the feelings they are demonstrating (which are real) and respond with verbal and physical expressions of comfort, support, and reassurance. Sometimes holding hands, touching, hugging, and praise will get the person to respond when all else fails.

9. Remember the good old days. Remembering the past is often a soothing and affirming activity. Many people with dementia may not remember what happened 45 minutes ago, but they can clearly recall their lives 45 years earlier. Therefore, avoid asking questions that rely on short-term memory, such as asking the person what they had for lunch. Instead, try asking general questions about the person's distant past—this information is more likely to be retained.

10. Maintain your sense of humor. Use humor whenever possible, though not at the person's expense. People with dementia tend to retain their social skills and are usually delighted to laugh along with you.

Handling Troubling Behavior

Some of the greatest challenges of caring for a loved one with dementia are the personality and behavior changes that often occur. You can best meet these challenges by using creativity, flexibility, patience, and compassion. It also helps to not take things personally and maintain your sense of humor.

To start, consider these ground rules:

We cannot change the person. The person you are caring for has a brain disorder that shapes who he has become. When you try to control or change his behavior, you'll most likely be unsuccessful or be met with resistance. It's important to:

- Try to accommodate the behavior, not control the behavior. For example, if the person insists on sleeping on the floor, place a mattress on the floor to make him more comfortable.

- Remember that we can change our behavior or the physical environment. Changing our own behavior will often result in a change in our loved one's behavior.

Check with the doctor first. Behavioral problems may have an underlying medical reason: perhaps the person is in pain or experiencing an adverse side effect from medications. In some cases, like incontinence or hallucinations, there may be some medication or treatment that can assist in managing the problem.

Behavior has a purpose. People with dementia typically cannot tell us what they want or need. They might do something, like take all the clothes out of the closet on a daily basis, and we wonder why. It is very likely that the person is fulfilling a need to be busy and productive. Always consider what need the person might be trying to meet with their behavior—and, when possible, try to accommodate them.

Behavior is triggered. It is important to understand that all behavior is triggered—it doesn't occur out of the blue. It might be something a person did or said that triggered a behavior or it could be a change in the physical environment. The root to changing behavior is disrupting the patterns that we create. Try a different approach, or try a different consequence.

What works today, may not tomorrow. The multiple factors that influence troubling behaviors and the natural progression of the disease process means that solutions that are effective today may need to be modified tomorrow—or may no longer work at all. The key to managing difficult behaviors is being creative and flexible in your strategies to address a given issue.

Get support from others. You are not alone—there are many others caring for someone with dementia. Call your local Area Agency on Aging, the local chapter of the Alzheimer's Association, a Caregiver Resource Center or one of the groups listed below in Resources to find support groups, organizations, and services that can help you. Expect that, like the loved one you are caring for, you will have good days and bad days.

The following is an overview of the most common dementia-associated behaviors with suggestions that may be useful in handling them.

Wandering

People with dementia walk, seemingly aimlessly, for a variety of reasons, such as boredom, medication side effects, or to look for "something" or someone. They also may be trying to fulfill a physical need—thirst, hunger, a need to use the toilet, or exercise. Discovering the triggers for wandering are not always easy, but they can provide insights to dealing with the behavior.

- Make time for regular exercise to minimize restlessness.

- Consider installing new locks that require a key. Position locks high or low on the door; many people with dementia will not think to look beyond eye level. Keep in mind fire and safety concerns for all family members; the locks must be accessible to others and not take more than a few seconds to open.

- Try a barrier like a curtain or colored streamer to mask the door. A "stop" sign or "do not enter" sign also may help.

- Place a black mat or paint a black space on your front porch; this may appear to be an impassable hole to the person with dementia.

- Add "child-safe" plastic covers to doorknobs.

- Consider installing a home security system or monitoring system designed to keep watch over someone with dementia. Also available are new digital devices that can be worn like a watch or clipped on a belt that use global positioning systems (GPS) or other technology to track a person's whereabouts or locate him if he wanders off.

- Put away essential items such as the confused person's coat, purse, or glasses. Some individuals will not go out without certain articles.

- Have your relative wear an ID bracelet and sew ID labels in their clothes. Always have a current photo available should you need to report your loved one missing. Consider leaving a copy on file at the police department or registering the person with the Alzheimer's Association Safe Return program.

- Tell neighbors about your relative's wandering behavior and make sure they have your phone number.

Incontinence

The loss of bladder or bowel control often occurs as dementia progresses. Sometimes accidents result from environmental factors; for example, someone can't remember where the bathroom is located or can't get to it in time. If an accident occurs, your understanding and reassurance will help the person maintain dignity and minimize embarrassment.

- Establish a routine for using the toilet. Try reminding the person or assisting her to the bathroom every two hours.

- Schedule fluid intake to ensure the confused person does not become dehydrated. However, avoid drinks with a diuretic effect like coffee, tea, cola, or beer. Limit fluid intake in the evening before bedtime.

- Use signs (with illustrations) to indicate which door leads to the bathroom.

- A commode, obtained at any medical supply store, can be left in the bedroom at night for easy access.

- Incontinence pads and products can be purchased at the pharmacy or supermarket. A urologist may be able to prescribe a special product or treatment.

- Use easy-to-remove clothing with elastic waistbands or Velcro closures, and provide clothes that are easily washable.

Agitation

Agitation refers to a range of behaviors associated with dementia, including irritability, sleeplessness, and verbal or physical aggression. Often these types of behavior problems progress with the stages of dementia, from mild to more severe. Agitation may be triggered by a variety of things, including environmental factors, fear, and fatigue. Most often, agitation is triggered when the person experiences "control" being taken from him.

- Reduce caffeine intake, sugar, and junk food.

- Reduce noise, clutter, or the number of persons in the room.

- Maintain structure by keeping the same routines. Keep household objects and furniture in the same places. Familiar objects and photographs offer a sense of security and can suggest pleasant memories.

- Try gentle touch, soothing music, reading, or walks to quell agitation. Speak in a reassuring voice. Do not try to restrain the person during a period of agitation.

- Keep dangerous objects out of reach.

- Allow the person to do as much for himself as possible—support his independence and ability to care for himself.

- Acknowledge the confused person's anger over the loss of control in his life. Tell him you understand his frustration.

- Distract the person with a snack or an activity. Allow him to forget the troubling incident. Confronting a confused person may increase anxiety.

Repetitive Speech or Actions (Perseveration)

People with dementia will often repeat a word, statement, question, or activity over and over. While this type of behavior is usually harmless for the person with dementia, it can be annoying and stressful to caregivers. Sometimes the behavior is triggered by anxiety, boredom, fear, or environmental factors.

- Provide plenty of reassurance and comfort, both in words and in touch.

- Try distracting with a snack or activity.

- Avoid reminding them that they just asked the same question. Try ignoring the behavior or question and distract the person into an activity.

- Don't discuss plans with a confused person until immediately prior to an event.

- You may want to try placing a sign on the kitchen table, such as, "Dinner is at 6:30" or "Lois comes home at 5:00" to remove anxiety and uncertainty about anticipated events.

- Learn to recognize certain behaviors. An agitated state or pulling at clothing, for example, could indicate a need to use the bathroom.

Paranoia

Seeing a loved one suddenly become suspicious, jealous, or accusatory is unsettling. Remember, what the person is experiencing is very real to them. It is best not to argue or disagree. This, too, is part of the dementia—try not to take it personally.

- If the confused person suspects money is "missing," allow her to keep small amounts of money in a pocket or handbag for easy inspection.

- Help them look for the object and then distract them into another activity. Try to learn where the confused person's favorite hiding places are for storing objects, which are frequently assumed to be "lost."

- Avoid arguing.

- Take time to explain to other family members and home-helpers that suspicious accusations are a part of the dementing illness.

- Try nonverbal reassurances like a gentle touch or hug. Respond to the feeling behind the accusation and then reassure the person. You might try saying, "I see this frightens you; stay with me, I won't let anything happen to you."

Sleeplessness/Sundowning

Restlessness, agitation, disorientation, and other troubling behavior in people with dementia often get worse at the end of the day and sometimes continue throughout the night. Experts believe this behavior, commonly called sundowning, is caused by a combination of factors, such as exhaustion from the day's events and changes in the person's biological clock that confuse day and night.

- Increase daytime activities, particularly physical exercise. Discourage inactivity and napping during the day.

- Watch out for dietary culprits, such as sugar, caffeine, and some types of junk food. Eliminate or restrict these types of foods and beverages to early in the day. Plan smaller meals throughout the day, including a light meal, such as half a sandwich, before bedtime.

- Plan for the afternoon and evening hours to be quiet and calm; however, structured, quiet activity is important. Perhaps take a stroll outdoors, play a simple card game, or listen to soothing music together.

- Turning on lights well before sunset and closing the curtains at dusk will minimize shadows and may help diminish confusion. At minimum, keep a nightlight in the person's room, hallway, and bathroom.

- Make sure the house is safe: block off stairs with gates, lock the kitchen door, and put away dangerous items.

- As a last resort, consider talking to the doctor about medication to help the agitated person relax and sleep. Be aware that sleeping pills and tranquilizers may solve one problem and create another, such as sleeping at night but being more confused the next day.

- It's essential that you, the caregiver, get enough sleep. If your loved one's nighttime activity keeps you awake, consider asking a friend or relative, or hiring someone, to take a turn so that you can get a good night's sleep. Catnaps during the day also might help.

Eating/Nutrition

Ensuring that your loved one is eating enough nutritious foods and drinking enough fluids is a challenge. People with dementia literally begin to forget that they need to eat and drink. Complicating the issue may be dental problems or medications that decrease appetite or make food taste "funny." The consequences of poor nutrition are many, including weight loss, irritability, sleeplessness, bladder or bowel problems, and disorientation.

- Make meal and snack times part of the daily routine and schedule them around the same time every day. Instead of three big meals, try five or six smaller ones.

- Make mealtimes a special time. Try flowers or soft music. Turn off loud radio programs and the TV.

- Eating independently should take precedence over eating neatly or with "proper" table manners. Finger foods support independence. Pre-cut and season the food. Try using a straw or a child's "sippy cup" if holding a glass has become difficult. Provide assistance only when necessary and allow plenty of time for meals.

- Sit down and eat with your loved one. Often they will mimic your actions and it makes the meal more pleasant to share it with someone.

- Prepare foods with your loved one in mind. If they have dentures or trouble chewing or swallowing, use soft foods or cut food into bite-size pieces.

- If chewing and swallowing are an issue, try gently moving the person's chin in a chewing motion or lightly stroking their throat to encourage them to swallow.

- If loss of weight is a problem, offer nutritious high-calorie snacks between meals. Breakfast foods high in carbohydrates are often preferred. On the other hand, if the problem is weight gain, keep high-calorie foods out of sight. Instead, keep handy fresh fruits, veggie trays, and other healthy low-calorie snacks.

Bathing

People with dementia often have difficulty remembering "good" hygiene, such as brushing teeth, toileting, bathing, and regularly changing their clothes. From childhood we are taught these are highly private and personal activities; to be undressed and cleaned by another can feel frightening, humiliating, and embarrassing. As a result, bathing often causes distress for both caregivers and their loved ones.

- Think historically of your loved one's hygiene routine—did she prefer baths or showers? Mornings or nights? Did she have her hair washed at the salon or do it herself? Was there a favorite scent, lotion, or talcum powder she always used? Adopting—as much as possible—her past bathing routine may provide some comfort. Remember that it may not be necessary to bathe every day—sometimes twice a week is sufficient.

- If your loved one has always been modest, enhance that feeling by making sure doors and curtains are closed. Whether in the shower or the bath, keep a towel over her front, lifting to wash as needed. Have towels and a robe or her clothes ready when she gets out.

- Be mindful of the environment, such as the temperature of the room and water (older adults are more sensitive to heat and cold) and the adequacy of lighting. It's a good idea to use safety features such as non-slip floor bath mats, grab-bars, and bath or shower seats. A hand-held shower might also be a good feature to install. Remember—people are often afraid of falling. Help them feel secure in the shower or tub.

- Never leave a person with dementia unattended in the bath or shower. Have all the bath things you need laid out beforehand. If giving a bath, draw the bath water first. Reassure the person that the water is warm—perhaps pour a cup of water over her hands before she steps in.

- If hair washing is a struggle, make it a separate activity. Or, use a dry shampoo.

- If bathing in the tub or shower is consistently traumatic, a towel bath provides a soothing alter-native. A bed bath has tradition-ally been done with only the most frail and bed-ridden patients, soaping up a bit at a time in their beds, rinsing off with a basin of water and drying with towels. A growing number of nurses in and out of facilities, however, are beginning to recognize its value and a variation—the "towel bath"—for others as well, including people with dementia who find bathing in the tub or shower un-comfortable or unpleasant. The towel bath uses a large bath towel and washcloths dampened in a plastic bag of warm water and no-rinse soap. Large bath-blankets are used to keep the patient cov-ered, dry and warm while the dampened towel and washcloths are massaged over the body.

Additional Problem Areas

- Dressing is difficult for most dementia patients. Choose loose-fitting, comfortable clothes with easy zippers or snaps and minimal buttons. Reduce the person's choices by removing seldom-worn clothes from the closet. To facilitate dressing and support independence, lay out one article of clothing at a time, in the order it is to be worn. Remove soiled clothes from the room. Don't argue if the person insists on wearing the same thing again.

- Hallucinations (seeing or hearing things that others don't) and delusions (false beliefs, such as someone is trying to hurt or kill another) may occur as the dementia progresses. State simply and calmly your perception of the situation, but avoid arguing or trying to convince the person their perceptions are wrong. Keep rooms well-lit to decrease shadows, and offer reassurance and a simple explanation if the curtains move from circulating air or a loud noise such as a plane or siren is heard. Distractions may help. Depending on the severity of symptoms, you might consider medication.

- Sexually inappropriate behavior, such as masturbating or undressing in public, lewd remarks, unreasonable sexual demands, even sexually aggressive or violent behavior, may occur during the course of the illness. Remember, this behavior is caused by the disease. Talk to the doctor about possible treatment plans. Develop an action plan to follow before the behavior occurs, that is, what you will say and do if the behavior happens at home, around other adults, or children. If you can, identify what triggers the behavior.

- Verbal outbursts such as cursing, arguing, and threatening often are expressions of anger or stress. React by staying calm and reassuring. Validate your loved one's feelings and then try to distract or redirect his attention to something else.

- "Shadowing" is when a person with dementia imitates and follows the caregiver, or constantly talks, asks questions and interrupts. Like sundowning, this behavior often occurs late in the day and can be irritating for caregivers. Comfort the person with verbal and physical reassurance. Distraction or redirection might also help. Giving your loved one a job such as folding laundry might help to make her feel needed and useful.

- People with dementia may become uncooperative and resistant to daily activities such as bathing, dressing, and eating. Often this is a response to feeling out of control, rushed, afraid, or confused by what you are asking of them. Break each task into steps and, in a reassuring voice, explain each step before you do it. Allow plenty of time. Find ways to have them assist to their ability in the process, or follow with an activity that they can perform.

Chapter 43

Understanding Alzheimer-Related Sleep Problems

Sleep and Alzheimer Disease

The problem with Alzheimer disease, as well as other forms of dementia, is that the disease has negative effects on the sleep/wake cycle. The greater the degree of dementia, the sleepier the patient is. With more severe forms of dementia, patients are often sleepier during the day, and their sleep at night tends to be fragmented and disrupted. Over a 24-hour period, for example, patients are rarely awake and rarely asleep for a full hour at a time. They are constantly waking up at night and falling asleep during the day. This pattern is fairly common in Alzheimer patients.

Many Alzheimer patients experience what is called "sundowning": agitated behavior that is thought to occur primarily after the sun goes down; for example, pacing, yelling out, or getting violent. This behavior is usually repetitive. Sundowning can include wandering around at night. Wandering and incontinence are the top two causes of institutionalization, because the family member has great difficultly taking care of a patient who displays one characteristic or the other.

This chapter begins with "Sleep and Alzheimer's Disease," by Sonia Ancoli-Israel, PhD, © 2001 National Sleep Foundation (www.sleepfoundation.org). All rights reserved. Reprinted with permission. Text under the heading "Caregivers Can Help Patients with Alzheimer's Disease Sleep Better by Using Behavioral Techniques," is reprinted with permission from the American Geriatrics Society Foundation for Health in Aging (http://www.healthinaging.org/) from the Aging in the Know website (http://www.healthinaging.org/agingintheknow/). For more information visit the AGS online at www.americangeriatrics.org.

393

It's important to realize that sundowning doesn't always occur after sundown; it can take place all day long and frequently peaks around 12:30–1:00 p.m. It is just easier for the family member to cope with a behavior like wandering during the day than at night, when it is more disruptive.

What can I do as a caregiver?

Unfortunately, there is no silver bullet. There are medications that are used to try to bring agitated behavior and sleep under control. Sometimes these medications make the patient better, sometimes worse. It is important to talk with the patient's physician about the advantages and disadvantages of medication in treating forms of dementia.

Fortunately, there are some things you can do at home to help improve the patient's behavior:

- Keep the patient on as regular a schedule as possible. Get her out of bed at the same time each morning, and put her to bed at the same time each night. Try to discourage her from taking multiple naps during the day—one nap in the afternoon is all right, as long as it lasts no more than an hour. During the day, keep the patient as active as possible.

- It's also important to get the patient to eat her meals at a regular time each day. In fact, the more routine there is in the schedule, the better the patient is able to cope with the effects of Alzheimer disease.

- It is important to expose the patient to as much bright light as possible. In a nursing home, most patients are exposed to bright light for only 10 minutes a day. Generally in the community, patients are exposed to about 30 minutes a day. Even this is not enough. It would be better if the patient were exposed to bright light for several hours a day. Take her outside whenever possible, especially in the morning. Morning light offers the best exposure, because in a patient with dementia, their circadian (biological) rhythm is out of sync with the rhythm of the environment. Bright light improves their functioning and makes them more alert.

- It is also important that the environment be dark at night. If the patient tends to wander at night and you are worried about her falling or bumping into furniture, you can keep a nightlight on. But understand that bright light interferes with circadian rhythms. Otherwise, keep the patient's bedroom as dark as possible. You should also keep the environment as quiet as possible during the night.

- Avoid caffeine products such as coffee, tea, chocolate, or soda, because they interfere with the circadian rhythm.

- Exercise is very important. Have her do whatever she is capable of doing: for example, take the patient on a short walk every day on a regular basis, and engage her in throwing a beach ball. Even if she has to use a wheelchair, encourage her to do arm exercises.

Are there other health problems I should look for?

One of the characteristics of dementia is sleep disordered breathing. More than 80 percent of dementia patients have sleep apnea. If we can treat them successfully for sleep apnea, we might be able to improve their sleep at night and their alertness during the day. Speak to the patient's physician about this possibility.

Improving sleep at night and functioning during the day helps to postpone institutionalization, which would be better for the patient and the family and would save tens of millions of dollars.

by Sonia Ancoli-Israel, PhD, Professor of Psychiatry at the University of California, San Diego. She is also Director of the Sleep Disorders Clinic at the Veterans Affairs San Diego Healthcare System. Dr. Ancoli-Israel is author of All I Want Is a Good Night's Sleep.

Caregivers Can Help Patients with Alzheimer Disease Sleep Better by Using Behavioral Techniques

Sleep problems are common among patients with Alzheimer disease (AD). Many AD patients sleep and nap during the day and wake up many times throughout the night. As many as 44% of patients with AD have sleep problems.

Problems sleeping at night can be very draining for the family members caring for AD patients living at home. Caregivers can be wakened at night by the AD patient who may get out of bed repeatedly, wander around, and talk while in bed. Such nighttime disturbances can lead to physical and psychological problems for caregivers and patients. Nighttime disturbances are also the reason many caregivers place AD patients into nursing homes.

New Research in the Journal of the American Geriatrics Society

The National Institutes of Health has called for more research into ways to improve the sleep/wake patterns of AD patients that do not involve drug therapy. Recently, researchers conducted a study designed to evaluate whether a comprehensive sleep education program called Nighttime Insomnia Treatment and Education for Alzheimer's Disease (NITE-AD) could improve the sleep patterns of AD patients living with family caregivers in the community.

The researchers worked with 36 AD patients and their caregivers. There were 17 assigned to receive the active treatment and 19 to receive general dementia education and usual caregiver support. All participants received written educational materials about age- and dementia-related changes in sleep and good sleep practices. In addition, the treatment group received specific information about setting up and performing a sleep hygiene program and training in behavior management skills. Patients in the treatment group also participated in walking exercise daily and increased their exposure to daytime light. This research study measured participants' sleep and mood before treatment began and again at two months and six months after treatment.

Patients and caregivers in both groups participated in six 1-hour sessions in the home with a psychologist about the behavioral interventions to be used. For all participants, the first session was spent learning about good sleep practices, sleep changes related to normal aging, and ideas to improve the sleep of patients with AD.

The researchers then helped caregivers in the treatment group develop an individual sleep hygiene program for the AD patient that included setting up a specified time to go to bed and wake up, no napping after 1:00 P.M., and no naps lasting more than 30 minutes. The researchers suggested ways to reduce nighttime waking, such as eliminating disruptions from outside noise and other causes of sleep disruptions in the home. AD patients in this group also began a program of walking for 30 minutes daily and receiving one hour of light exposure from a light box.

Two months after the study began, the researchers found that the treatment group spent 32% less time awake at night and had 32% fewer nighttime awakenings than before the study began. This translates into 36 minutes more nighttime sleep than the non-treatment group and 5.3 fewer nighttime awakenings than the control group. At the six month follow-up, significant differences remained between the treatment group and the control group for patient time awake at night, exercise days, and depression. In addition, patients in the treatment group had significantly fewer awakenings per hour and stayed awake for less time than patients in the non-treatment group.

This study showed that AD patients can improve their sleep patterns after participating in a treatment program that trains caregivers about behavioral strategies to improve sleep. Improvements found at the 2-month follow-up were maintained at the 6-month follow-up.

This study was small, and not all participants completed the study. Yet, it shows that patients with AD living in the home can benefit from behavioral techniques to improve sleep, which can be an alternative or addition to medication. Improvements in sleep benefit the quality of life for both the AD patient and the caregiver. Larger studies in the future may be able to determine whether such treatment programs that improve sleep can delay nursing home placement.

The summary above is from the full report entitled "Nighttime Insomnia Treatment and Education for Alzheimer Disease (NITE-AD): A Randomized Controlled Trial." It is in the May 2005 issue of the *Journal of the American Geriatrics Society* (Volume 53, Issue 5, pages 609-618). The report is authored by Susan M. McCurry, PhD, Laura E. Gibbons, PhD, Rebecca G. Logsdon, PhD, Michael V. Vitiello, PhD, and Linda Teri, PhD.

Chapter 44

Coping with Problems Related to Sexual Behaviors

Alzheimer disease changes the functioning of a person's brain. When that happens, the person's sexual behavior can change. Some people may forget appropriate public behavior and undress or fondle themselves. Some may use vulgar words or act sexually aggressive toward a spouse or others. Still others may lose interest in sex altogether. It's important to remember that changes in sexual behavior are not reflections of the person's character—they're symptoms of the disease. As a caregiver, it's also important to get the support you need to deal with your own feelings about such behavior.

Understand Causes of Behavior

- Get a medical evaluation for a person who shows either an excessive interest or no interest in sex.

- Realize that sexuality and the need for touching are human drives.

- Explore the possibility that the person craves affection and affirmation.

"Sexuality" is reprinted with permission of the Alzheimer's Association. For additional information, call the Alzheimer's Association toll-free helpline, 800-272-2900, or visit their website at www.alz.org. © 2006 Alzheimer's Association. All rights reserved.

- Consider possible reasons for inappropriate undressing:
  - Time of day. The person may simply want to get ready for sleep.
  - Clothing that's too tight.
  - Hot weather or an overheated room.
  - The person may need to use the toilet.
- Consider possible reasons for sexual displays and inappropriate or aggressive advances:
  - Loss of inhibition due to changes in the brain.
  - Insatiable desire due to changes in the brain.
  - Misunderstood circumstances.
  - Mistaking someone for one's partner.
  - Forgetfulness.
  - Boredom.
- Consider the possible reasons for reduced sexual desire:
  - Physical illness.
  - Hormonal imbalance.
  - Side effect of medication.
  - Depression.
  - Sensing a partner's emotional withdrawal.

Be Matter-of-Fact

- Do not overreact or express shock.
- Avoid becoming angry or arguing.
- Don't shame or ridicule the person.
- Try gently reminding the person when a behavior is inappropriate.
- Remember to be sensitive and reassuring. Acknowledge that masturbation feels good before distracting the person or gently relocating him or her to a private area.

Distract or Redirect

- Be aware of conditions that may provoke excessive sexual interest.

- Firmly set clear limits for behavior.

- Redirect the person to a meaningful or favorite activity.

- Postpone. Tell the person, "Later. Right now we must do ..."

- Provide a reality check. For example, the daughter of a man who often mistakes her for his wife, always greets him by saying, "Hi Dad."

- Respond to feelings of rejection, loneliness, or a need for closeness with gentle talk, a caring pat, or a hug. Establish a balance; over responding may encourage unwanted sexual behavior.

Adjust to Changes in Desire

- Come to terms with the knowledge that your sexual relationship will change.

- Adjust to your partner's excessive desire. Redirect the person to masturbation. Consider separate bedrooms.

- Adjust to your partner's reduced desire. Get a medical evaluation for your partner. Lack of desire could stem from physical problems or be a side effect of medication.

- Retain a sense of intimacy by sharing touch and reminiscing together.

- Prepare yourself for the time when your partner no longer recognizes you. Try not to take this change personally. It's normal to feel lonely and rejected.

- Know that it's common, if sexual relations continue, for the caregiver to feel a sense of guilt.

- Know that it may be possible to continue a caring sexual relationship if you take the lead.

- Realize that it's common for a caregiver to lose sexual desire because of the demands of caregiving, the changing role from intimate partner to caregiver, and changes taking place in the person's personality.

Take Care of Yourself

- Do what feels best for you.

- Do not feel guilty if you are no longer attracted to your partner and want to end the sexual relationship. Find new ways to connect with each other.

- Consider dating, if it feels right for you.

- Know that there is no right or wrong approach.

- Join a support group.

Chapter 45

Hiring In-Home Help

Most family caregivers reach a point when they realize they need help at home. Tell-tale signs include recognizing that your loved one requires constant supervision or assistance with everyday activities, such as bathing and dressing. Caregivers also find that certain housekeeping routines and regular errands are accomplished with great difficulty or are left undone. It may become apparent that in order to take care of any business outside the home, more than one caregiver is required.

Assessing Your Home-Care Needs

A number of options are available for finding help at home. It is often best to start by assessing both your needs as a caregiver and the needs of the person you are caring for. There are a variety of checklists to help you evaluate what types of help are needed. In general, consider the following areas:

- **Personal care:** bathing, eating, dressing, toileting

- **Household care:** cooking, cleaning, laundry, shopping

- **Health care:** medication management, physician's appointments, physical therapy

- **Emotional care:** companionship, meaningful activities, conversation

It is also important to evaluate the values and preferences of the person receiving care. He or she may be more comfortable with a home care worker who shares his or her cultural background and language. The care recipient may also have a preference between male and female caregivers, particularly if the worker will be helping with personal care.

This assessment may also enable you to include alternative (and possibly less expensive) approaches to care such as adult day care, friendly visiting services, home grocery delivery, pharmacy delivery services, and meals-on-wheels programs.

Writing a Job Description

Once you have identified the types of help you need, writing a job description can be fairly straightforward. In addition to including the tasks you have identified from your assessment, be sure to include the following when and if appropriate:

- Health care training (what level and what type—CNA, LVN, RN)

- Driving (car needed or only valid driver's license)

- Ability to lift care recipient or operate special equipment

- Experience with people with memory impairments or other disabilities

- Language skills

- Any other special skills needed

At this point, you have the option of hiring an individual or going through a home care or home health care agency. In some states, publicly-funded programs may allow you to hire another family member to

Table 45.1. Checklists

A number of checklists are available to help in evaluating what types of help are needed. Here are some recommended ones:

- *Needs Assessment Worksheet* from Family Care America, available at www.familycareamerica.com or 804-342-2337

- *Helping My Parents: How Do I Know If They Need Help* from AARP, available at http://www.aarp.org/families/caregiving/caring_parents/a2003-10-27-caregiving-needhelp.html or 800-424-3410

assist you in providing care at home. In making that decision, consider the following:

Home Care Agency

Pros

- Screening, hiring/firing, pay, and taxes are handled by the agency. (Note: There are also some agencies that will handle the paperwork, like taxes and social security, if you hire a home care worker on your own.)

- If the worker is sick, a substitute can be sent.

- Can provide individuals with a variety of skills to meet varying needs (for example, skilled nursing care, physical therapy, occupational therapy).

- May be partially covered by Medicaid or private insurance.

Cons

- Often several workers are used which can be confusing or distressing for the person receiving care.

- Less individual choice in workers.

- More expensive than privately hiring an individual.

Privately Hired Home Care Worker

Pros

- A strong one-on-one relationship can develop between the worker and the person receiving care, although this can also happen through an agency when there is a commitment to continuity.

- Usually less expensive than going through an agency.

- You get to choose the person you think will be the best to provide care to your loved one.

Cons

- If the home care worker is sick, no substitute is readily available.

- Screening, hiring/firing, pay, and taxes must be handled by you.

- May not be covered by Medicaid or private insurance.

Developing a Job Contract

The job contract is based upon the job description. It formalizes the agreement between you, the employer, and the employee, and is signed by both of you. Should questions or problems come up later, either party can refer to the written agreement. A good work contract should include the following:

- Name of employer and "household employee"

- Wages (including tax withholding) and benefits (for example, mileage, meals, vacation, holidays)

- When and how payment will be made

- Hours of work

- Employee's Social Security number

- Duties to be performed (the job description)

- Unacceptable behavior (for example, smoking, abusive language, tardiness)

- Termination (how much notice, reasons for termination without notice)

- Dated signatures of employee and employer

Finding the Right Home Care Worker

Set aside some time as you approach this critical next step: finding the appropriate person to fit the job description. One of the best ways to find a helper is to get a personal recommendation from a trusted relative or friend. Churches, synagogues, senior centers, Independent Living Centers, and local college career centers, especially those which have nursing or social work programs, are good places to advertise for in-home help. Listings for these places can be found in your local phone book.

Most communities have attendant registries that can be an excellent resource for finding in-home help because they typically provide some initial screening of applicants. When calling an attendant registry (generally listed under Nurses and Nurse Registries in the phone book), it is important to inquire about their particular screening process and training requirements as well as about any fees charged. While some are free, fees for using a registry can vary greatly. It is a good idea to shop around and obtain the best service at an affordable price. There are also nonprofit community agencies (generally listed under *Social & Human Services for Individuals & Families* in the phone book) that maintain lists of individuals available to perform all kinds of household tasks, from cleaning and laundry to repairs and gardening.

If all of these sources fail to produce an in-home worker, you may choose to advertise in the "Help Wanted" classified section of a community college, local paper, or neighborhood newsletter. The advertisement, at the minimum, should include hours, a brief description of duties, telephone number, and best time to call, for example: "Home Care Assistant needed to provide supervision and companionship to older adult with memory loss. Must be compassionate, reliable, and able to assist with bathing, dressing, and eating. References required. Call to apply."

Locating Resources in Your Community

One place to begin your search is with your local Area Agency on Aging (AAA). To find the AAA nearest to you, call the Eldercare Locator at 800-677-1116 or visit the AAA website at www.n4a.org. Your AAA can provide the following:

- Information about attendant registries
- Lists of home care agencies
- Tax help for seniors
- Suggestions for places to advertise in your community

Interviewing the Applicant

You do not have to hold a face-to-face interview with every person who applies for the job. Some screening over the telephone is appropriate. In screening applicants over the telephone, caregivers should describe the job in detail and state specific expectations listed in the work contract as well as information about the hours and wages. At this time, it is also important to ask about the applicant's past experience and whether he/she has references. If the applicant sounds acceptable, then an interview should be scheduled. Consider having another family member, the care recipient (if appropriate), or friend sit in on the interview to provide a second opinion.

In preparation for the interview, the caregiver should have a list of questions pertinent to the job description and a sample work contract ready for the applicant to read. The following are some suggested questions for the interview:

- Where have you worked before?

- What were your duties?

- How do you feel about caring for a disabled person? Or a person with memory problems?

- Have you had experience cooking for other people?

- How do you handle people who are angry, stubborn, or fearful?

- Do you have a car? Would you be able to transfer someone from a wheelchair into a car or into a bed?

- What days and hours would you be available? How many hours per week?

- Is there anything in the job description that you are uncomfortable doing?

- Can you give me two work-related and one personal reference?

Consider what qualities/skills you require and what you can train a good candidate to do.

Be sure that you have a chance to watch the interactions between the in-home worker and the family member for whom he or she will be providing care. You may want to do this at the end of the interview with individuals you feel are good candidates, or you may want to invite the top two candidates back to meet with your family member. If your family member is able, he or she should be included in the interview process and in making the final decision.

Immediately after the interview, it is important for you to write down first impressions, and if possible, discuss these with another family member or friend. Consider the person most qualified for the job and with whom you feel most comfortable. Always check the references of at least two final applicants. Don't wait too long to make an offer, as good applicants may find another job. If the job offer is accepted, you and the in-home helper should set a date to sign the contract and begin work. Both employer and employee should keep a copy of the contract.

Using the Internet in Your Search

Several websites have listings of home care agencies and additional information on finding and evaluating home care services:

- Homecare Online: www.nahc.org
- Extended Care Information Network: www.extendedcare.com

What Are the Employer's Responsibilities?

As an employer of a "household employee," there are several legal considerations. First, household employers should verify that their household insurance (renter's or homeowner's) covers household employees in case of an accident. It is also imperative that the employer be fully informed of the legal responsibility of paying taxes for household employees.

As the employer, you may also be responsible for withholding Social Security taxes, Medicare taxes or federal unemployment tax, and filing them with the Internal Revenue Service annually or quarterly. Social Security taxes are owed by both the employer and the employee. Rules governing the amount(s) to be withheld and payment schedules can change annually. For information on paying federal taxes for household employees, call (800) TAX-FORM and ask for Publication 926 or view it on the web at www.irs.gov/formspubs/index.html.

There are also state regulations. Some states require that employers pay state tax and/or state disability insurance. To find out the regulations in your state, call the state employment department listed in the government section of your local phonebook. The penalties for not paying taxes on household employees include paying the back taxes and paying interest and penalty fines.

There is one other requirement that every employer should know. Each employee is required to fill out an Employment Eligibility Verification form I-9 and a record of this should be kept on file. This form verifies that the person is legally entitled to work in the United States. The form can be downloaded from the web at www.irs.gov/formspubs/index.html or ordered by calling (800) TAX-FORM.

The Family Caregiver Alliance (FCA) advises that household employers and employees stay informed and comply with state and federal tax laws. There are often local services available to seniors who need assistance in filing tax statements for household employees.

Making Your Home Care Situation Work

The relationships between the family, the person who requires assistance, and the in-home worker are very important. Consequently, it is imperative that you take the time to go carefully through the selection process. Good communication is essential for a good relationship.

Schedule regular times to meet and discuss concerns, problems, and changes. It is also important to make expectations clear and to provide adequate training to meet those expectations. If you hire a home care worker on your own, it is important you feel comfortable both providing training and firing the worker if necessary. If the person you have hired is doing a great job, be sure to tell him or her. A smile and well-deserved praise can make a big difference. None of us likes to feel that our work is not appreciated.

Chapter 46

Handling Hospitalizations

Hospitalization Happens: A Guide to Hospital Visits for Loved Ones with Memory Disorders

A trip to the hospital with a loved one who has a memory disorder can be stressful for both of you. This chapter can relieve some of that stress by helping you prepare for both unexpected and planned hospital visits. In it you will find steps you can take now to make hospital visits as easy as possible, tips on making your loved one more comfortable once you arrive at the hospital, and advice on working with hospital staff and doctors.

Share this information with family and friends, keep this information in a handy spot and prepare now for the future.

Hospital Emergencies: What You Can Do Now

Planning ahead is the key to making either an unexpected or a planned trip to the hospital easier for you and your loved one. Here is what you should do now:

- Register your relative for a SAFE RETURN bracelet through your local Alzheimer's Association chapter. People who are lost

This chapter includes "Hospitalization Happens: A Guide to Hospital Visits for Loved Ones with Memory Disorders," and "Acute Hospitalization and Alzheimer's Disease: A Special Kind of Care," © 2006 North Carolina Department of Health and Human Services, Division of Aging and Adult Services (www.ncdhhs.gov/aging). Reprinted with permission.

may be taken to an emergency room. The bracelet will speed the process of reconnecting you and your loved one.

- Know who you can count on. You need a family member or trusted friend to stay with your loved one when he or she is admitted to the emergency room or hospital. Have at least two dependable family members, neighbors, or friends you can call on to go with you or meet you at the hospital at a moment's notice so that one of you can take care of the paperwork and the other can stay with your loved one.

- Pack an "Emergency Bag" containing the following:

  - A sheet of paper listing: the person's name, nickname, address, insurance companies (include policy numbers and pre-authorization phone numbers), Medicare and Medicaid card numbers, doctors (include addresses).

  - A list of important phone numbers such as doctors, key family members, minister, and helpful friends.

  - A list of all current medicines and dosage instructions. This list should be updated when there is any change.

  - A list of medicines taken that have ever caused a bad reaction and a list of any allergies to medicines and foods.

  - Copies of important papers such as Durable Power of Attorney, Health Care Power of Attorney, Living Will.

  - Extra adult briefs (for example, Depends) if the person usually wears them. These may not be easy to get in the emergency room if you need them.

  - A change of clothes in case the person's clothes become soiled or torn and a plastic bag for the soiled clothing.

  - A card that says, "Please Understand—My companion has a memory disorder. Let me help with specific questions." You should avoid talking about your relative's memory changes or behaviors in front of him. This can be upsetting and embarrassing to your relative.

  - Moist hand wipes such as Wet Ones.

  - A reassuring object, a Walkman with a favorite tape or a portable radio.

- A writing pad and pen so that you can jot down information and directions given to you by hospital staff. You will also want to write down your loved one's symptoms and problems. You might be asked the same questions by many people. Show them what you have written instead of repeating your answers.

- Pain medicine such as Advil, Tylenol, or aspirin. This is for you, the caregiver. A trip to the ER may take longer than you think. Stress can lead to a headache or other symptoms.

- A sealed snack such as a pack of crackers and a bottle of water or juice for you and your loved one. You could wait for quite a while.

- A small amount of cash.

- If you have a cellular phone, put a note on the outside of the "Emergency Bag" to take the phone with you.

By taking these steps in advance you will greatly reduce the stress and confusion that can often accompany a hospital visit particularly if the visit is an unplanned trip to the emergency room.

At the Emergency Room

A trip to the emergency room may tire or even frighten your loved one. There are some important things to remember:

- Be patient. It could be a long wait if the reason for your visit is not life-threatening. Know that results from lab tests take time.

- Offer physical comfort and verbal reassurance to your relative. Stay calm and confident.

- Realize that just because you do not see staff at work, does not mean they are not working.

- Be aware that emergency room staff often has little training in Alzheimer disease so help them understand your loved one.

- Do not assume your loved one will be admitted to the hospital.

- Do not leave the ER to go home without a follow-up plan. If you are sent home, make sure you have all instructions for follow-up care.

Before a Hospital Stay

If your loved one is going to the hospital for a planned stay, you have time to prepare and ask your doctor questions. Ask your doctor if the procedure can be done as an outpatient visit. If not, ask if tests can be done before going to the hospital to shorten the hospital stay. Ask if your doctor plans to talk with other doctors. If so, find out if your relative can see these specialists before going into the hospital.

You should also ask questions about anesthesia, catheters, and IVs. General anesthesia can have side effects. Ask if local anesthesia is an option and if you will be allowed in the recovery room.

Before Going to the Hospital

- If your insurance allows, ask for a private room if possible. It is more quiet and calm.

- Let your loved one take part in the planning for the hospital stay as much as possible.

- Don't talk about the hospital stay in front of your relative as if s/he is not there.

- Plan ahead. Make a schedule with family and friends to take turns sitting with your relative during the entire hospital stay.

- Shortly before going to the hospital, decide the best way to tell your loved one that the two of you are going to spend a short time in the hospital.

- When packing, include a copy of important papers such as a living will and health care power of attorney.

Pack comfort items. Things to help your loved one feel safe and secure such as favorite clothes or blankets and photos.

During the Hospital Stay

- Have someone with your loved one at all times if possible— even during medical tests. This may be hard to do, but it will help keep your loved one calm and make the hospital stay easier for him.

- Ask doctors to limit their questions to your relative who may not be able to answer. Instead, answer questions from the doctor outside your relative's room.

- Ask the staff to avoid using physical restraints.

- Help your relative fill out menu requests.

- Open food containers and remove trays.

- Talk with your loved one in the way he will best understand.

- Remind your relative to drink fluids. Offer fluids and have him make regular trips to the bathroom.

- Know that a strange place, medicines, tests, and surgery will make a person with Alzheimer disease more confused. S/he will need more help with personal care.

- Assume your relative will have problems finding the bathroom and using his/her call button.

Sudden confusion can be caused by a medical problem. Ask the doctor if your loved one seems suddenly worse.

If Anxiety or Agitation Occurs

Try some of the following:

- Remove street clothes from sight.

- Post reminders or cues if this comforts your relative.

- Turn off the television, the telephone ringer, and the intercom.

- Talk in a calm voice and offer reassurance. Repeat answers to questions.

- Give a comforting touch or distract your loved one with offers of snacks.

- Listen to soothing music or try comforting rituals.

- Slow down, try not to rush your loved one.

Working with Hospital Staff

Remember that not everyone in the hospital knows the same basic facts about memory loss and Alzheimer disease. You may be their best teacher of what works with your family member.

You can help the staff by giving them a list of your loved one's normal routine; personal habits; likes and dislikes; possible behaviors, what might cause them and how you handle them; and signs of pain or discomfort.

You should:

- Make the list easy to read with headings and short, simple statements. Have a copy with the chart and at the nurse's station.

- Decide with the hospital staff who will do what for your loved one. For example, you may want to be the one who helps your family member get a bath, eat, or use the toilet.

- Think about placing a poster above the head of the bed with key information, including names of people important to your loved one and the relationship (spouse, cousin, friend).

- Tell the staff about any unusual behaviors, hearing problems, or communication problems your relative may have and offer ideas for what works best in those instances.

- Make sure your family member is safe, tell the staff about any previous problems with wandering, getting lost, suspiciousness, or falls.

- Not assume the staff knows your loved one's needs. Tell them in a nice, calm manner.

- Ask questions when you don't understand hospital procedures, tests, or when you have a concern.

- Realize that hospital staff are caring for many people and practice the art of patience.

Make Contact with National Resources

The following agencies can provide you with information about Alzheimer disease, assist you through caregiver support groups or connect you with community resources:

- Alzheimer's Association: 800-272-3900 www.alz.org

- Eldercare Locator: 800-677-1116 www.eldercare.gov

- For educational and training materials, contact the Alzheimer's Disease Education and Referral (ADEAR) Center at 800-438-4380 or visit them on the internet at www.alzheimers.nia.nih .gov

Acute Hospitalization and Alzheimer Disease: A Special Kind of Care

A new environment filled with strange sights, odors, and sounds, a change in the daily routine, medications, and tests, and the disease process itself can all be factors that increase confusion, anxiety, and agitation in a hospitalized individual with Alzheimer disease. This information will help you to meet the needs of these patients. In it you will find facts about communication tips, personal care techniques, suggestions for working with behaviors, and environmental factors to consider in the ER and in the hospital room.

When hospitalization occurs, the best option for the individual with Alzheimer disease is the constant presence of a family member or a trusted friend. Because this may not always be possible, this section hopes to serve as a guide in helping you understand and practice the many facets of care for your patient with memory disorder.

Remember, family members are your most valuable resource for information about the individual and the caregiving techniques that work best.

More Than Just Words: Effective Communication Techniques

Communicating with an Alzheimer disease patient can be challenging, but remember, decreased verbal communication does not mean decreased awareness. Most patients are very aware and feel a great deal of distress about their increased loss of ability.

General Rules of Thumb

Reality orientation does not work. Instead, use memory aids such as labeling objects (for example, closet, bathroom). Be aware that as Alzheimer disease progresses, an individual's ability to name objects and use words decreases.

Simplify the environment for Alzheimer patients. Eliminate distracting noises such as the radio or TV, or loud conversation.

Do not use the in-room intercom to communicate. The patient may be frightened or confused by hearing a voice only.

Communication Tips

- Always begin by identifying yourself and calling the patient's name.

417

- Always approach from the front.

- Maintain good eye contact.

- Use short, simple sentences.

- Speak slowly.

- Be specific. Use the name of the person or object instead of "this" or "they."

- Keep tone of voice low and pleasant.

- Keep facial expression warm and friendly.

- Use non-verbal cues: a reassuring touch, a smile, a demonstration stating the emotion.

- Give the person plenty of time to respond to your question (20 seconds).

- Always repeat your question exactly the same way.

- Use concrete language.

- State in positive terms. Constant use of "no" or commands increases resistance.

- Don't test the patient's memory. Erase the words, "Don't you remember?" from your vocabulary.

- Give directions simply and one at a time.

- When helping with personal care, tell the patient what you are doing each step of the way. Add occasional social or reassuring comments to avoid "task-focused talk" only.

- Do not appear rushed or tense. The patient will become tense and agitated.

- Listen to the patient. Try to find the key thought and take note of the feeling or emotion being expressed along with the spoken word.

- Reassure through words. Remind the patient who you are and that you will take care of him.

- Sometimes asking a "Why" question can get to the reason behind a repetitive question and decrease its occurrence (for example, "Why are you concerned about what time it is?").

In the Emergency Room: Assessment Tips

- Do not leave the patient alone. A family member, trusted caregiver, or friend should be present at all times.

- Continuous cueing to the environment (place) and activity may be necessary. A family member can assist with this and offer reassurance as well.

- Obtain patient's history from a close relative or caregiver.

- Pay close attention to the caregiver's description of the patient's usual level of consciousness. Increased dementia or the onset of delirium can be a sign of acute physical illness or metabolic distress.

- Perform a complete head to toe assessment. The patient may not be able to automatically identify painful or affected areas to you.

- Before every communication with the patient, make sure you have his attention by calling his name and making direct eye contact with him. Your eyes should be level with the patient's eyes.

- Ask simple "yes" and "no" questions. Allow ample response time (at least 20 seconds).

- Watch for non-verbal communication of pain or discomfort such as grimacing, guarding, or anger.

- Apologize each time you cause pain and avoid repeating painful exams.

- In short, simple statements, tell the patient what you are doing, why and that you will be finished soon. Repeat this throughout the examination.

- Never talk about the patient to others as if he is not in the room.

General Guidelines for Hospital Staff

For an Alzheimer disease patient, the trauma or ailment that preceded hospitalization, the strange new environment, the disrupted daily routine, and the influence of medications can all be factors for increased confusion and decreased ability.

There are a number of things you can do to reassure your patient. You should:

- Provide a consistent, predictable routine. Ask the primary caregiver for the patient's usual routine and follow it as closely as possible.

- Encourage the use of security objects from home (favorite pillow or quilt).

- Provide care by the same nurses and nursing assistants as much as possible.

- Avoid surrounding the patient with several doctors and medical students at one time.

- Evaluate the patient for sources of potential pain and discomfort. Even though he may be experiencing pain, the patient will probably not verbally complain.

- When possible, schedule tests at a time of day when the patient is at his best and not fatigued.

- Discontinue asking orientation questions once the patient's level of comprehension is established.

- Use good communication techniques.

- Schedule at least two rest periods: A half hour after morning care and an hour in early afternoon. Rest is important!

- Post rest period times on the patient's door. Use a big "Resting" or "Do Not Disturb" sign during the actual rest period.

- Limit visitors to one or two at a time.

- Cue the patient for sleep by darkening and quieting the room.

- Avoid using physical restraints. They do not prevent falls. Injuries from falls while the patient is restrained are often more serious.

Room Service: Assessing the Environment

- Avoid numerous room changes. Change increases confusion and anxiety.

- Avoid placing the patient in a room located in a high noise, high traffic area.

- Keep the television off until the patient turns it on or requests it.

- Remove artwork containing people or animals if the patient interprets them as real-life intruders.

- Keep lighting as free of shadows and glare as possible.

- Avoid clutter. It can increase confusion, agitation, and the risk of falls.

- If the patient can understand written words, then large, bold lettered signs can serve as cues to the bathroom, closet, and personal items.

Providing the Essentials: Comfort and Safety

Comfort

- Always communicate a sense of security, caring, and respect.

- Each staff/patient interaction should include: touch, eye contact, orienting information, and an activity the patient can successfully perform.

- Eyeglasses, dentures, and hearing aids can enhance the patient's communication. Offer to assist the patient with placement of these devices. Be aware in some instances the patient is more comfortable without them.

- If the patient has a comfort item, something that makes him feel secure, make sure it is within reach.

Safety

- Provide a safe, structured environment.

- Provide consistent staff to attend the patient.

- Place the patient in a room that allows easy and careful observation.

- Place bed in low position.

- Don't leave anything at the bedside that might harm the patient.

- Elopement precautions: Place the patient in a room where he has to pass the nursing station in order to reach an exit. Have a photo of the patient on file.

Positive Approaches to Personal Care: Activities of Daily Living

Eating

- Do not ask the patient to fill out a menu. Ask the family about food preferences.

- Simplify the food tray. Keep small, colored dishes on the unit to allow for smaller portions and the ability to offer one or two food items at a time.

- Smaller, more frequent meals may work better for the patient than the standard three large meals.

- Cueing the patient to eat by using verbal reminders along with a light touch to the forearm increases food intake.

- Finger foods, cups with lids, and broad-handled utensils may make mealtime easier for the patient.

- Late stage patients may chew, but need frequent reminders to swallow.

- Plate guards and bibs with pockets catch spills and protect the patient's clothing.

- Offer the patient fluids frequently throughout the day. Ask the caregiver what the patient prefers to drink and the type of drinking container used at home.

Oral Hygiene

- Brush the patient's teeth at least twice a day.

- For less impaired patients, apples and other fresh fruits aid with oral hygiene.

Bathing

- Bathe the patient at his "best" time of day.

- If possible, bathe the patient at the time he normally bathes at home.

- Avoid using the shower. A hand-held showerhead provides better control of the water.

- Allow the patient to do as much as possible. Break down the task into simple steps using verbal and visual cues.

- When assisting the patient, give the bath slowly. To avoid agitation, tell the patient what you are going to do one step at a time.

- Use soft music, talking, or snacks as pleasant distractions.

- Keep the patient warm! During a bed bath, cover body parts except the parts that are being washed.

- Sounds amplify off tile walls. Running water can sound frightening.

- Be flexible. A "bird bath" may be more acceptable to the patient.

Toileting

- Clear a path to the toilet or commode.

- Place bed in view of toilet.

- To help cue the patient, place a picture of a toilet or a written sign on bathroom door.

- Place your patient on a two-hour toileting schedule.

- Use a nightlight to make it easier for the patient to find the toilet in the middle of the night.

- Observe your patient for constipation. Ask questions about abdominal discomfort. Watch for non-verbal signs of discomfort such as grimacing or clutching. Do not ask the patient if he has had a bowel movement.

The Art of Camouflage: Protecting Tubes and Dressings

Reduce the number of tubes as quickly as possible while considering patient safety. Make remaining tubes as unobtrusive as possible.

- **Nasogastric tubes (of small diameter):** Tape to the side of the face, place tube behind patient's ear and fasten to shoulder area of the gown with a safety pin.

- **Central venous pressure lines:** Can remain under the gown with a point of departure through the sleeve.

- **Peripheral intravenous line:** 1. Can be wrapped in bandage gauze to prevent access or, 2. Can be place high on dominant arm. Dress patient in long sleeve gown with cuff (like an operating room gown), run tubing up the arm and out the neck of the gown.

- **Foley catheters:** Should be run directly from the area of insertion to the end of the bed to prevent accidental pulling by the patient. Patient should wear undergarments to minimize access to the catheter.

- **Foley catheter in men:** Should be taped to the abdomen.

- **Picks at dressing:** Consult with your occupational therapist to develop hand splints (like those used for patients with burns or rheumatoid arthritis) that maintain alignment and mobility but eliminate the pincer grasp, thus eliminating the ability to pick at the dressing.

What Do I Do When...? Tips for Working with Behaviors

General Guidelines

- Think of behaviors (no matter how unusual) as communication signals from the patient that there is a problem or unmet need. Try to figure out that signal.

- Remain calm.

- Protect the patient both physically and from embarrassment.

- Offer reassurance and appropriate assistance.

Changes In Sleep Patterns

Possible Causes

- Medications
- Pain
- Not enough activity during the day
- Can't find the bathroom
- Too hot or too cold
- May be hungry

Possible Strategies

- Review medications for possible side effect of restlessness.

- Evaluate your patient for pain and treat if needed.

- Provide nightlights to aid the patient in finding the bathroom. Make sure the pathway is clear and well lit.

- Attend to toilet needs right before bedtime.

- Continue the patient's at-home bedtime routine as much as possible.

- Limit beverages containing caffeine in the afternoon and evening.

- If the patient wakes up at night, let him walk around (in sight) or sit at the nursing station until he is tired.

Confusion

Possible Causes

- Unfamiliar environment

- Medications

- Environment too noisy

- Unfamiliar or difficult task

- Unable to understand directions

Possible Strategies

- Identify any potential dangers in the environment.

- Use pictures (symbols) instead of written signs to assist the patient with locating his room and bathroom.

- Decrease noise level if possible by avoiding paging systems and buzzing call lights.

- Place the patient's name in large block letters on the door to his room.

- Review medications for side effect of confusion.

- Simplify tasks. Break them down into smaller steps.

- Simplify communication. Use short sentences and avoid lengthy explanations.

- Ask the family member/caregiver about the comfort strategies used at home.

Wandering

Possible Causes

- Patient is stressed and anxious
- Lifestyle related—previous work role or habits
- Looking for security
- Pain
- Searching for something familiar

Possible Strategies

- Ask the caregiver where and when the patient usually wanders. Find out what strategies have worked at home.
- Place the patient in a room that is convenient for you to keep a watchful eye on and that is away from stairs or elevator.
- Keep the patient's suitcase, street shoes, and street clothes out of sight.
- Assess the patient for pain and treat if needed.
- Plan walks with the patient.
- Use distractions such as a snack or music.
- Take time to talk with the patient.
- Offer a simple, meaningful activity.

Catastrophic Reactions: Patient Feels Overwhelmed and Overreacts to a Situation

Possible Causes

- Fatigue
- Environment is too stimulating
- Patient is asked too many questions at a time
- Too many strangers in a noisy, crowded atmosphere

- Patient is asked to perform a task beyond his abilities
- Fails at a simple task
- Encounters irritable, impatient staff

Possible Strategies

- Remain calm.
- Use a low tone of voice.
- Do not argue with the patient.
- Try the activity or task again later.
- Refrain from forcing or restraining the patient.
- Offer reassurance and try distraction.
- Move the patient to a quieter area.
- Simplify the task for the patient.
- Build in rest periods.
- Simplify communication.
- Be aware of your own body language and what it is saying.

Preventing Catastrophic Reactions

- Maintain a simple, structured, secure environment.
- Follow routines and schedules.
- Limit choices—choose between two items instead of five or six.
- Introduce new treatments slowly.
- Give step by step directions.

Disruptive Vocalizations: Calling Out or Screaming

Possible Causes

- Fear
- Pain
- Loneliness
- Self-stimulation

Possible Strategies

- Offer the patient reassurance.

- Place the patient where he can see a nurse.

- Spend time with the patient.

- Assess the patient for pain.

- Provide a range of textures in the environment for stimulation.

Sources

Alzheimer's Disease Fact Sheet, National Alzheimer's Association, Chicago, IL, 1994.

Effective Communication with Patients with Dementia, Zimmermann, Polly G., RN, MS, MBA, CEN, *Journal of Emergency Nursing*, Vol. 24, Number 5, October, 1998, pp. 412–415.

Managing the Care of Patients with Irreversible Dementia During Hospitalization for Comorbidities, Stolley, Jacqueline M., Hall, Geri R., MA, RN, CS, Collins, Judith, RN, CS, et al, *Nursing Clinics of America*, Vol. 28, Number 4, December, 1993, pp. 774–775.

Nursing the Hospitalized Dementia Patient, Evans, Lois K., DNSc, RN, *Journal of Advanced Medical-Surgical Nursing*, March, 1989, pp. 22, 24–26, 28–29.

The Person With Dementia: ED Assessment Tips for This At-Risk Patient, Royer, Mark, RN, MSW, CSW, *Journal of Emergency Nursing*, Volume 24, Number 4, August, 1998, pp. 331–332.

This Hospital Patient Has Alzheimer's, Hall, Geri R., MA, RN, CS, *American Journal of Nursing*, October, 1991, pp. 45–50.

When Your Patient Has Alzheimer's Disease, Stolley, Jacqueline M., RN, C, MA, *American Journal of Nursing*, August, 1994, p.38.

Information on The Art of Camouflage: Protecting Tubes and Dressings from Managing the Care of Patients with Irreversible Dementia During Hospitalization for Comorbidities, Stolley, Jacqueline M., Hall, Geri R., MA, RN, CS, Collins, Judith, MA, RN, et al, *Nursing Clinics of America*, Vol. 28, Number 4, December, 1993, pp. 774–775.

Chapter 47

Late-Stage Care for Alzheimer Patients

The late stage of Alzheimer disease and related dementias may last from several weeks to several years. Intensive, around-the-clock assistance is usually required.

A person with late-stage Alzheimer disease usually:

- has difficulty eating and swallowing;
- needs assistance walking and eventually becomes bedridden or chair-bound;
- needs full-time help with personal care, including toileting;
- is vulnerable to infections and pneumonia;
- loses the ability to communicate with words.

For the person with late-stage Alzheimer disease, it is important to focus on preserving quality of life and dignity. The person should always be treated with compassion and respect.

Body and Skin

A person with late-stage Alzheimer disease can become bedridden or chair-bound. This inability to move around can cause skin breakdown, pressure sores, and the "freezing" of joints.

"Late-Stage Care," is reprinted with permission of the Alzheimer's Association. For additional information, call the Alzheimer's Association toll-free helpline, 800-272-2900, or visit their website at www.alz.org. © 2005 Alzheimer's Association. All rights reserved.

To keep skin and body healthy:

Relieve body pressure: Change the person's position at least every two hours to relieve pressure and improve skin moisture. Make sure the person is comfortable and that their body is kept properly aligned. Use pillows to support arms and legs. To avoid injury to your loved one and yourself, see a health care professional about the proper way to lift and turn the person.

Keep the skin clean and dry: The person's skin can tear or bruise easily. Use gentle motions and avoid friction when cleaning fragile skin. Wash the skin with mild soap and blot dry. Check the skin daily for rashes, sores, or breakdowns.

Protect bony areas: Use pillows or pads to protect elbows, knees, hips, and other bony areas. If you use moisturizer on the person's skin, apply it gently over bony areas; do not massage the lotion into these areas.

Prevent "freezing" of joints: "Freezing" of the joints (limb contractures) can occur when a person is confined to a chair or bed. To maintain the person's range of motion in the joints, carefully and slowly move his or her arms and legs two to three times a day. Do these exercises when the person's skin and muscles are warm, like right after bathing. See a physical therapist to learn the proper method for range-of-motion exercises. Call your local Alzheimer's Association office to find a health care professional in your area.

Bowel and Bladder Function

A person with late-stage Alzheimer disease may experience incontinence for a number of reasons, including a urinary tract infection or fecal impaction.

First, see the doctor to rule out any medical problems.

To maintain bowel and bladder function:

Set a toileting schedule: Keep a written record of when the person goes to the bathroom, and when and how much the person eats and drinks. This will help you verify the person's natural toileting routine. If the person is not able to get to the toilet, use a bedside commode.

Eliminate drinks that have caffeine: Coffee, cola, tea, and other drinks with caffeine tend to increase the flow of urine.

Limit liquids before bedtime: Limit liquids at least two hours before bedtime, but be sure to provide adequate fluids for the person to drink throughout the day.

Use absorbent and protective products: Adult briefs and bed pads at night can serve as a backup to the daytime toileting schedule.

Monitor bowel movements: It is not necessary for the person to have a bowel movement every day. If the person goes three days without a bowel movement, however, he or she may be constipated. It may help to add natural laxatives to the person's diet, like prunes, or fiber-rich foods, such as bran or whole-grain breads.

Food and Fluids

Everyone needs to eat nutritious foods and drink enough fluids to be healthy. But a person with late-stage Alzheimer disease may have trouble swallowing, which may cause food or drink to be breathed into the airway and lungs. This can lead to pneumonia.

To help the person eat and drink safely:

Keep surroundings quiet and calm: Serve meals away from the TV and other distractions. If the person can eat at the table, use a simple setting with a plate or bowl, place mat, cup, and utensils.

Allow enough time for meals: Mealtimes may last longer now. Allow at least one hour for meals. Don't rush the person or force him or her to eat. Find out what the person prefers. He or she may do better with smaller meals or snacks throughout the day rather than three bigger meals.

Comfortably seat the person: Make sure the person is in a comfortable, upright position. To aid digestion, keep the person upright for 30 minutes after eating.

Adapt foods to the person's needs: Choose soft foods that can be chewed and swallowed easily. The person may prefer bite-sized finger foods, like slices of cheese, Tater Tots, or chicken nuggets. If he or she can no longer eat solid food, mash or puree it in a blender.

Encourage self-feeding: Sometimes a person needs cues to get started. Lift the spoon to your mouth as a reminder of how it's done. Or get the person started by putting food on the spoon, gently putting his or her hand on the spoon, and guiding it to the person's mouth.

Assist the person with feeding, if needed: Offer food or drink slowly. Make sure it's all swallowed before continuing. Alternate small bites of food with a drink. You may have to remind the person to chew or swallow. Don't put your fingers in the person's mouth; he or she could bite down.

Encourage the person to drink fluids: The person may not always realize that he or she is thirsty and could forget to drink. If the person has trouble swallowing water, try fruit juice, gelatin, sherbet, or soup. Check the temperature of warm or hot liquids before serving them to avoid burns.

Thicken liquids: Swallowing problems put a person with dementia at higher risk for choking. To make liquids thicker, add cornstarch or unflavored gelatin to water, juice, milk, broth, and soup. Or buy food thickeners at a pharmacy or health care supply store. Try pudding or ice cream, or substitute milk with plain yogurt.

Monitor weight: While weight loss during the end of life is to be expected, it may also be a sign of inadequate nutrition, another illness, or medication side effects. See the doctor to have weight loss evaluated.

Know what to do if the person chokes: Difficulty swallowing can lead to coughing and choking. Be prepared for an emergency, and learn the Heimlich maneuver. Check for classes at your local hospital or community center.

Infections and Pneumonia

The inability to move around in late-stage Alzheimer disease can make a person more vulnerable to infections.

To help prevent infections and pneumonia:

Keep the teeth and mouth clean: Good oral health reduces the risk of bacteria in the mouth that can lead to infection. Brush the person's teeth after each meal. If the person wears dentures, remove and clean them every night.

Clean all soft tissues of the mouth: Use a soft toothbrush or moistened gauze pad to clean the gums, tongue, and other soft mouth tissues. Doing this cleaning at least once a day helps prevent tooth decay and gingivitis (inflammation of the gums).

Treat cuts and scrapes immediately: Clean cuts with warm soapy water and apply an antibiotic ointment. If the cut is deep, seek professional medical help.

Protect against the flu and pneumonia: The flu (influenza) can lead to pneumonia (infection in the lungs). That's why it's vital for the person as well as the caregivers to get flu vaccines every year to help reduce the risk. Also, a person can receive a vaccine every five years to guard against pneumococcal pneumonia (a severe lung infection caused by bacteria).

Pain and Illness

Promoting quality of life means keeping the person with late-stage Alzheimer disease comfortable. This becomes more challenging for the caregiver in this stage because the person with the disease has more difficulty communicating his or her pain.

If you suspect pain or illness, see a doctor as soon as possible to find the cause. In some cases, pain medication may be prescribed.

To recognize pain and illness:

Look for physical signs: Pale skin tone; flushed skin tone; dry, pale gums; mouth sores; vomiting; feverish skin; or swelling of any part of the body can indicate illness.

Pay attention to nonverbal signs: Keep track of the person's gestures, spoken sounds, and the expressions on his or her face (wincing, for example) that may signal pain or discomfort.

Be alert to changes in behavior: Anxiety, agitation, shouting, and sleeping problems can all be signs of pain.

Personal Connection

Because of the loss of brain function, people with late-stage Alzheimer disease experience the world through their senses.

While you may not be able to communicate with the person through words, you can use many other ways to show the person reassurance and love.

To keep the personal connection:

Comfort the person with touch: Touch can be a powerful connector. Hold your loved one's hand. Give a gentle massage to the hands, legs, or feet. Give a kiss. Gently brush his or her hair.

Stimulate the senses: The person may find joy in the smell of a favorite perfume, flower, food, or scented lotion. He or she may enjoy how it feels to stroke a beloved pet or fabrics with different textures. If the person can walk with assistance or uses a wheelchair, he or she may benefit from going outside to see a garden or watch the birds. You can also place the person in a spot where he or she can gaze out the window; avoid places where sunlight is too bright or too warm.

Use your voice to soothe: It doesn't matter so much what you say—it's how you say it. Speak gently and with affection. Your tone can help the person feel safe and relaxed.

Play music and videos: Choose music your loved one enjoyed when he or she was young. Or use music related to the person's ethnic or spiritual background. Videos can also be relaxing. Choose one with scenes of nature with soft, calming sounds.

Read to the person: The tone and rhythm of your voice can be soothing, even if the person does not understand the words. Read a favorite story, poem, spiritual passage, or blessing.

Reminisce and share: Fill a box with photographs and other items that represent the person's interests, favorite activities, or past work or military history. Have the person take out an item and share with him or her a story about the item. Examples include a family photograph from a favorite vacation, a holiday recipe card with a traditional family dish, or a military medal.

Residential Care

By the time your loved one reaches late-stage Alzheimer disease, you have likely been caring for him or her for many years. During this time, challenges may arise that lead to moving a person to a residential care setting.

The amount of time needed to care for the person is one reason for deciding to make the move to a new care setting. A person with late-stage Alzheimer disease often requires 24-hour assistance. This round-the-clock care can be too difficult, especially for a sole caregiver.

If you are thinking about moving your loved one to a long-term care setting, call your local Alzheimer's Association office. Their staff can answer your questions, refer you to support groups and help you through the transition.

10 Quick Tips: Caring for a Person with Late-Stage Alzheimer Disease

1. Focus on what the person can still do and enjoy.

2. Learn how to safely lift and move the person.

3. If the person refuses to eat, find out why.

4. Use a bendable straw to help encourage drinking.

5. Ask the doctor if a food supplement is needed.

6. If the person is losing weight, contact the doctor.

7. Get help from family and friends or professional home care nurses or aides.

8. Encourage the person to interact with loved ones.

9. Use sights, sounds, smells and touch to communicate.

10. Treat the person with compassion and respect.

Chapter 48

End-of-Life Decisions

Dementia is a general term for the loss of decision-making, memory, and other mental abilities serious enough to interfere with daily life. Alzheimer disease, the most common form of dementia, is a physical and terminal illness.

When a person with late-stage Alzheimer disease nears the end of life and is no longer able to make decisions, families must make choices.

In ideal circumstances, the person with dementia has put advance directives into place to specifically spell out his or her wishes. Without such directives, or if certain issues were not addressed, families must make decisions based on what they believe the person would want.

End-of-life decisions should respect the person's values and wishes while maintaining comfort and dignity.

The Alzheimer's Association can help you prepare for making end-of-life choices such as:

- advocating for the kind of care that is based on the expressed wishes of the person with dementia;
- refusing, starting, limiting, or ending medical treatments;
- making the change from treatment to care that is focused on comfort;
- arranging for a brain autopsy.

"End-of-Life Decisions" is reprinted with permission of the Alzheimer's Association. For additional information, call the Alzheimer's Association toll-free helpline, 800-272-2900, or visit their website at www.alz.org. © 2006 Alzheimer's Association. All rights reserved.

Honoring the Person's Wishes

Advance Directives

A person with dementia has the legal right to limit, refuse or stop medical treatments. These wishes are usually expressed through advance directives—legal papers that specify the type of medical care a person wants to receive once he or she can no longer make such decisions due to incapacity.

If advance directives are not in place, the family must be prepared to make decisions consistent with what they believe the person would have wanted while acting in that person's best interest.

Advance directives should be made when the person with dementia still has legal capacity—the level of judgment and decision-making ability needed to sign official documents. These documents should be developed as soon as possible following a diagnosis of dementia. Contact the Alzheimer's Association for information about making legal plans.

Types of Advance Directives

Living will: A living will is a set of written instructions that provides specific preferences about the kind of medical treatment that a person would or would not want to have.

A living will does not designate someone to make medical decisions on the person's behalf. Instead, it allows the person to communicate wishes about future care.

Durable power of attorney for health care: This document allows a person to choose a partner, family member, or trusted friend to make decisions about care and treatment when the person with dementia is no longer able.

Use the forms for advance directives that are recognized in the state where care is, or will be, provided. Your local Alzheimer's Association can assist you with these forms.

Take Action to Make Sure Advance Directives Are Followed

Give copies of advance directives to all those involved in decisions:

- Family members
- Doctors
- Other health care providers

Have advance directives placed in the individual's medical record. If the person is transferred to a new setting, provide copies to those newly involved in caregiving.

Discuss advance directives: Family members should understand, respect, and abide by the person's wishes. Discuss these wishes together as a family to work out any disagreements. This helps prevent future conflict or crisis decision-making.

Discuss advance directives with the doctors and other health care providers to ensure they're aware of their patient's wishes.

If a conflict develops between members of the family or with health care providers, residential care facilities, and hospitals often have ethics committees that can help.

Stay involved in medical decisions: Work with the health care team to create and follow a care plan based on the advance directives. Make sure you are kept informed of any changes in your loved one's condition that may prompt the need for new decisions.

Understanding Levels of Care

Be aware of the range of medical care available when making decisions to use, withdraw, limit, or refuse treatment for the person with Alzheimer disease.

Aggressive Medical Care

Aggressive medical care is a term used to describe measures to be taken to keep a person alive and may include:

- respirators;
- feeding tubes;
- IV hydration;
- antibiotics;
- CPR.

Respirators: If a person with Alzheimer disease is no longer able to breathe independently, a respirator may be used to help the individual breathe. However, this treatment may cause the person's body to undergo unneeded stress and can cause greater discomfort.

439

Feeding tubes: Feeding tubes are sometimes used if a person has a hard time eating or swallowing, which often happens in late-stage Alzheimer disease. However, there is no proof that tube feeding has any significant benefits or extends life.

Tube feeding can also result in:

- infections;

- need for physical restraints (the person may try to pull out the tube, causing injury).

There are other ways to feed a person with late-stage Alzheimer disease, such as a carefully monitored, assisted-feeding program. For someone who can no longer swallow, an approach focusing on comfort in dying is most appropriate.

IV hydration: Liquid given to a person through a needle in a vein, IV hydration may temporarily provide fluid when a person can no longer drink, but it cannot supply the nutrition needed to stay alive.

Increased hydration may also make the person less comfortable because it can cause difficulty breathing.

Lack of hydration is a normal part of the dying process and allows a more comfortable death over a period of days. Using IV hydration can draw out dying for weeks and physically burden the person.

If artificial nutrition and hydration are used, families will eventually need to decide if or when these treatments should be stopped.

Antibiotics: Several types of infections, such as pneumonia and urinary tract infections, are common in late-stage Alzheimer disease. Antibiotics may be prescribed to treat an infection, but they might not improve the person's condition.

Cardiopulmonary resuscitation (CPR): A family may have to decide whether medical professionals should try to revive a person with CPR.

CPR is a group of treatments used to restore function when a person's heart or breathing stops. It may include mouth-to-mouth breathing or pressing on the chest to mimic heart function and cause blood to circulate.

Consider that CPR:

- may be painful and traumatic;

- may leave the person in worse condition;

- may not prolong life;

- is not recommended by many experts when a person is terminally ill.

The family can ask the doctor to sign a "do not resuscitate" (DNR)
order and place it in the medical chart. A DNR states that no attempts
will be made to revive the person.

Comfort or Palliative Care

Instead of seeking a cure or trying to prolong life, comfort care focuses on dignity and quality of life. It aims to keep the person comfortable and pain-free until life ends naturally.

Comfort care covers a variety of care options and does not mean
withholding all treatments.

A person can continue to receive any necessary medications, for
example, for chronic conditions such as diabetes or high blood pressure, as well as those that prevent pain and discomfort.

Through comfort care, the person avoids medical treatments, tests,
and procedures that may do more harm than good. Comfort care focuses on the quality of remaining life.

Hospice care: Hospice programs provide comfort care and preserve the dignity of those in the last stages of terminal illness while
also offering support services to families. It can be provided at home
or in a hospital or residential care facility.

A hospice team includes a doctor, nurse, social worker, dietitian,
clergy, and trained volunteers. They work together to address the
physical, emotional, and spiritual care of the person as well as the
family.

For Medicare to cover hospice care, a doctor must estimate that
the person has six or fewer months to live. Hospice benefit may be
extended if the person lives longer than expected.

Your local Alzheimer's Association can refer you to hospice services
in your area.

Making Informed Decisions

Consider the factors below when making choices about your loved
one's end-of-life care. Follow instructions given in advance directives,
if available.

Focus on the person's wishes: Compare any recommended treatments or actions with the person's wishes for care, or with what you believe he or she would have wanted. For example:

- Did the person want all available treatment measures or only certain ones?
- Did the person want medication to fight pain but not infection?

Stay true to their values and beliefs: Consider all factors that would influence the person's decisions about treatments, as well as definitions of quality of life and death, like:

- cultural background;
- spirituality;
- religious beliefs;
- family values.

Be aware of the differences between your values and beliefs and those of your loved one—and make sure it is the person's values and beliefs that are guiding your decision.

Weigh pros and cons of treatments: Talk with the medical care team about the impact of using or refusing specific care treatments, for example:

- Will the treatment improve the person's condition or comfort?
- If so, how long will the treatment benefit the person's condition or comfort?
- Will the treatment create physical or emotional burdens?

Compare any recommended treatments with your loved one's wishes for end-of-life care.

Consider where care will be given: Discuss with the care team if and when moving someone to a different setting is best. Find out if the treatment or care:

- can be provided in familiar surroundings;
- requires transfer to another setting.

Sometimes the temporary transfer to a hospital for a procedure—such as putting in a feeding tube—is disorienting and may be harmful to the person with dementia.

The Difference between Withholding Treatment and Assisted Suicide

You should not think that any refusal or withdrawal of treatment—including tube feeding, antibiotics, CPR, or other treatments—is considered assisted suicide (euthanasia). Limiting treatments lets the disease take its natural course and supports the person's comfort and dignity. If treatment is refused or withdrawn, the care team will still provide good care.

Resolving Family Conflicts

Family members need to take part in ongoing discussions when making decisions on behalf of their loved one. Some may disagree about a recommended treatment and get angry or defensive. Or, they may refuse to engage in discussions because they feel the family is "planning for death."

These guidelines may be helpful when dealing with family conflict:

Listen to each family member with respect: Family members may have different opinions about end-of-life preferences and quality of care. And they may not fully accept that the person is approaching death. Help family members avoid blaming or attacking each other as this will only cause more hurt.

Involve a third party: A physician, nurse, social worker, hospital ethics committee member, or spiritual leader can be asked to facilitate family meetings and help work through difficult issues.

Cope with your feelings together: The approaching death of a family member is an emotional time for everyone and may cause people to act in unusual ways. Caregivers and their families may want to seek emotional support, particularly during the last stage of the disease.

Contact the Alzheimer's Association about support groups that can assist you and your family members in working through emotions, including:

- stress;

- grief;
- guilt;
- anger;
- depression.

Arranging for a Brain Autopsy

A brain autopsy involves a researcher or physician to examine the brain after death to look for the plaques and tangles found in Alzheimer-affected brains. It is the definitive way to confirm a diagnosis of Alzheimer disease. And, it may provide information researchers can use to better understand the disease.

A brain autopsy may involve cost and special arrangements. Some brain donation programs provide a free autopsy report. Make the decision before the person's death. To learn more about getting a brain autopsy, contact the Alzheimer's Association.

10 Questions about End-of-Life Care: What to Ask the Doctor

1. What is the treatment for?

2. How will it help?

3. What are the physical risks or discomforts?

4. What are the emotional risks or discomforts?

5. Does the treatment match what the person would have wanted?

6. Are we doing all we can to uphold dignity?

7. Are we doing all we can to give the person the best quality of life?

8. Is he or she in pain?

9. What can be done to ease the pain?

10. When is the best time to ask for hospice care?

Part Five

Alzheimer Disease and Dementia-Related Research

Chapter 49

Alzheimer Disease Clinical Trials

AD Clinical Trials: Questions and Answers

Rapid advances in our knowledge about AD have led to the development of many new drugs and treatment strategies. However, before these new strategies can be adopted, they must be shown to work in patients. This means that clinical trials—studies in people to rigorously test how well a treatment works—have become an increasingly important part of AD research. Advances in treatment are only possible through the participation of patients and family members in clinical trials.

Clinical trials are the primary way that researchers find out if a promising treatment is safe and effective for patients. Clinical trials also tell researchers which treatments are more effective than others. Trials take place at private research facilities, teaching hospitals, specialized AD research centers, and doctors' offices.

Participating in a clinical trial is a big step for people with AD and their caregivers. That's why physicians and clinical trials staff spend lots of time talking with participants about what it's like to be in a trial and the pros and cons of participating. Here are some things that potential participants might want to know about clinical trials.

This chapter includes "AD Clinical Trials: Questions and Answers," National Institute on Aging, August 2006; and "New Alzheimer's Clinical Trials to Be Undertaken by NIA Nationwide Consortium," National Institute on Aging, October 2006.

What kind of trials are there?

- Treatment trials with existing drugs assess whether an already approved drug or compound is useful for other purposes. For example, one current trial is testing whether anti-inflammatory drugs already used to treat arthritis might help to prevent AD.

- Treatment trials with experimental drugs or strategies find out whether a brand new drug or treatment strategy can help improve cognitive function or lessen symptoms in people with AD, slow the progression to AD, or prevent it. Potential drugs tested in these trials are developed from knowledge about the mechanisms involved in the AD disease process. These compounds are rigorously tested in tissue culture and in animals for their action. Safety and effectiveness studies are also conducted in animals before the compounds are tested in humans.

What are the phases of clinical trials?

- During Phase I trials, a study team gives the treatment to a small number of volunteers and examines its action in the body, its safety, and its effects at various doses. Phase I trials generally last only a few months.

- If results show that the treatment appears safe, it will be tested in Phase II and Phase III clinical trials. These trials involve larger numbers of people over longer periods of time. In these trials, the study team wants to know whether the treatment is safe and effective and what side effects it might have.

After these phases are complete and investigators are satisfied that the treatment is safe and effective, the study team may submit its data to the Food and Drug Administration (FDA) for approval. The FDA reviews the data and decides whether to approve the drug or treatment for use in patients.

What happens when a person signs up for a clinical trial?

First it is important to learn about the study. Study staff explain the trial in detail to potential research participants and describe possible risks and benefits. Staff also talk about the participants' rights as research volunteers, including their right to leave the study at any time. Participants and their family members are entitled to have this information repeated and explained until they feel they understand the nature of the study and any potential risks.

Once all questions have been answered and if there is still interest in being a part of the study, a patient participant is asked to sign an informed consent form. Laws and regulations regarding informed consent differ across states and research institutions, but all are intended to ensure that patient participants are protected and well cared for.

In some cases, a patient participant may no longer be able to provide informed consent because of problems with memory and confusion. In such cases, it is still possible for an authorized representative (usually a family member) to give permission for the patient to participate. For example, the patient participant may have previously included research participation as part of his or her durable power of attorney.

The person (proxy) exercising the durable power of attorney can decide to let the patient participate in a trial if they are convinced that the patient would have wanted to consent if able to do so. Even so, it is still important that patients assent to be in the study, even if they can no longer formally consent to it. Different states have different laws about who is a legal representative. These laws are in a state of flux as researchers and the public grapple with the ethical issues of proxy consent.

Next, patients go through a screening process to see if they qualify to participate in the study. If they qualify and can safely participate, they can proceed with the other parts of the study.

What happens during a trial?

If participants agree to join the study and the screening process shows they're a good match, they have a "baseline" visit with the study staff. This visit generally involves a full physical exam and extensive cognitive and physical tests. This give the study team information against which to measure future mental and physical changes. Participants also receive the test drug or treatment. As the study progresses, participating patients and family members usually must follow strict medication or treatment instructions and keep detailed records of symptoms.

Every so often, participants visit the clinic or research center to have physical and cognitive exams, give blood and urine samples, and talk with study staff. These visits allow the investigators to assess the effects of the test drug or treatment, see how the disease is progressing, and see how the participant and the caregiver are doing.

In most clinical trials, participants are randomly assigned to a study group. One group, the test group, receives the experimental drug. Other groups may receive a different drug or a placebo (an inactive substance that looks like the study drug). Having the different groups is important because only by comparing them can researchers be confident that changes in the test group are the result of the experimental treatment and not some other factor.

In many trials, no one—not even the study team—knows who is getting the experimental drug and who is getting the placebo or other drug. This is called "masking" meaning that the patient or family member and the staff are "blind" to the treatment being received.

What should people consider before participating in a clinical trial?

Expectations and motivations: Clinical trials generally don't have miraculous results. The test drug or treatment may relieve a symptom, change a clinical measurement, or reduce the risk of death. With a complex disease like AD, it is unlikely that one drug will cure or prevent the disease. Some people choose not to participate or drop out of a study because this reality doesn't meet their expectations. Others participate because they realize that even if the benefit to them may be slight, they are making a valuable contribution to knowledge that will help future patients.

Uncertainty: Some families have a hard time with the uncertainties of participation—not knowing whether the person is on the test drug or the placebo, not being able to choose which study group to be in, not knowing for a long time whether the study was successful or not. Ongoing and open communication with study staff can help to counter this frustration.

Finding the right clinical trial: Some clinical trials want participants who are cognitively healthy or have only mild symptoms because they are testing a drug that might delay the decline in cognitive function. Other trials are interested in working with participants who have more advanced AD because they are testing a drug that might lessen behavioral symptoms, or they are testing new strategies to help caregivers. Even though a participant may not be eligible for one trial, another trial may be just right.

The biggest benefit of all: Many families find that the biggest benefit of participating in a clinical trial is the regular contact with the study team. These visits provide an opportunity to get state-of-the-art

AD care and also to talk on an ongoing basis with experts in AD who have lots of practical experience and a broad perspective on the disease. The study team understands and can provide advice on the emotional and physical aspects of the person with AD and the caregivers' experience. They can suggest ways to cope with the present and give insights into what to expect in the future. They also can share information about support groups and other helpful resources.

For More Information

For a list of clinical trials on Alzheimer disease and dementia currently in progress at centers throughout the U.S., go to the Alzheimer's Disease Education and Referral (ADEAR) Clinical Trials Database (http://www.nia.nih.gov/Alzheimers/ResearchInformation/ClinicalTrials/).

You may also wish to visit these clinical trials websites:

* National Institutes of Health: www.clinicaltrials.gov

* Alzheimer's Association: www.alz.org/Resources/FactSheets.asp

New Alzheimer Clinical Trials to Be Undertaken by NIA Nationwide Consortium

The Alzheimer's Disease Cooperative Study (ADCS), a federally established consortium conducting clinical trials on Alzheimer disease (AD), will receive $52 million over six years to conduct several new trials, the National Institutes of Health (NIH) announced today. The award is a cooperative agreement between the NIH's National Institute on Aging (NIA) and the University of California, San Diego (UCSD), which coordinates the consortium of nearly 70 sites in the United States and Canada.

The purpose of the award is to test drugs for their effectiveness in slowing down the progression or treating the symptoms of AD, as well as to investigate new methods for conducting dementia research. Specifically, researchers will focus on possible therapies aimed at affecting the beta amyloid peptide and the tau protein, both involved in the development of AD.

"We have learned a great deal from basic and observational research about how Alzheimer disease and other neurodegenerative diseases develop," says Richard J. Hodes, M.D., Director of the NIA. "The consortium's work will translate this knowledge in clinical trials of interventions that target the mechanisms underlying Alzheimer's disease."

Among the new studies to be undertaken are:

- **Docosahexaenoic acid (DHA):** This trial will examine whether treatment with DHA, an omega-3 fatty acid found in fish, will slow decline in AD. Observational studies associate high fish consumption with reduced risk of AD in people, and studies in mouse models of AD show that dietary DHA reduces brain levels of beta amyloid, oxidative damage associated with beta amyloid, and neurotoxicity.

- **Intravenous immunoglobulin (IVIg):** There is increased interest in passive immunization strategies against AD. IVIg contains naturally occurring antibodies against beta amyloid, and preliminary studies have shown that IVIg may improve cognition. In addition, research has demonstrated that IVIg increased levels of anti-beta amyloid antibodies in plasma and promoted clearance of beta amyloid from cerebrospinal fluid. The new ADCS trial will more definitively demonstrate whether IVIg is useful clinically for treating AD.

- **Lithium:** The biological activity of lithium, which has been shown in animal models to block abnormal changes in tau, has created interest in lithium as a novel treatment for AD. ADCS investigators will undertake a pilot biomarker study to see whether the drug can lower tau and beta amyloid levels in cerebrospinal fluid and be safely tolerated in older AD patients.

- **Home-based assessment:** Older individuals, particularly the very elderly, may have physical, social and health limitations that make it difficult for them to take part in research trials. This study, conducted in people aged 75 and older, will examine the use of mail-in questionnaires, automated telephone technology and computerized data collection to assess cognitive, functional, and other factors in the home environment to see how home-based assessments might be used in primary prevention trials. Such an approach could significantly reduce the cost and increase the feasibility of participation in these long-term, costly clinical trials.

These projects join ongoing ADCS trials testing whether statins and high-dose folate/B6/B12 supplements can slow the clinical signs of AD, as well as a study of valproate to determine whether this drug can either slow decline or help delay the agitation and psychosis that often emerge in AD patients.

Leon Thal, M.D., chair of the Department of Neurosciences at the UCSD School of Medicine and principal investigator of the ADCS, notes that the selection of compounds for testing was enhanced by seeking ideas from the biotechnology sector as well as from individual investigators and the consortium's members. "We have been able to bring together a larger universe of people studying therapies for Alzheimer's, and I think this group of studies reflects new thinking in how to approach the disease," he says.

This ADCS consortium was first established in 1991 as an infrastructure of leading researchers to carry out clinical trials for promising new therapies for AD. Investigators have tested such compounds as vitamin E, the anti-Parkinson disease drug selegiline, estrogen, anti-inflammatories and donepezil for their potential in slowing down or preventing cognitive impairment or dementia. Recently, positive but limited effects have been shown in slowing the development of dementia with donepezil.

To date, approximately 4,600 people have participated in the ADCS studies. Neil Buckholtz, Ph.D., who leads the federal government's partnership with the consortium as chief of the Dementias of Aging Branch of the NIA, recognized the efforts of the study participants and their families. "Participating in research takes time and dedication, and the efforts of the participants and their families stand out," Buckholtz notes. "We are deeply grateful for their help in finding new and better ways to treat and prevent Alzheimer's disease." As the new round of trials gets underway, stepped up public participation will be essential for their success, Buckholtz says, and he urges the public to learn more about how to take part in such research.

Alzheimer disease affects an estimated 4.5 million people in the U.S. It increases dramatically with age, affecting approximately 40–50 percent of people age 85 and older. The numbers of people with AD are expected to rise dramatically with the aging of the population over the next few decades.

The NIA, one of 27 institutes and centers at the NIH, is part of the U.S. Department of Health and Human Services. It leads the federal effort to support and conduct basic, clinical, and social and behavioral studies on aging generally and AD specifically. NIA supports the Alzheimer's Disease Education and Referral (ADEAR) Center, which provides information on clinical studies and other research to the public, health professionals, and the media. ADEAR can be contacted toll-free at 800-438-4380 or by viewing www.nia.nih.gov/alzheimers.

As the studies mentioned above move forward, more information will be available at the ADEAR website about participation. NIA invites the public to sign up for e-mail alerts, which will let subscribers know when trials begin recruitment and generally when new information about AD is available.

Chapter 50

Studies to Detect and Monitor Alzheimer Disease

Getting a Jump on Alzheimer Disease

The hallmarks of mid-stage Alzheimer disease are all too readily apparent, including severe memory loss, wandering and getting lost, and inability to perform daily functions like dressing, eating, and bathing without assistance. Unfortunately, by the time the disease has progressed this far, the few treatment strategies available for Alzheimer disease are of little help. The fight against Alzheimer disease, therefore, needs improved methods of diagnosing the disease at its earliest stages, before overt symptoms have appeared.

Today's Testing Challenges

Currently, the primary method of diagnosing Alzheimer disease in living patients involves taking detailed patient histories, administering memory and psychological tests, and ruling out other explanations for memory loss, including temporary conditions like depression or vitamin B_{12} deficiency or permanent ones like stroke. These clinical diagnostic methods, however, are not foolproof.

This chapter begins with "Getting a Jump on Alzheimer's Disease," by Lisa Chippendale, reprinted with permission from the American Federation for Aging Research, © 2003. For additional information, visit www.infoaging.org. It continues with excerpts from "New Study Demonstrates Combined Techniques to Detect, Monitor Alzheimer's Disease," National Institute on Aging (NIA), December 21, 2005; and excerpts from "New Brain Imaging Compound Shows Promise for Earlier Detection of Alzheimer's Disease," NIA, December 20, 2006.

One obstacle to diagnosis is pinpointing the type of dementia; Alzheimer disease is only one of many different forms of dementia. Because of this, Alzheimer disease cannot be diagnosed with complete accuracy until after death, when autopsy reveals the disease's characteristic amyloid plaques and neurofibrillary tangles in a patient's brain. In addition, clinical diagnostic procedures are only helpful after patients have begun displaying significant, abnormal memory loss or personality changes. By then, a patient has likely had Alzheimer disease for years.

New Tests Under Development

Recognizing the need for earlier and more accurate detection of Alzheimer disease, scientists are devising new brain imaging technologies and blood, urine, or spinal fluid tests that could improve diagnosis. Dr. John Trojanowski, Professor of Pathology and Laboratory Medicine at the University of Pennsylvania Medical Center, is a member of the National Institute on Aging's Biological Markers Working Group, which is part of the National Institute of Health's Alzheimer's Disease Prevention Initiative.

"We need a way to diagnose Alzheimer's disease in the prodromal, or presymptomatic, phase of Alzheimer's disease, where intervention will have the greatest benefit," he explains. "If using these tests helps a physician make a secure diagnosis in the first year rather than after two years, then that's good for the patient."

The Biological Markers Working Group recently released a discussion of the status of biomarker research in Alzheimer disease. Biomarkers are substances in a person's biological fluids—blood, urine, or cerebrospinal fluid—that can be measured to indicate whether a person has or is likely to develop Alzheimer disease.

Amyloid beta and tau: Perhaps the most well-researched of these markers are amyloid beta and tau, measured in cerebrospinal fluid. Research has shown that tau, released as neurons degenerate, is higher than normal in the spinal fluids of Alzheimer patients, whereas beta amyloid is low, presumably because it is trapped in the brain in the form of amyloid plaques.

In April 2003 a study and review of the scientific literature, published in the *Journal of the American Medical Association*, concluded that by measuring levels of these substances, scientists could distinguish patients with Alzheimer disease from normal controls with about 90% accuracy. Commercial tests are already available for doctors to measure cerebrospinal amyloid beta and tau levels, but the tests are not likely to gain widespread use—or be covered by insurers—until further, large-scale studies show the benefit of the new diagnostic tool.

Isoprostanes: One significant hurdle to acceptance of an amyloid beta and tau test by patients is that it requires a spinal tap, a potentially frightening and painful procedure. Dr. Trojanowski, Dr. Domenico Pratico and colleagues at the University of Pennsylvania, therefore, have sought another biomarker that not only accurately diagnoses Alzheimer disease, but can be obtained through blood or even urine: isoprostanes.

Isoprostanes are markers of oxidative damage, caused by substances called free radicals released as a byproduct of oxygen metabolism. Alzheimer disease is associated with an increased level of oxidative damage in the brain, and persons with Alzheimer disease have increased levels of isoprostanes in cerebrospinal fluid, blood, and urine. In 2001, Dr. Trojanowski and colleagues authored a paper reporting studies led by Dr. Pratico that showed evidence that heightened oxidative damage is one of the earliest signs of Alzheimer disease, occurring even before the formation of plaques and tangles. A year later, they demonstrated that persons with mild cognitive impairment—often a precursor to Alzheimer disease—have increased levels of isoprostanes in their bodily fluids, as compared to normal controls. More recent research led by Dr. Pratico indicates that the isoprostane urine test may also be able to help physicians rule out certain non-Alzheimer forms of dementia when diagnosing patients.

Advances in brain imaging: Just as important as work on biomarkers are new advances in brain imaging technology. "There are three general approaches to using imaging for early detection of Alzheimer's disease," says Dr. Scott Small, Assistant Professor of Neurology at Columbia University. "However, none of them has yet moved from the laboratory into the clinical realm."

Among the most promising technologies is using magnetic resonance imaging (MRI) to examine brain shrinkage, or atrophy, in Alzheimer patients. Scientific evidence shows that persons with Alzheimer disease experience an accelerated rate of brain shrinkage: 2.5% a year, as compared to 0.4% for normal persons the same age. Work published in the April 2, 2002, issue of the *Proceedings of the National Academy of Science* by a group of researchers at the Institute of Neurology at the University College London suggests that brain atrophy begins before the onset of symptoms of memory loss in Alzheimer disease, and that the brain locations showing the most atrophy vary as the disease progresses. This may mean that using MRI to measure brain atrophy will be useful not only as an early detection tool, but also as a means to track disease progression.

Another technology being adapted for Alzheimer diagnosis is positron emission topography, or PET. Researchers are developing ways to use PET scanning to image the plaques and tangles of Alzheimer disease in living patients. Scientists have developed several substances, called ligands, that when injected into the body travel into the brain and bind to plaques and tangles. The scientists tag the ligand with a radioactive marker, permitting them to image the radiolabeled plaques and tangles with a PET scan. This technique could not only assist doctors with making certain that memory-impaired patients truly have Alzheimer disease rather than another type of dementia, but could also be used during clinical trials to monitor whether treatments designed to attack plaques and tangles are having an effect. The approach may not be the best method for early detection, however, as most scientists agree that brain dysfunction precedes the development of plaques and tangles in Alzheimer disease.

The third technology, a variant of MRI called functional MRI (fMRI), may allow the earliest diagnosis of Alzheimer disease. Dr. Small has been refining fMRI technology to differentiate between patients with normal age-related memory loss and those in the earliest stages of Alzheimer disease. Measuring oxygen levels in the blood in the hippocampus—the brain's memory center—while the brain is at rest, Dr. Small has been able to pinpoint differences in brain activity in different subregions of the hippocampus. In 1999, he found that older adults with mild memory loss have one of two different patterns of dysfunction in the hippocampus. The first matches the pattern seen in patients with confirmed Alzheimer disease and likely indicates early Alzheimer disease; the other pattern seems to be associated with normal aging.

Since then, Dr. Small has been working to demonstrate that fMRI scans of the hippocampus could be a valuable and accurate tool for early identification of Alzheimer disease. Animal studies in rhesus monkeys—who never get Alzheimer disease—and transgenic mouse models of Alzheimer disease—who always develop Alzheimer symptoms—support Dr. Small's theory.

The rhesus monkeys show a pattern of hippocampal function consistent with normal aging, whereas the Alzheimer mice show the Alzheimer-like pattern of hippocampal dysfunction. The next step, says Dr. Small, is to do a long-term study of the technology in humans.

"We want to image hundreds, or hopefully thousands, of people to be sure about diagnostic specificity and sensitivity," he says. "We plan to test our hypothesis that anyone over 60 with an Alzheimer-like pattern in the hippocampus is more likely to develop Alzheimer's disease."

A Complement to Existing Techniques

None of these new imaging techniques or biomarkers is likely to become a stand-alone method of diagnosing Alzheimer disease. Instead, they will complement existing clinical tests and criteria to help patients obtain earlier and more accurate diagnoses. "Most conditions and diseases are not easily diagnosed with one test or marker," notes Dr. Trojanowski. "I think a combination of imaging and biomarkers will help physicians nail down a diagnosis with much greater accuracy than they can now." And perhaps most important, these new techniques should help patients suffering from Alzheimer disease obtain treatment sooner, allowing them to prolong their health and sustain their quality of life.

References

Frank RA, Galasko D, Hampel H, Hardy J, de Leon MJ, Mehta PD, Rogers J, Siemers E, Trojanowski JQ; National Institute on Aging Biological Markers Working Group. Biological markers for therapeutic trials in Alzheimer's disease. Proceedings of the biological markers working group; NIA initiative on neuroimaging in Alzheimer's disease. *Neurobiol Aging* 2003; 24: 521-36.

Pratico D, Clark CM, Liun F, Rokach J, Lee VY, Trojanowski JQ. Increase of brain oxidative stress in mild cognitive impairment: a possible predictor of Alzheimer disease. *Arch Neurol* 2002; 59: 972-6.

Pratico D, Uryu K, Leight S, Trojanowski JQ, Lee VM. Increased lipid peroxidation precedes amyloid plaque formation in an animal model of Alzheimer amyloidosis. *J Neurosc.* 2001; 21: 4183-7.

Scahill RI, Schott JM, Stevens JM, Rossor MN, Fox NC. Mapping the evolution of regional atrophy in Alzheimer's disease: unbiased analysis of fluid-registered serial MRI. *Proc Natl Acad Sci USA* 2002; 99: 4703-7.

Small SA, Perera GM, DeLaPaz R, Mayeux R, Stern Y. Differential regional dysfunction of the hippocampal formation among elderly with memory decline and Alzheimer's disease. *Ann Neurol* 1999; 45: 466-72.

New Study Demonstrates Combined Techniques to Detect, Monitor Alzheimer Disease

The search for new measures, or "biomarkers," to detect Alzheimer disease (AD) before signs of memory loss appear has advanced an important step in a study by researchers at Washington University in St. Louis, MO, and the University of Pittsburgh.

The researchers combined high-tech brain imaging with measurement of beta-amyloid protein fragments in cerebrospinal fluid (CSF). They found that greater amounts of beta-amyloid containing plaques in the brain were associated with lower levels of a specific protein fragment, amyloid-beta 1-42, in CSF. Prior research indicates that amyloid-beta 1-42 is central to AD development. The fragment is a major component of amyloid plaques in the brain, which are believed to influence cell-to-cell communication and are considered a hallmark of the Alzheimer brain.

The study, published online December 21, 2005, by the *Annals of Neurology*, is the first to examine the relationship between levels of amyloid plaque deposits in the brain and different forms of beta-amyloid in CSF in living humans. It was supported by the National Institute on Aging (NIA), a component of the National Institutes of Health (NIH) at the U.S. Department of Health and Human Services, and by the Washington University General Clinical Research Center, funded by the NIH.

The method studied might one day help to more accurately diagnose AD, even before the appearance of cognitive symptoms, and to monitor disease progression. In the near term, the findings could be useful in a research context, allowing scientists to track the effects of potential beta-amyloid lowering treatments in clinical trials.

New Brain Imaging Compound Shows Promise for Earlier Detection of Alzheimer Disease

A new imaging molecule that can detect and map plaques and tangles in the brains of people with Alzheimer disease could eventually lead to earlier diagnosis of the devastating disease, researchers at the University of California, Los Angeles (UCLA) report in the December 21, 2006, issue of the *New England Journal of Medicine*. The compound, developed by UCLA and called FDDNP, also holds promise as a research tool to evaluate new treatments for Alzheimer disease. The study was funded in part by the National Institute on Aging (NIA), one of the National Institutes of Health (NIH).

FDDNP binds to plaques and tangles, enabling researchers to see these abnormal deposits that form in the brains of people with Alzheimer disease on PET (positron emission tomography) scans. PET scans display maps of the brain that scientists use to understand brain function. In a clinical trial with volunteers who reported memory problems, results of PET scans using FDDNP correlated well with the volunteers' clinical diagnoses measured by performance on memory tests.

In this study, Gary Small, MD, of UCLA, led a research team that compared PET scans using FDDNP, PET scans using another molecule (FDG) to measure brain activity, and magnetic resonance imaging (MRI), which can show areas losing brain tissue in Alzheimer disease. Of 83 people who volunteered for the trial, researchers classified 25 as having Alzheimer disease, 28 as having mild cognitive impairment, and 30 as healthy. The FDDNP PET scans were more accurate than FDG PET scans or MRI at detecting differences among the groups of volunteers, the study found. Two years later, follow-up testing on a subset of the volunteers showed that FDDNP PET scans continued to correlate well with their clinical symptoms and diagnoses.

Reference: G.W. Small et al. PET of Brain Amyloid and Tau in Mild Cognitive Impairment. *The New England Journal of Medicine.* Vol:355;25. pp:2652-63. Dec. 21, 2006.

Chapter 51

New Genetic Clues Regarding Dementia

Scientists Find New Genetic Clue to Cause of Alzheimer Disease

Variations in a gene known as SORL1 may be a factor in the development of late-onset Alzheimer disease, an international team of researchers has discovered. The genetic clue, which could lead to a better understanding of one cause of Alzheimer disease, is reported in *Nature Genetics* online, January 14, 2007, and was supported in part by the National Institutes of Health (NIH).

The researchers suggest that faulty versions of the SORL1 gene contribute to formation of amyloid plaques, a hallmark sign of Alzheimer disease in the brains of people with the disease. They identified 29 variants that mark relatively short segments of DNA where disease-causing changes could lie. The study did not, however, identify specific genetic changes that result in Alzheimer disease.

Richard Mayeux, M.D., of Columbia University, Lindsay Farrer, Ph.D., of Boston University, and Peter St. George-Hyslop, M.D., of the University of Toronto, led the study, which involved 14 collaborating institutions in North America, Europe, and Asia, and 6,000 individuals who donated blood for genetic typing. The work was funded by

This chapter includes text from three documents produced by the National Institute on Aging (http://www.nia.nih.gov): "Scientists Find New Genetic Clue to Cause of Alzheimer's Disease," January 2007; "Scientists Discover New Frontotemporal Dementia Gene," July 2006; and "Twins Comparison Suggests Genetic Risk for Dementia," December 2005.

NIH's National Institute on Aging (NIA) and National Human Genome Research Institute (NHGRI), as well as by 18 other international public and private organizations.

"We do not fully understand what causes Alzheimer disease, but we know that genetic factors can play a role," says NIA director Richard J. Hodes, M.D. "Scientists have previously identified three genes, variants of which can cause early-onset Alzheimer disease, and one that increases risk for the late-onset form. This discovery provides a completely new genetic clue about the late-onset forms of this very complex disease. We are eager to investigate the role of this gene further."

Scientists think that in Alzheimer disease, amyloid precursor protein, or APP, is processed into amyloid beta protein fragments that make up plaques in the brain. The researchers began their search for genetic influences amid a group of proteins that transport APP within cells, looking for small changes, or "misspellings," in seven genes involved in moving APP within cells.

To start, the scientists combed two large data sets of genetic information from families in which more than one person has Alzheimer disease. They were soon able to see that many of the families with Alzheimer disease had variations in the SORL1 gene but not consistently in any of the other six genes.

They then expanded their search to genetic data sets from families of Northern European, Caribbean Hispanic, Caucasian, African American, and Israeli Arab heritage for changes in the SORL1 gene. Again, they found the same association between SORL1 variations and Alzheimer disease. Searching additional data sets provided by Steven Younkin, M.D., Ph.D., of the Mayo Clinic further confirmed the association of SORL1 variations and Alzheimer disease.

"We are seeing the gene implicated in multiple data sets, across ethnic and racial groups," says Farrer. He adds that the group was "encouraged and excited" by cell biology experiments that demonstrate SORL1's role in production of beta amyloid fragments.

Examining blood cells from people with and without Alzheimer disease, the researchers found less than half the level of SORL1 protein in people with Alzheimer disease compared to people without the disease. In laboratory experiments, they found that altering the levels of SORL1 changed the way APP was moved around in cells, with low levels of SORL1 resulting in increased production of amyloid beta fragments while high levels decreased production. However, the researchers note, other genetic and non-genetic factors are likely to affect SORL1 production in people, and more research is needed to determine how different versions of the SORL1 gene influence production of the harmful protein fragments.

NIA and NHGRI support a number of studies looking at genetic factors that may be involved in Alzheimer disease. For information on the NIA Alzheimer's Disease Genetics Study, which is currently recruiting volunteers from families with two or more siblings affected by late-onset Alzheimer disease, visit the study website, http://www .ncrad.org, call 800-526-2839, or e-mail alzstudy@iupui.edu.

Scientists Discover New Frontotemporal Dementia Gene

Scientists have discovered genetic mutations that cause a form of familial frontotemporal dementia (FTD), a finding that provides clues to the underlying mechanism of this devastating disease and that may provide insight for future approaches to developing therapies. The mutations are contained in a single gene that scientists can now identify as responsible for a large portion of inherited FTD. A rare brain disorder, FTD usually affects people between ages 40 and 64 with symptoms that include personality changes and inappropriate social behavior. Published online July 16, 2006, in *Nature*, the research was funded by the National Institute on Aging (NIA), part of the National Institutes of Health (NIH).

The discovery builds on a 1998 finding of mutations in another gene that is responsible for a smaller proportion of inherited FTD cases. Amazingly, both the gene found in 1998 and the newly found gene were found on the same region of chromosome 17. Today's discovery appears to explain all the remaining inherited FTD cases linked to genes on chromosome 17 and may provide new insights into the causes of the overall disease process. Geneticist Michael Hutton, Ph.D., of the Mayo Clinic College of Medicine, Jacksonville, Florida, led an international scientific team to discover the new gene.

"This new finding is an important advance in our understanding of frontotemporal dementia," says NIA director Richard J. Hodes. "It identifies a mutation in the gene producing a growth factor that helps neurons survive, and it suggests that lack of this growth factor may be involved in this form of frontotemporal dementia."

FTD encompasses a set of rare brain disorders. While most cases are sporadic, an estimated 20 to 50 percent has a family history of dementia, according to the Association for Frontotemporal Dementias. FTD affects the frontal and temporal lobes of the brain. People with FTD may exhibit uninhibited and socially inappropriate behavior, changes in personality, and, in late stages, loss of memory, motor skills, and speech. There is no treatment.

Hutton and colleagues began looking for genetic causes of FTD after a 1996 NIA-funded conference on the disorder. The conference, he recalls, encouraged researchers to cooperate, rather than compete, to find the FTD gene. At the start, they knew only that the inherited changes were linked to chromosome 17. Two years later, Hutton along with other researchers discovered that mutations in a particular gene on chromosome 17 were responsible for a subset of inherited FTD cases. That gene, called MAPT, contains instructions for a protein known as tau.

But, the researchers also knew there were many other families where FTD was inherited but without mutations in the tau gene. Further searching of chromosome 17 in the families without tau mutations finally turned up what is reported today—another set of mutations in another gene, this one containing instructions for the assembly of a protein known as progranulin. The progranulin, or PGRN, gene makes a growth factor protein that stimulates cell division and motility during multiple processes including embryonic development, wound repair, and inflammation. Scientists say it is unclear what role progranulin plays in the normal brain. In the FTD families, they explain, the progranulin mutations appear to cut short the assembly process for the protein in brain nerve cells (neurons), and the lack of progranulin eventually causes neurons to die.

Understanding how the mutations of the two different genes on chromosome 17 cause neuronal death might help scientists better understand the different pathways that cause dementia. The findings also suggest that PGRN may play a role in other neurodegenerative diseases, such as ALS (amyotrophic lateral sclerosis) or Lou Gehrig's disease, the researchers noted.

The study was conducted as part of the NIA-supported Alzheimer's Disease Center at the Mayo Medical Center. In addition to NIA funding, the researchers were supported by several other entities in the United States, Belgium, Great Britain and Canada, including, in the United States, the Mayo Foundation, the Robert and Clarice Smith Fellowship program and the Alzheimer's Association.

Twins Comparison Suggests Genetic Risk for Dementia

On average, twins of people who have been diagnosed with dementia score lower on cognitive tests than do the twins of people without dementia, new research has found. The study, which included more than 100 Swedish twins age 65 and older, also found that, on average, identical twins of people with dementia have poorer cognitive skills than do fraternal (non-identical) twins of people with dementia.

The researchers suggest that these differences in thinking skills reflect a genetic risk for dementia. However, they emphasize that cognitive changes and elevated genetic risk do not always predict that twins or siblings of people with dementia will eventually develop dementia themselves.

The research, reported in the December 2005 issue of the *Journal of Geriatric Psychiatry and Neurology*, was led by Margaret Gatz, Ph.D., of the University of Southern California and the Karolinska Institute in Sweden. The study was funded by the National Institute on Aging (NIA), a component of the National Institutes of Health, U.S. Department of Health and Human Services, and a Zenith Award from the Alzheimer's Association. The University of Southern California Alzheimer's Disease Center is one of more than 30 Alzheimer's Disease Centers nationwide supported by the NIA.

"This research is intriguing because it associates genetic risk for dementia with twins' cognitive deficits, even in the absence of dementia," says Neil Buckholtz, Ph.D., chief of the Dementias of Aging Branch of NIA's Neuroscience and Neuropsychology of Aging Program. "The differences in cognitive deficits between identical and fraternal twins are also important, suggesting that the twins who were more similar genetically had the greater risk."

The study included 112 members of the Swedish Twin Registry who were at least 65 years old in 1998. The registry, established in 1961, includes all twins born in Sweden. Of the study participants, 23 were identical twins and 62 were fraternal twins whose co-twins had dementia but who did not have dementia themselves. A comparison group included 27 non-demented twins whose co-twins did not have dementia. The comparison group was similar to the other participants in terms of age, gender, and level of education.

All of the study participants took a series of neuropsychological tests that assessed their attention, memory, verbal recall, verbal fluency, ability to copy simple drawings, comprehension, and other cognitive skills. The test results for twins of people with dementia were weighed against those of the comparison group.

Twins whose twin siblings had dementia had significantly lower overall scores on the cognitive-skills tests than those of the comparison group. The twins of demented co-twins and the comparison group differed most on the tests of memory and "executive functioning," such as verbal fluency and remembering patterns that include symbols and numbers. Gatz and her colleagues say this finding suggests that the twins of people with dementia are at higher risk for developing dementia in the future, although they had already lived without dementia for an average of nearly 8 years beyond their co-twins' dementia onset.

"Identical twins of dementia cases had a strikingly poorer cognitive performance profile," Gatz notes. "It could be that these twins are more likely to progress to dementia, but we don't know that. We might be seeing a difference in performance that could already have persisted for a long time without getting worse or it could be a signal that the currently non-demented twin is at greater risk for progressing."

Gatz and her co-authors point out, however, that the study included only a "modest number" of twins. They also did not gather long-term data that would show changes or stability in cognitive performance over time or whether participants would develop dementia in the future.

"While there may be a genetic risk for dementia, it is important to recognize that not everyone with a genetic risk factor will develop dementia," Buckholtz comments. "More research is needed to help us understand who will and will not develop dementia, even if they are at risk. Beyond genetics, environmental and life style factors also play a role."

The Gatz article is one of several in the December 2005 *Journal of Geriatric Psychiatry and Neurology* focusing on children of Alzheimer parents (http://jgpn.sagepub.com). The papers, including a number reporting on studies funded by the NIA, are based on presentations at a workshop held in conjunction with the American Association for Geriatric Psychiatry Annual Conference in March 2005.

In other recent NIA-supported research, Gatz and her colleagues focused on lifestyle prevention factors. They found that twins who are involved in complex work—particularly complex work with people—are at lower risk of dementia and Alzheimer disease than are their co-twins who are not involved in complex work, even when age, gender, and level of education are considered. That study, which included more than 10,000 members of the Swedish Twin Registry, was published in the September 2005 issue of the *Journal of Gerontology: Psychological Sciences*.

The NIA supports several research projects on the genetic factors that may influence the risk of developing Alzheimer disease or dementia, including the Alzheimer's Disease Genetics Study. For information on participating in that study or in an AD clinical trial, visit www.clinicaltrials.gov (search for Alzheimer disease trials), or the

Alzheimer's Disease Education and Referral (ADEAR) Center website at www.alzheimers.org. ADEAR may also be contacted toll free at 800-438-4380. The ADEAR Center is sponsored by the NIA to provide information to the public and health professionals about AD and age-related cognitive change and may be contacted at the website and phone number above for a variety of publications and fact sheets, as well as information on clinical trials.

References

E Rogaeva et al. The neuronal sortilin receptor SORL1 is genetically associated with Alzheimer's Disease. *Nature Genetics* (2006). DOI: 10.1038/ng1943

M Hutton et al. Nature, 2006. Mutations in Progranulin cause tau-negative frontotemporal dementia linked to chromosome 17. *Nature* 2006. DOI: 10.1038/nature05016.

Chapter 52

Anti-Inflammatory Drugs Do Not Prevent Alzheimer Disease

NIA Statement: Data Published on Safety Review of Anti-Inflammatory Drugs in ADAPT Alzheimer's Disease Clinical Trial

On December 17, 2004, the Alzheimer's Disease Anti-Inflammatory Prevention Trial (ADAPT) steering committee suspended treatments with two non-steroidal anti-inflammatory drugs (NSAIDs) in a large, three-arm, national Alzheimer disease prevention trial. ADAPT, sponsored by the NIH's National Institute on Aging (NIA), was designed to test the potential benefit of long-term use of naproxen sodium (220 mg twice a day) and celecoxib (200 mg twice a day) in decreasing risk of Alzheimer disease and cognitive decline in non-symptomatic people 70 and older who were at elevated risk because of family history of the disease.

The ADAPT steering committee halted the Alzheimer trial medications following a report earlier in the day linking use of celecoxib to increased risk of cardiovascular disease in an unrelated clinical trial for cancer prevention (APC: Adenoma Prevention with Celecoxib) and after a preliminary review of data from ADAPT signaled a possible

---

This chapter includes excerpts from two documents produced by the National Institute on Aging (http://www.nia.nih.gov): "NIA Statement: Data Published on Safety Review of Anti-Inflammatory Drugs in ADAPT Alzheimer's Disease Clinical Trial," November 2006, and "NIA Statement: Early Findings from ADAPT Indicate NSAIDs Do Not Prevent Alzheimer's Disease," April 2007.

increased risk for heart disease and stroke among participants taking naproxen. While the naproxen data were not considered sufficient in themselves to warrant interruption of treatment, they raised substantial concerns about the practicality or wisdom of continuing ADAPT as a two-arm trial comparing naproxen and placebo. The ADAPT data did not suggest a similarly increased risk of cardiovascular disease related to celecoxib.

At the time the ADAPT medications were halted, the investigators and the NIH promised to notify the public and health professionals as soon as their data became available in a peer-reviewed publication. Those data appear in the November 17, 2006, issue of *PLoS Clinical Trials*, a journal of the Public Library of Science, reported by the ADAPT Research Group, with Barbara K. Martin, Ph.D., of the Johns Hopkins Bloomberg School of Public Health as corresponding author.

According to the journal report, "For celecoxib, the ADAPT data do not show the same level of risk as those of the APC trial. The data for naproxen, although not definitive, are suggestive of increased cardiovascular and cerebrovascular risk." The researchers emphasize that the results are not definitive because of the relatively small numbers of heart attacks and strokes during the trial. The risk analysis is also limited because the study was intended to measure cognitive symptoms and dementia, not heart disease and stroke, as the primary outcomes of drug treatment.

"The ADAPT researchers and the NIH felt it important to follow up with a thorough review of the safety data and to then make that review available to the scientific community and the broader public," says Richard J. Hodes, MD, director of NIA. "Though the results of the review did not produce definitive answers on the risks and benefits of NSAIDs in patients at risk of Alzheimer disease, they add to the body of information on the safety of these anti-inflammatory drugs."

Several recent reports have summarized available data from multiple studies related to the safety of specific NSAID agents and provide a broad perspective on this important and complex issue, Hodes noted. These include recent systematic reviews and meta-analyses of cyclooxygenase 2 (COX-2) inhibitors and an editorial on NSAIDs in the October 4, 2006, *Journal of the American Medical Association*.

The ADAPT trial began in 2001 and was conducted in six U.S. cities: Tampa, Florida; Rochester, New York; Baltimore, Maryland; Sun City, Arizona; Seattle, Washington; and, Boston, Massachusetts. Approximately 2,500 people were enrolled in ADAPT when the medications were suspended. About 1,100 enrollees were assigned to a control group, while about 700 received celecoxib and another 700 received naproxen. In their safety analysis, researchers counted participants who experienced death due to heart disease or stroke, non-fatal heart attack or stroke, congestive heart failure and transient ischemic attack (brief stroke), or who started high blood pressure treatment during the trial.

Investigators are continuing to follow volunteers in the trial for cardiovascular and cognitive symptoms, and dementia.

NIA Statement: Early Findings from ADAPT Indicate NSAIDs Do Not Prevent Alzheimer Disease

The drugs naproxen and celecoxib did not reduce risk for Alzheimer disease in an analysis of data from a clinical trial sponsored by the National Institute on Aging (NIA), part of the National Institutes of Health. The trial researchers noted that the results are contrary to those of earlier observational studies on non-steroidal anti-inflammatory drugs (NSAIDs) and Alzheimer risk, and that more time may be needed to see protective effects in this trial.

The findings, published April 26, 2007 in _Neurology_, come from the Alzheimer's Disease Anti-inflammatory Prevention Trial (ADAPT) which was designed to test whether long-term use of naproxen or celecoxib can prevent Alzheimer disease in individuals at risk for the disease because of a family history of Alzheimer disease. ADAPT is a multicenter trial administered through the University of Washington, with clinical centers in Baltimore, Boston, Rochester, New York, Sun City, Arizona, Tampa and Seattle, and a coordinating center in Baltimore. The trial began enrolling volunteers in 2001. Treatment was suspended in December 2004 (see statement at http://www.nia.nih .gov/NewsAndEvents/PressReleases/PR20061117ADAPTData.htm).

Researchers have continued to follow participants closely since that time to assess whether the medications produced any changes in their risk for Alzheimer disease and to further evaluate their risk for cardiovascular disease.

Although this early analysis suggests that naproxen and celecoxib do not reduce risk for developing Alzheimer disease, the researchers note that a different picture could emerge after following the ADAPT participants for a few more years. They recommend continued follow-up to see whether the timing of the drug treatments relative to onset of dementia has important bearing on their effect.

In the *Neurology* paper, the ADAPT investigators consider possible explanations for the differences in treatment effects in ADAPT and earlier observational studies. They note that protection against Alzheimer disease might be limited to certain NSAIDs that were not the drugs used in ADAPT. But they also speculate that NSAIDs' influence on Alzheimer disease could differ with the stage of disease progression, noting that the drugs might have a protective effect only if given several years before symptoms appear. By the time symptoms begin to emerge, NSAIDs appear to have no effect, or may even inhibit the brain's ability to clear abnormal protein deposits.

An analysis of the cardiovascular risks of the ADAPT study medications appeared in the November. 17, 2006, issue of *PLoS Clinical Trials*, a journal of the Public Library of Science. Additional information on ADAPT is available on the ADAPT website, http://www.jhucct .com/adapt/default.htm.

References

ADAPT Research Group. Naproxen and celecoxib do not prevent AD in early results from a randomized controlled trial. *Neurology*, DOI: 10.1212/01.wnl.0000260269.93245.d2

Chapter 53

Loss of Body Mass Linked to Development of Alzheimer Disease

Loss of body mass over time appears to be strongly linked to older adults' risk of developing Alzheimer disease (AD), and the greater the loss the greater the chance of a person developing the disease, new research has found. The findings are the first to associate decline in body mass index (BMI) with the eventual onset of AD. The researchers suggest that the loss of body mass reflects disease processes and that change in BMI might be a clinical predictor of the development of AD.

The research, reported in the September 27, 2005, issue of *Neurology*, was conducted by Aron S. Buchman, MD, David A. Bennett, MD, and colleagues at Rush University Medical Center in Chicago, IL, as part of the Religious Orders Study. The Religious Orders Study is a comprehensive, long-term look at aging and AD among Catholic nuns, priests, and brothers nationwide that has been funded by the National Institute on Aging (NIA), a component of the National Institutes of Health, U.S. Department of Health and Human Services, since 1993. Rush University Medical Center is one of more than 30 Alzheimer Disease Centers supported by the NIA.

"People with Alzheimer's disease are known to lose weight and body mass after they have the disease," says Dallas W. Anderson, Ph.D., program director for population studies in the Dementias of Aging Branch of NIA's Neuroscience and Neuropsychology of Aging Program. "This study is significant in that it looks at body mass changes in the

---

"Loss of Body Mass Linked to Development of Alzheimer's Disease, Study Finds," National Institute on Aging, September 2005.

years preceding dementia and cognitive decline. Other studies have looked at BMI at only one point in time or studied body mass loss in people who already have AD."

Each of the 820 study participants took part in yearly clinical evaluations that included a medical history, neurologic examination, and extensive cognitive function testing. The participants' weights and heights were also measured to determine their BMI, a widely used measure of body composition that is calculated by dividing weight in kilograms by height in meters squared. They completed an average of 6.6 annual evaluations, with a 95 percent follow-up rate. All of the participants were older than 65 years, and the vast majority of them were white and of European ancestry.

When the study began, none of the participants had dementia, and their average BMI was 27.4. During the follow-up period, 151 of the participants (18.4 percent) developed AD. Both baseline BMI and the annual rate of change in BMI were linked to the risk of developing AD.

People who lost approximately one unit of BMI per year had a 35 percent greater risk of developing AD than that of people with no change in BMI over the course of the study. Those with no change in BMI had a 20 percent greater risk of developing the disease than that of people who gained six-tenths of a unit of BMI per year.

The findings held true even after adjusting for factors such as chronic health problems, age, sex, and education. They also held true when those who developed AD in the first four years of follow-up—and might have had mild, undiagnosed AD early in the study—were excluded from the analysis.

The investigators found a similar relationship between changes in BMI and rate of cognitive decline, which is the clinical hallmark of AD. Even when controlling for baseline cognitive function, baseline BMI, age, sex, and education, the rate of cognitive decline among people losing approximately one unit of BMI per year was more than 35 percent higher than that of people with no change in BMI and 80 percent higher than that of people who gained six-tenths of a unit of BMI per year.

Further analyses showed that depressive symptoms, participants' physical activity levels, and female participants' use of estrogen replacement did not explain the link between BMI loss and development of AD.

In addition, when the researchers looked at changes in weight rather than BMI, they found that a loss of one pound per year was associated with a five percent increase in the risk of AD.

"These findings suggest that subtle, unexplained body mass and weight loss in an older person may be an early sign of AD and can precede the development of obvious memory problems," explains Bennett, who directs the Rush Alzheimer's Disease Center. "The most likely explanation is that there is something about these individuals or about this disease that affects BMI before the clinical syndrome becomes apparent—that loss of BMI reflects the disease process itself."

"Our understanding of Alzheimer's disease is changing as we get more information, particularly as we look at the pathology of the disease," adds Buchman, the lead investigator for the study. "It turns out that Alzheimer's disease not only results in cognitive dysfunction, but also may have a variety of other symptoms, depending on which brain regions are affected. If the disease pathology affects a region of the brain that controls weight, your body mass may decline prior to loss of cognition."

Based on the Religious Orders Study findings and other evidence, the researchers suggest that loss of body mass could be added to the "relatively short list" of signs doctors can use to predict a person's risk of developing AD.

"There are actually very few predictors of Alzheimer's disease," Bennett explains. "This study makes us think about the spectrum of clinical signs of AD beyond changes in memory and behavior and motor skills. Changes in BMI are easy to measure in a doctor's office without an expensive scan," he says.

Bennett and colleagues acknowledge that the study participants were limited to Catholic clergy living in communal settings and recommend replication of the research with more diverse groups of people. They also note that the group's homogeneity strengthened their research because they knew that all of the participants had access to ample, nutritious food. The authors are indebted to the altruism and support of the participants in the Religious Orders Study.

The researchers note that the Religious Orders Study research complements recently published findings of the Honolulu-Asia Aging Study, a 32-year population-based study funded jointly by NIA and the National Heart, Lung, and Blood Institute, NIH. Those findings, released in the January 2005 Archives of Neurology, show that dementia-associated weight loss in Japanese-American men begins before the onset of dementia and accelerates by the time of diagnosis.

For more information on participation in an AD clinical trial, visit www.clinicaltrials.gov (search for "Alzheimer disease trials") or the Alzheimer's Disease Education and Referral (ADEAR) Center website. ADEAR may also be contacted toll free at 800-438-4380. The ADEAR Center is sponsored by the NIA to provide information to the public and health professionals about AD and age-related cognitive change and may be contacted at the website and phone number above for a variety of publications and fact sheets, as well as information on clinical trials.

Chapter 54

Studying the Effects of Mental Exercise on Seniors' Thinking Skills

Certain mental exercises can offset some of the expected decline in older adults' thinking skills and show promise for maintaining cognitive abilities needed to do everyday tasks such as shopping, making meals, and handling finances, according to a new study. The research, funded by the National Institutes of Health (NIH) and published in the December 20, 2006, *Journal of the American Medical Association*, showed that some of the benefits of short-term cognitive training persisted for as long as five years.

The Advanced Cognitive Training for Independent and Vital Elderly, or ACTIVE, Study is the first randomized, controlled trial to demonstrate long-lasting, positive effects of brief cognitive training in older adults. However, testing indicated that the training did not improve the participants' ability to tackle everyday tasks, and more research is needed to translate the findings from the laboratory into interventions that prove effective at home.

The ACTIVE trial was funded by the National Institute on Aging (NIA) and the National Institute of Nursing Research (NINR), both components of NIH. Sherry L. Willis, PhD, of Pennsylvania State University in State College, Pennsylvania, and co-authors report the findings on behalf of ACTIVE investigators at the study's six sites: Hebrew SeniorLife, Boston; Indiana University School of Medicine, Indianapolis; Johns Hopkins University, Baltimore; Pennsylvania

"Mental Exercise Helps Maintain Some Seniors' Thinking Skills," National Institute on Aging, December 2006.

State University; University of Alabama at Birmingham; and University of Florida, Gainesville (in collaboration with Wayne State University, Detroit), and the data coordinating center at the New England Research Institutes, Watertown, Massachusetts.

"This large trial found that community-dwelling seniors who received cognitive training had less of a decline in certain thinking skills than their peers who did not have training. The study addresses a very important hypothesis—that interventions can be designed to maintain cognitive function," says NIA Director Richard J. Hodes, MD. "The challenge now is to further examine these interventions and others to see how they can be employed in real-world settings."

"Cognitive decline is known to precede loss of functional ability in older adults. It affects everyday activities such as driving or following instructions on a medicine bottle," says NINR Director Patricia A. Grady, PhD, RN. "Research to identify effective ways of delaying this decline is important because it may help individuals, and our aging citizenry, maintain greater independence as they grow older."

The ACTIVE Study included 2,802 adults aged 65 and older who were living independently and had normal cognitive and functional status at the beginning of the study. Participants were randomly assigned to four groups. Three groups took part in training that targeted a specific cognitive ability—memory, reasoning, or speed of processing. The fourth group received no cognitive training.

People in the three intervention groups attended up to 10 training sessions lasting 60 to 75 minutes each, over a five- to six-week time period. The memory group learned strategies for remembering word lists and sequences of items, text, and story ideas and details. The reasoning group learned strategies for finding the pattern in a letter or word series and identifying the next item in a series. The speed-of-processing group learned ways to identify an object on a computer screen at increasingly brief exposures, while quickly noting where another object was located on the screen.

After the initial training, 60 percent of those who completed the initial training took part in 75-minute "booster" sessions designed to maintain improvements gained from the initial sessions.

The investigators tested the participants at baseline, after the intervention, and annually over five years. They found the following:

• Immediately after the initial training, 87 percent of the speed-training group, 74 percent of the reasoning group and 26 percent of the memory group showed improvement in the skills taught.

- After five years, people in each group performed better on tests in their respective areas of training than did people in the control group. The reasoning-training and speed-training groups who received booster training had the greatest benefit.

"The improvements seen after the training roughly counteract the degree of decline in cognitive performance that we would expect to see over a seven- to fourteen-year period among older people without dementia," says Dr. Willis.

The researchers also looked at the training's effects on participants' everyday lives. After five years, all three intervention groups reported less difficulty than the control group in tasks such as preparing meals, managing money, and doing housework. Only the effect of reasoning training on self-reported performance of daily tasks was statistically significant. Those who received speed-of-processing training and follow-up booster training scored better on how quickly and accurately they could find items on a pantry shelf, make change, read medicine dosing instructions, place telephone calls, and react to road traffic signs.

"Beyond middle age, people worry about their mental sharpness getting 'rusty.' This study offers hope that cognitive training may be useful," notes Richard Suzman, PhD, director of the NIA's Behavioral and Social Research Program, which sponsored the work. "ACTIVE has shown that relatively brief targeted cognitive exercises can produce durable changes in the skills taught. I would now like to see studies aimed at producing more generalized changes, perhaps through more intensive and broader interventions."

The NIA leads the federal effort supporting and conducting research on aging and the medical, social and behavioral issues of older people. For more information on research and aging, go to www.nia.nih .gov. Publications on research and on a variety of topics of interest on health and aging can be viewed and ordered by visiting the NIA website or can be ordered by calling toll-free 800-222-2225.

The primary mission of the NINR is to support clinical and basic research to establish a scientific basis for the care of individuals across the life span. For additional information, visit the NINR website at www.ninr.nih.gov.

The NIH—the nation's medical research agency—includes 27 institutes and centers and is a component of the U.S. Department of Health and Human Services. It is the primary federal agency for conducting and supporting basic, clinical and translational medical research, and it investigates the causes, treatments and cures for both common and rare diseases. For more information about NIH and its programs, visit www.nih.gov.

Chapter 55

Study Finds Mix of Disease Processes at Work in Brains of Most People with Dementia

Few older people die with brains untouched by a pathological process, however, an individual's likelihood of having clinical signs of dementia increases with the number of different disease processes present in the brain, according to a new study. The research was funded by the National Institute on Aging (NIA), part of the National Institutes of Health, and conducted at the Rush Alzheimer's Disease Center at Rush University Medical Center in Chicago. Julie Schneider, MD, and colleagues report the findings in the journal *Neurology* online today.

Among their findings is the observation that the combination of Alzheimer disease and cerebral infarcts (strokes) is the most common mix of pathologies in the brains of people with dementia. The implication of these findings is that public health efforts to prevent and treat vascular disease could potentially reduce the occurrence of dementia, the researchers say in the paper.

The researchers used data from the Rush Memory and Aging Project—an ongoing study of 1,200 elderly volunteers who have agreed to be evaluated every year and to donate their brains upon death. The current study compared clinical and autopsy data on the first 141 participants who have died.

Annual physical and psychological exams showed that, while they were alive, 50 of the 141 had dementia. Upon death, a neuropathologist, who was unaware of the results of the clinical evaluation, analyzed

"Study Finds Mix of Disease Processes at Work in Brains of Most People with Dementia," National Institutes of Health, press release dated June 13, 2007.

each person's brain. The autopsies showed that about 85 percent of the individuals had evidence of at least one chronic disease process, such as Alzheimer disease, strokes, Parkinson disease, hemorrhages, tumors, traumatic brain injury, or others.

Comparison of the clinical and autopsy results showed that only 30 percent of people with signs of dementia had Alzheimer disease alone. By contrast, 42 percent of the people with dementia had Alzheimer disease with infarcts and 16 percent had Alzheimer disease with Parkinson disease (including two people with all three conditions). Infarcts alone caused another 12 percent of the cases. Also, 80 of the 141 volunteers who died had sufficient Alzheimer disease pathology in their brains to fulfill accepted neuropathologic criteria for Alzheimer disease, although in life only 47 were clinically diagnosed with probable or possible Alzheimer disease.

"We know that people can have Alzheimer pathology without having symptoms," says Dallas Anderson, PhD, population studies program director in the NIA Neuroscience and Neuropsychology of Aging Program. "The finding that Alzheimer pathology with cerebral infarcts is a very common combination in people with dementia adds to emerging evidence that we might be able to reduce some of the risk of dementia with the same tools we use for cardiovascular disease such as control of blood cholesterol levels and hypertension."

NIA is conducting clinical trials to determine whether interventions for cardiovascular disease can prevent or slow the progress of Alzheimer disease. On-going trials cover a range of interventions such as statin drugs, vitamins, and exercise.

NIA leads the federal effort supporting and conducting research on aging and the medical, social, and behavioral issues of older people, including Alzheimer disease and age-related cognitive decline. For information on dementia and aging, please visit NIA's Alzheimer's Disease Education and Referral Center at www.nia.nih.gov/alzheimers, or call 800-438-4380.

Chapter 56

Cardiovascular Risks May Also Increase Risk for Alzheimer Disease

High cholesterol, high blood pressure, diabetes, and smoking—long considered serious risk factors for heart disease—may also increase your long-term risk for Alzheimer disease, a new study of nearly 9,000 Californians shows. Middle-aged men and women who had one or more of these risk factors during their early 40s were much more likely to develop Alzheimer disease and other forms of dementia years down the road.

Researchers found that having any one of these risk factors in your early 40s increases your risk of dementia in later life by some 20 to 40 percent. Having two or more, though, was especially hazardous to your long-term mental acuity. Compared to individuals who had none of these risk factors for heart disease, those with two of the factors were 70 percent more likely to be diagnosed with dementia in later life. Those with three were more than twice as likely to develop dementia. And those with all four were at 2.37 times greater risk.

This study is important because it looked at a large number of people and charted their progress over several decades, solidifying earlier evidence that what's good for the heart is good for the brain. "The real strength of our study is the large, multiethnic cohort of men and women, followed up for 27 years, all with equal access to medical care," said study author Rachel Whitmer, PhD, of Kaiser Permanente,

485

a non-profit HMO [health maintenance organization] in Oakland, California. Participants included men and women of various ethnic groups, including whites, blacks, and Asians. All belonged to an HMO and had equal access to doctors and medical care. The study appeared in the January 25, 2005 issue of *Neurology*, the scientific journal of the American Academy of Neurology.

Here's how the individual risk factors broke down:

Diabetes: People who had diabetes in their middle years were at highest risk of developing Alzheimer disease later in life. Diabetes increased the risk by 46 percent. Other studies indicate that those who develop diabetes late in life are also at increased risk of developing dementia. Doctors believe this may occur because diabetes damages blood vessels throughout the body, including those that feed the brain. Additional studies are needed to determine whether proper treatment and control of blood sugar throughout middle age and beyond can lower the risk of Alzheimer disease.

High cholesterol: Those with high cholesterol levels in their mid-years were 42 percent more likely to develop Alzheimer disease as seniors. Doctors suspect that high cholesterol may lead to high levels of beta-amyloid, the toxic substance that builds up in the brains of those with Alzheimer disease, killing off healthy brain cells. Other studies suggest that taking medications such as statin drugs that lower cholesterol may help to keep the memory intact, though more research into these medicines is needed.

High blood pressure: Men and women who had high blood pressure in their forties were 24 percent more likely to develop dementia later in life. Recent research have found that treating high blood pressure as we age may lower the risk of developing memory problems and dementia.

Smoking: Research on the effects of smoking on Alzheimer disease have been mixed. In this study, middle-aged smokers were 26 percent more likely to develop dementia with age. Some research suggests that the nicotine in tobacco smoke may actually lower the risk of Alzheimer disease, because nicotine may help to stem the development of plaques that accumulate in the brains of those with the disease. However, other population studies suggest that smoking increases the risk of Alzheimer disease and other forms of dementia.

Experts are hopeful that a sound diet, lots of exercise, other healthy lifestyle measures, and proper medical treatment—all good for the heart—may help to protect against Alzheimer disease as well. This and other studies suggest that may be so. Alzheimer disease, however, is a complex disease with genetic and various environmental factors all playing a role. No one measure can guarantee you'll stay sharp into old age, but at the least, a healthy lifestyle may help.

References

R.A. Whitmer, PhD, S. Sidney, MD, J. Selby, MD, et al: Midlife Cardiovascular Risk Factors and Risk of Dementia in Late Life. *Neurology* 2005; 64, pages 277–281.

Chapter 57

Diabetes Linked to Increased Risk of Alzheimer Disease

Diabetes mellitus was linked to a 65 percent increased risk of developing Alzheimer disease (AD), appearing to affect some aspects of cognitive function differently than others in a new study supported by the National Institute on Aging (NIA) at the National Institutes of Health. The findings, from the Rush Alzheimer's Disease Center's Religious Orders Study, add to a developing body of research examining a possible link between diabetes and cognitive decline. The results reported today are among the first to examine how certain cognitive "systems"—memory for words and events, the speed of processing information, and the ability to recognize spatial patterns—may be affected selectively in people with diabetes.

The research, by Zoe Arvanitakis, MD, David Bennett, MD, and colleagues at the Rush University Medical Center in Chicago, IL, appears in the May 2004 issue of the *Archives of Neurology*. The investigators are part of the institution's Rush Alzheimer's Disease Center, headed by Dr. Bennett. The AD Center is one of 30 across the U.S. supported by the NIA to study and care for Alzheimer patients.

"The research on a possible link between diabetes and increased risk of AD is intriguing, and this study gives us important additional insights," says Neil Buckholtz, PhD, head of the Dementias of Aging Branch in the NIA's neurosciences program. "Further research, some currently underway, will tell us whether therapies for diabetes may in fact play a role in lowering risk of AD or cognitive decline."

"Diabetes Linked to Increased Risk of Alzheimer's in Long-Term Study," National Institute on Aging (http://www.nia.nih.gov), May 2004.

Some 824 Catholic nuns, priests, and brothers participating in the Religious Orders Study were followed for an average of 5.5 years. They received detailed clinical evaluations annually, including neuropsychological testing of five cognitive "systems" commonly affected by aging, AD, and other dementias—episodic memory (memory of specific life events), semantic memory (general knowledge), working memory (ability to hold and mentally rearrange information), perceptual speed (the speed with which simple perceptual comparisons can be made, such as whether two strings of numbers are the same or different), and visuospatial ability (the ability to recognize spatial patterns).

Over the study period, 151 of the participants had a clinical diagnosis of AD, including 31 who had diabetes. The researchers found a 65 percent increase in the risk of developing AD among those with diabetes compared with people who did not have diabetes.

In measures of cognitive function, only in the area of perceptual speed was there an association with an increased rate of decline over time, by about 44%, when comparing the diabetes and non-diabetes groups. Since stroke-related changes in the brain were found in a previous study to be tied to a decline in perceptual speed, the researchers could not say whether the link between cognitive decline and diabetes appeared because of the changes in the brain associated with Alzheimer disease or those of some other common age-related condition like stroke or other vascular complications. Studies looking at pathological or brain imaging data would be needed to address these possibilities.

In other areas of cognition, the rate of change over the time period of the study was no different in the two groups. However, at the start of the study, the baseline cognitive function scores of people with diabetes were lower than those of people without diabetes.

"We found that diabetes was related to decline in some cognitive systems but not in others," says Dr. Arvanitakis of Rush, the lead author of the report. "Since all participants have agreed to brain donation at their deaths, we will have the opportunity to examine the pathologic basis of the association of diabetes to cognitive decline." The Rush researchers also expressed their indebtedness to the more than 1,000 nuns, priests, and brothers from across the U.S. participating in the Religious Orders Study.

Chapter 58

Dementia and Amyotrophic Lateral Sclerosis (ALS) May Share a Common Pathological Process

Scientists have identified a misfolded, or incorrectly formed, protein common to two devastating neurological diseases, frontotemporal dementia (FTD) and amyotrophic lateral sclerosis (ALS, also known as Lou Gehrig disease), according to a report in the October 6, 2006, issue of *Science*. The findings suggest that certain forms of FTD, ALS, and possibly other neurological diseases might share a common pathological process.

Virginia Lee, PhD, and John Trojanowski, MD, PhD, of the University of Pennsylvania, led an international team of scientists in this discovery. The work was funded by the National Institute on Aging (NIA), part of the National Institutes of Health (NIH), and was done at the NIA-funded Alzheimer's Disease Center at the University of Pennsylvania School of Medicine Institute on Aging.

"This exciting basic science discovery provides the first molecular link between a dementia—FTD—and a motor neuron disease—ALS. It will advance understanding of the pathological processes of FTD and ALS, and possibly of other neurological disorders," says NIA director Richard J. Hodes, MD. Improved understanding of underlying disease processes is critically important in pointing researchers toward the development of therapies for FTD, ALS and other neurodegenerative diseases, Hodes and the study authors note.

"Researchers Discover Misfolded Protein Clumps Common to Dementia, Lou Gehrig's Disease," National Institute on Aging (http://www.nia.nih.gov), October 2006.

FTD affects the frontal and temporal lobes of the brain. People with FTD may exhibit uninhibited and socially inappropriate behavior, changes in personality, and, in late stages, loss of memory, motor skills, and speech. After Alzheimer disease, it is the most common cause of dementia in people under age 65.

ALS is a progressive disease of brain and spinal cord motor neurons that control movement. Over time, walking, eating, speaking, and breathing become more difficult in this fatal disease. Some people with ALS also have FTD, and some with FTD also develop ALS, suggesting that common mechanisms might underlie these two diseases.

In certain neurodegenerative diseases, including ALS and some forms of FTD, scientists have identified clumps of protein—or inclusion bodies—that accumulate in brain cells and neurons. However, understanding why they form and what they contain has been elusive. Lee and Trojanowski have long sought to solve that mystery.

Following years of research, they have now identified TDP-43 as a constituent part of the clumps that form in ALS and in the most common form of FTD. Although its precise role is not well understood, TDP-43 is involved in the complex process of transcribing and regulating genetic information in the nucleus of the cell.

"There is much more to learn about how this nuclear protein is clumped in the cytoplasm of cells and about the mechanism by which it is implicated in two distinctly different diseases," says Stephen Snyder, PhD, program director, etiology of Alzheimer disease, NIA Neuroscience and Neuropsychology of Aging Program. "It is possible that the TDP-43 protein will be a key to a more complete understanding of both FTD and ALS."

References

M Neumann et al. Ubiquinated TDP-43 in Frontotemporal Lobar Degeneration and Amyotrophic Lateral Sclerosis. *Science* DOI:10.1126/science.1134108 (2006).

Chapter 59

Clinical Antipsychotic Trials of Intervention Effectiveness (CATIE): Phase I Results

Questions and Answers About the NIMH Clinical Antipsychotic Trials of Intervention Effectiveness (CATIE) Alzheimer's Disease Study—Phase I Results

What is the CATIE Alzheimer disease study?

The CATIE Alzheimer disease trial was a large-scale public health study using newer, atypical antipsychotic medications for the treatment of delusions, hallucinations, aggression, and agitation that often accompany Alzheimer disease. Such symptoms affect more than 75 percent of the people who have Alzheimer disease.

The $16.9 million CATIE Alzheimer disease study was conducted at 42 sites with 421 participants and is one of two large-scale nationwide clinical trials funded by the National Institutes of Health (NIH)'s National Institute of Mental Health (NIMH) to examine the effectiveness of atypical antipsychotic medications. These medications were developed originally to treat symptoms (such as hallucinations and delusions) associated with schizophrenia, but they are widely used to treat similar symptoms in Alzheimer disease.

This chapter includes text from "Questions and Answers about the NIMH Clinical Antipsychotic Trials of Intervention Effectiveness (CATIE) Alzheimer's Disease Study—Phase I Results," "NIMH Perspective on Treating Alzheimer's Patients with Antipsychotic Medications," and "Antipsychotic Medications Used to Treat Alzheimer's Patients Found Lacking," National Institute of Mental Health (http://www.nimh.nih.gov), October 2006.

Why is the CATIE Alzheimer study important?

Memory loss and disorientation are the most common symptoms of Alzheimer disease, but many people with the disease experience symptoms such as delusions, hallucinations, aggressive behavior, or agitation. These symptoms are associated with a rapid worsening of the illness and often result in the patient being placed in a nursing home or other specialized care institution.

The U.S. Food and Drug Administration (FDA) has not specifically approved antipsychotic medications for use in treating people with Alzheimer disease, but many doctors prescribe these medications "off label" when they believe a patient may benefit. Although many different antipsychotic medications have been used to treat these thinking and behavior symptoms in people with Alzheimer disease, doctors do not have data about how well they work, if some work better than others, and if they are safe. About 25 percent of Alzheimer patients living in nursing homes receive atypical antipsychotics.[1] However, no data exist that indicate how many Alzheimer patients living outside of nursing home currently receive these medications.

The CATIE Alzheimer disease study was designed to evaluate the overall effectiveness of the newer antipsychotic medications in treating hallucinations, aggression, and related symptoms. Specifically, it aimed to determine if these medications—overall—are beneficial, tolerable, and safe for use by Alzheimer patients. The study is unique for several reasons. Although studies of antipsychotic medications have been conducted, nearly all of those studies were conducted in nursing homes and therefore, are less relevant to the many people with Alzheimer disease cared for by family members in their own homes or in assisted-living facilities. Further, none of these earlier studies followed participants for longer than 12 weeks. Lastly, these earlier studies did not compare different antipsychotic medications to each other.

In contrast, the CATIE Alzheimer disease study included three of the most widely used antipsychotic medications and placebo (inactive pill) among patients in non-nursing home settings, who were experiencing delusions, hallucinations, aggression, or agitation. The study followed the participants over nine months and also included the involvement of caregivers.

Who participated in the study?

The 421 participants all had Alzheimer disease, and were geographically dispersed at 42 clinical sites across the United States. All were experiencing delusions, hallucinations, aggression, or agitation that disrupted their daily functioning, such that an antipsychotic medication was determined to be appropriate treatment. Participants were ambulatory and still living at home or in assisted living facilities. A family member, caregiver, or study partner who had regular contact with the patient also participated in the study to help with monitoring and assessments. Study staff worked closely with participants' regular doctors to monitor co-occurring medical illnesses.

Patient Characteristics

- Patients Enrolled: 421

- Gender: 56 percent female

- Average age: 78 years

- Race: 21 percent non-white

- Residence: 73 percent in own home; 16 percent in family member's home; 10 percent in assisted living

Caregiver Characteristics

Among caregivers, 71 percent were women; 52 percent of caregivers were spouses and 33 percent were children or sons-in-law or daughters-in-law. The average ages of caregivers were 73.5 years for spouses and 51.2 years for children or their spouses. They spent 5.2 hours per day in specific caregiving activities.

What treatments were given in the CATIE Alzheimer study and how was treatment chosen for each participant?

The CATIE Alzheimer study was designed with several phases. In phase 1, participants were randomly assigned to one of four treatment groups—three antipsychotic medications (olanzapine, quetiapine, and risperidone) or placebo (inactive pill). This means that they, their caregivers, and their doctors could not choose which one of the four treatments they would receive. Further, the study was "double-blinded," meaning that neither the participant or caregiver, nor the medical staff knew which treatment the participant was taking. This type of "placebo-controlled, double-blind, randomized clinical trial" helps to ensure objective results because researchers, participants, and caregivers will not be biased by their expectations about how well a medication may work.

During Phase 1, doctors could adjust a participant's dose based on the participant's individual needs. Participants who benefited from their assigned treatment could continue on this treatment for up to 36 weeks. However, if after two weeks the participant was not benefiting from the treatment, then he or she could discontinue the medication and enter Phase 2 of the study, where he or she could receive on a random basis a different antipsychotic medication or citalopram, an antidepressant medication, also on a "double-blind" basis. Participants could leave the study at any time.

In addition to the medications in the study, patients and their caregivers received basic information about Alzheimer disease. The caregivers were offered two counseling sessions during the study and could speak with study staff as needed.

What were the results of phase 1?

To determine both the benefits and the risks associated with each treatment, the researchers used the length of time patients stayed on their assigned treatments as the primary measure of treatment success. After a minimum two-week period, a medication could be discontinued if it was not benefiting the patient, if he or she was experiencing intolerable side effects, such as dizziness, or for any other reason. This "all cause discontinuation" or "time in treatment" benchmark integrated patients', caregivers', and clinicians' judgments of efficacy, safety, and tolerability into an overall measure of effectiveness that reflected therapeutic benefits in relation to undesirable effects.

In phase 1, there were no differences in the length of time in treatment among any of the four treatment groups. Patients stayed on their assigned medication for an average of about eight weeks, regardless of their specific treatments. In other words, the participants who took placebo benefited just as much as those who took any of the three antipsychotic medications.

When the researchers examined the reasons for discontinuation, they found some differences between placebo and the medications. Those taking olanzapine and risperidone were less likely to cite lack of benefit as a reason to discontinue use. However, those taking any of the three antipsychotic medications were more likely to discontinue use because of intolerable side effects than those taking placebo.

The dosage levels of olanzapine and risperidone used in this study were similar to those used in previous studies, but the quetiapine dose was lower than what was used in other studies. It is possible that the quetiapine dose was too low to have a therapeutic effect, but the physicians were free to raise it, and the dose was still high enough to cause side effects.

Were there differences in side effects among the treatment groups?

Although some participants in the study benefited from the treatments, those who received the antipsychotic medications experienced more side effects and discontinued their treatment because of side effects more than those who received placebo. All three antipsychotic medications were more likely to cause sleepiness and weight gain than placebo. There were some differences among the three medication treatments with respect to movement problems (less likely with quetiapine), confusion (more likely with olanzapine), and psychotic symptoms (more likely with olanzapine).

What do these results mean for clinicians who treat people affected by Alzheimer disease, and their caregivers?

For the first time, doctors, patients, and their caregivers have extensive and clinically relevant information on antipsychotic medications from a large, long-term study directly comparing the medications to each other and to placebo. The results from this first phase of the study indicate that the overall benefit of these medications is offset by intolerability to associated side effects. Doctors pondering whether to prescribe atypical antipsychotic medications for their Alzheimer patients need to consider the risks, benefits, and individual needs of a given patient. Although some patients may benefit greatly from these medications, the evidence from this study suggests these medications hold limited value for the majority of patients. These results further emphasize the challenge of managing behavioral problems in Alzheimer patients. Prior to prescribing these medications, clinicians must ensure that agitation or aggression in their Alzheimer patients are not related to medical, social, or environmental factors (for example, fever from an infection, side effects from another medication) which might be mitigated without resorting to psychotropic medications.

The results from subsequent phases of the study will provide further information to help guide practice.

What other information will doctors and patients be able to learn from CATIE-AD in the future?

CATIE-AD will determine whether people who discontinue treatment during phase I can be helped by switching to a different antipsychotic or to an antidepressant. The study will also show which treatments, if any, will help improve symptoms, quality of life, and functioning, as well as caregiver burden, thereby delaying nursing home placement.

Who conducted the CATIE Alzheimer disease study?

The CATIE AD study was led by Drs. Lon Schneider at the University of Southern California (USC), Los Angeles and Pierre Tariot (Banner Alzheimer's Institute in Phoenix, AZ). Co-authors included: Karen Dagerman (USC Los Angeles); Sonia Davis (Quintiles, Research Triangle Park, NC); M. Saleem Ismail and J. Michael Ryan (University of Rochester, NY); John K. Hsiao (NIMH) and Barry D. Lebowitz (University of California, San Diego; formerly NIMH); Constantine G. Lyketsos (Johns Hopkins University, Baltimore, MD); T. Scott Stroup (The University of North Carolina (UNC), Chapel Hill); David L. Sultzer (Veteran's Affairs Greater Los Angeles Healthcare System, University of California, Los Angeles); Daniel Weintraub (University of Pennsylvania, Philadelphia); and Jeffrey A. Lieberman (College of Physicians and Surgeons, Columbia University, NY).

The University of North Carolina was the primary contractor for the CATIE project, led by Dr. Jeffrey Lieberman, (formerly of UNC, Chapel Hill). Quintiles, a private contract research organization (CRO), assisted with study implementation and data analysis of the trial.

What role did the pharmaceutical companies have in CATIE?

The pharmaceutical companies donated the medications used in this study. They had no input into the planning of the study but were presented with an overview of the design. They had no input into its implementation or conducting of the data analysis, and did not participate in preparing manuscripts for publication. The medications used in the study and their manufacturers included:

- Olanzapine (Zyprexa®), manufactured by Eli Lilly and Company

- Quetiapine (Seroquel®), manufactured by Astra Zeneca Corporation

- Risperidone (Risperdal®), manufactured by Janssen Pharmaceuticals

- Citalopram (Celexa®), manufactured by Forest Laboratories in the United States, was used in phase 2 of the study to be reported later.

NIMH Perspective on Treating Alzheimer Patients with Antipsychotic Medications

The recent publication of phase 1 results from the NIMH-funded Clinical Antipsychotic Trials in Intervention Effectiveness for Alzheimer disease (CATIE-AD) in the *New England Journal of Medicine* provides new information about the use of several "atypical" antipsychotic medications for the treatment of psychotic symptoms in patients with Alzheimer disease.

Approximately 75 percent of Alzheimer patients experience psychotic symptoms such as hallucinations, and behavioral symptoms such as aggression and agitation.[2] The U.S. Food and Drug Administration has not approved the use of antipsychotic medications for treating psychosis or agitation among Alzheimer patients, citing safety concerns. In the absence of a better pharmacological alternative, however, antipsychotic medications are widely used on an off-label basis. In fact, it is estimated that 25 percent of Medicare beneficiaries in nursing homes receive these medications.[3]

The extent to which these medications benefit patients is unclear, and opinions vary as to whether they are safe for this population. The results of phase 1 of CATIE-AD provide a first set of real-world effectiveness data where little existed before. Overall, data from this trial suggest:

- Although some atypical antipsychotic medications are modestly helpful for some patients, they are not effective for the majority of Alzheimer patients with psychotic symptoms.

- Good clinical practice requires that medical or environmental causes for Alzheimer-related agitation and aggression be ruled out and that behavioral interventions be considered before turning to antipsychotic medications.

- If an antipsychotic medication then is warranted, clinicians should closely monitor their Alzheimer patients for intolerable side effects and potential safety concerns.

- Clinicians should be mindful of the limitations of these medications and weigh the risks against potential benefits.

Clinical research data indicate that other medications—such as antidepressants, anxiety medications, sedatives, and mood stabilizers—that are commonly used to manage psychotic symptoms in Alzheimer patients, also have significant limitations and risks. Therefore, developing policy that could severely limit physician and patient use of atypical antipsychotic medications would not be in the best interest of these patients. More research is needed to identify the subset of patients who will most likely benefit from and tolerate these medications, and to develop better treatments for this vulnerable population.

Antipsychotic Medications Used to Treat Alzheimer Patients Found Lacking

Commonly prescribed antipsychotic medications used to treat Alzheimer patients with delusions, aggression, hallucinations, and other similar symptoms can benefit some patients, but they appear to be no more effective than a placebo when adverse side effects are considered, according to the first phase of the large-scale clinical trial CATIE-AD funded by the National Institutes of Health's National Institute of Mental Health (NIMH).

"Antipsychotic medications have been used extensively for Alzheimer patients without enough solid evidence of whether they are effective," said NIMH Director Thomas R. Insel, MD. "The study has vital public health implications because it provides physicians and patients with information to more accurately weigh the medications' benefits against their drawbacks, with the needs and unique reactions of their individual patients."

In this first phase of the trial, patients were randomized to olanzapine (Zyprexa), quetiapine (Seroquel), risperidone (Risperdal)—all newer antipsychotic medications—or to an inactive pill known as a placebo. Lead author Lon Schneider, MD, of the University of Southern California Keck School of Medicine and colleagues judged each medication's overall benefits and risks by measuring how long a patient stayed on the medication before discontinuing for any reason. On average, patients discontinued their medication after about eight weeks, regardless of whether they were taking an active medication or placebo, indicating no significant differences in effectiveness between the active medications and placebo.

Some participants did benefit from the treatment; 26 to 32 percent of those taking the active medications improved, compared to 21 percent of those taking placebo. But the antipsychotic medications also were more often associated with troubling side effects, such as sedation, confusion, and weight gain, compared to placebo. Fifteen to 24 percent of those taking active medications discontinued use because of side effects, while only 5 percent of those taking placebo discontinued use citing side effects.

The study investigators determined the medications' effectiveness by balancing their associated benefits with their associated risks. "The antipsychotic medications may be effective against some symptoms in Alzheimer patients compared to placebo, but their tendency to cause intolerable adverse side effects in this vulnerable population offsets their benefits," concluded Schneider.

Those who discontinued their medications in Phase 1—82 percent—went on to subsequent phases of the CATIE-AD trial in which they were randomized to one of the other study medications that they had not yet taken, or to citalopram, an antidepressant medication. Results of these phases are being analyzed and will be published later.

The flexible design and implementation of the CATIE-AD trial reflects real-world practices, in which newer antipsychotic medications often are used to treat delusions, aggression, hallucinations, and agitation in Alzheimer patients. Study physicians determined medication dosage levels according to their patients' individual needs, and consulted with the patient and caregivers when determining if and when a patient should discontinue. Patients represented a broad range of ages (average age was 80 years), diversity, level of disability, and cognitive difficulties.

"In many cases, the moderate to severe thinking and behavioral symptoms of Alzheimer's precipitate placement in a nursing home, at which point the economic and social costs associated with Alzheimer's care skyrocket," said co-lead author Pierre Tariot, MD, of the Banner Alzheimer's Institute in Phoenix, AZ. "By identifying the limitations of existing treatment options, this study is an important step toward finding a treatment that can delay full-time nursing home confinements, and reduce the suffering of patients and their families."

References

1. The Quality of Antipsychotic Drug Prescribing in Nursing Homes, Becky A. Briesacher; M. Rhona Limcangco; Linda Simoni-Wastila; Jalpa A. Doshi; Suzi R. Levens; Dennis G. Shea; Bruce Stuart, *Arch Intern Med.* 2005;165:1280-1285.

2. Devanand DP, Jacobs DM, Tang MX, et al. The course of psychopathologic features in mild to moderate Alzheimer disease. *Archives of General Psychiatry* 1997; 54:257–63.

3. The Quality of Antipsychotic Drug Prescribing in Nursing Homes, Becky A. Briesacher; M. Rhona Limcangco; Linda Simoni-Wastila; Jalpa A. Doshi; Suzi R. Levens; Dennis G. Shea; Bruce Stuart, *Arch Intern Med.* 2005;165:1280–12.

Additional Sources

Schneider L, Tariot P, Dagerman K, Davis S, Hsiao J, Ismail MS, Lebowitz B, Lyketsos C, Ryan M, Stroup TS, Sultzer D, Weintraub D, Lieberman J. Effectiveness of Atypical Antipsychotic Drugs in Patients with Alzheimer's Disease. *New England Journal of Medicine.* 2006; 355:1525–38.

Schneider L, Tariot PN, Lyketsos CG, et al. NIMH Clinical Antipsychotic Trials of Intervention Effectiveness (CATIE): Alzheimer disease trial methodology. *American Journal of Geriatric Psychiatry* 2001; 9: 346–60.

Chapter 60

Study Suggests New Treatments for Alzheimer Disease

While several treatments are currently available for Alzheimer disease (AD), none of them can slow or halt the course of this devastating disorder. In a new study, researchers have now identified three compounds that inhibit an enzyme believed to be involved in the process that leads to AD. This discovery may lead to new treatments that can stop the disease process in its tracks.

"Because of recent advances in understanding Alzheimer disease, we are now moving strongly toward devising therapies that will treat the disease," says Kenneth Kosik, MD, of the Neuroscience Research Institute at the University of California, Santa Barbara (UCSB), who led the new study. Dr. Kosik and his colleagues tested thousands of compounds to learn if any of them could interfere with an enzyme called Cdk5. This enzyme helps to form bundles of twisted filaments found within neurons, called neurofibrillary tangles, which are a hallmark of AD. The study was funded in part by the National Institute of Neurological Disorders and Stroke (NINDS) and appeared in the July 22, 2005, issue of *Chemistry & Biology*.

Neurofibrillary tangles are composed largely of a protein called tau. In healthy neurons, tau is a component of microtubules, which form part of the cell's structural support and deliver substances throughout the nerve cell. However, in AD, tau gets attached to many molecules called phosphate groups. These phosphate groups change the protein's structure

"Drug Screening Study Suggests New Treatments for Alzheimer's," National Institute of Neurological Disorders and Stroke (http://www.ninds.nih.gov), September 2006.

and function and cause it to form tangles. Previous studies have shown that Cdk5 helps the phosphate groups attach to tau. Therefore, researchers hypothesize that inhibiting Cdk5 might stop neurofibrillary tangles from forming and prevent some of the neuron loss in AD.

The investigators tested drug-like molecules that are small enough to enter the brain and penetrate neurons. With additional development, these molecules could serve as the basis for future drugs to treat neurodegenerative disorders such as AD, Niemann-Pick disease, and Parkinson diseases. Using a new "high-throughput" screening test, the researchers rapidly tested 58,000 molecules from a chemical library to see if any of them would prevent Cdk5 from adding phosphate groups to tau—a process called phosphorylation. They identified three compounds that worked. One of the compounds was similar to other, previously identified inhibitor compounds. However, the other two compounds worked in previously undescribed ways.

The researchers are particularly interested in one of the compounds because it binds to Cdk5 and prevents tau phosphorylation in a manner that is unlikely to interfere with other activities of the enzyme. Since Cdk5 and similar enzymes have many different roles in the body, stopping their activity completely could cause many side effects. Therefore, researchers want to find a drug that can selectively inhibit Cdk5's ability to modify tau without interfering with its other functions.

While none of the three compounds identified in this study works well enough to be a strong drug candidate for AD, learning how these compounds work could help biochemists modify them in ways that would increase their effectiveness, Dr. Kosik says. They also might be able to use this knowledge to identify or design new, more effective compounds.

In addition to AD, Cdk5 has been linked to development of Parkinson disease, amyotrophic lateral sclerosis, and Niemann-Pick disease type C. While it is not yet clear exactly how the enzyme contributes to these diseases, a Cdk5-blocking drug developed to treat AD might also be useful for treating them, the researchers say.

This drug screening project is unique in that it was conducted by a group of university researchers rather than at a pharmaceutical company. Early-stage drug discovery can sometimes proceed more rapidly in academic settings because university researchers don't share the same market-driven concerns as companies, Dr. Kosik comments. He also credits the success of this project to "extraordinary collaborators" from Harvard Medical School in Boston, the Massachusetts Institute of Technology in Cambridge, and Italy. The project began while Dr. Kosik worked at Harvard.

The researchers are continuing their drug screening efforts and they have now tested about 100,000 compounds, Dr. Kosik says. They also are exploring ways to modify the Cdk5-blocking compounds they've identified and they are looking to biochemistry and to natural substances to find new compounds to screen. He hopes they might eventually identify compounds that can specifically inhibit the transfer of phosphate groups to tau, instead of interfering with Cdk5. Such compounds would allow a much more precise way of treating AD, he adds.

The NINDS is a component of the National Institutes of Health (NIH) within the Department of Health and Human Services and is the nation's primary supporter of biomedical research on the brain and nervous system. The NIH is comprised of 27 Institutes and Centers and is a component of the U.S. Department of Health and Human Services. It is the primary Federal agency for conducting and supporting basic, clinical, and translational medical research, and investigates the causes, treatments, and cures for both common and rare diseases. For more information about NIH and its programs, visit http://www.nih.gov.

References

Ahn JS, Radhakrishnan ML, Mapelli M, Choi S, Tidor B, Cuny GD, Musacchio A, Yrh L-A, Kosik KS. "Defining Cdk5 Ligand Chemical Space with Small Molecule Inhibitors of Tau Phosphorylation." *Chemistry & Biology*, July 2005, Vol. 12, No. 7, pp. 811–823.

Chapter 61

Study Identifies Predictors of Alzheimer Disease Longevity

It's among the first questions asked after someone is diagnosed with Alzheimer disease: "What can we expect?" It's a tough question that has been difficult to answer. But a new study suggests that assessing several key clinical aspects of the disease soon after diagnosis could help families and physicians better predict long-term survival in individuals with Alzheimer disease (AD). These insights also could help public health officials refine cost projections and plan services for the growing number of older Americans at risk for the disease.

The study, funded by the National Institute on Aging (NIA) of the National Institutes of Health (NIH), appears in the April 6, 2004 issue of the journal *Annals of Internal Medicine.*

The researchers from Seattle's Group Health Cooperative and the University of Washington found that in the years following diagnosis, people with AD survived about half as long as those of similar age in the U.S. population. Women tended to live longer than men, surviving about 6 years compared to men who lived for about 4 years after diagnosis. But this gender gap narrowed with age. Age at diagnosis was also a factor. Those who were diagnosed with AD in their 70s had longer survival times than those diagnosed at age 85 or older.

"This finding moves us toward a more precise vision of the course that Alzheimer disease may take in people with certain clinical characteristics," says Eric B. Larson, MD, MPH, director of Group Health

"Study Identifies Predictors of Alzheimer's Disease Longevity," National Institute on Aging (http://www.nia.nih.gov), April 2004.

Cooperative's Center for Health Studies in Seattle and former medical director at the University of Washington Medical Center. "For doctors, this provides very useful data for gauging the prognosis of an AD patient. For patients and their caregivers, as difficult as this may be to hear, it can help in making appropriate plans for the future."

During the study, Dr. Larson and his colleagues followed 521 community-dwelling men and women aged 60 and older who had been recently diagnosed with Alzheimer disease. They were recruited from a database of 23,000 people listed in an Alzheimer's Disease Patient Registry in the Seattle area. The average follow-up period was about 5 years, with an approximate range from 2½ months to 14 years.

As they entered the study, each person was evaluated for cognitive and memory problems and examined for other conditions including heart disease, heart failure, diabetes, stroke, depression, and urinary incontinence. They were also assessed for a history of agitation, wandering, paranoia, falls, and walking difficulties. Survival was measured from the time of initial diagnosis until death or when the study ended in 2001.

When compared to the life expectancy of the general U.S. population, overall survival was lower for people with AD in all age groups. For instance, median survival was 8 years for women aged 70 diagnosed with AD, which is about half the life expectancy of similarly aged American women who do not have the disease (median is the middle value in the set of numbers; in this case, it means an equal number of AD patients lived for longer and shorter times than the median survival cited in this study). Similar trends were found among 70-year old men with AD who had a median survival time of 4.4 years compared with 9.3 years for the U.S. population.

Survival was poorest among those aged 85 and older who wandered, had walking problems, and had histories of diabetes and congestive heart failure. However, the difference in the life expectancy between those who were diagnosed with AD and the general population progressively diminished with age. At 85, for example, median life expectancy for women with AD was 3.9 years after diagnosis compared to about 6 years for women who didn't have the disease. Similarly, 85-year-old men with newly diagnosed AD had a median life expectancy of 3.3 years compared to 4.7 for men of the same age who didn't have AD.

Poor scores on the initial tests of memory and cognitive performance predicted shorter survival time after diagnosis. In fact, a five-point drop in one key test, the Mini-Mental State Exam, during the first year following diagnosis predicted up to a 66 percent increase in the risk of death after that initial year. Walking problems, congestive heart failure, and a history of falls, diabetes and ischemic heart disease were other important predictors of reduced life expectancy after AD diagnosis.

"This study suggests that several critical factors can be evaluated to help answer some of the important questions posed by Alzheimer disease patients and their families," says Neil Buckholtz, PhD, chief of the NIA's Dementias of Aging Branch. "These conversations are never easy. But these findings could help clarify what patients and families can expect. And ultimately, families who have more precise information on the likely course of the disease should be better prepared to deal with it as it progresses."

AD is an irreversible disorder of the brain, robbing those who have it of memory, and eventually, overall mental and physical function, leading to death. It is the most common cause of dementia among people over age 65. Recent studies estimate that up to 4.5 million people currently have the disease, and the prevalence (the number of people with the disease at any one time) doubles every 5 years after the age of 65. By 2050, if current population trends continue and no preventive treatments become available, some 13.5 million Americans will have Alzheimer disease.

The annual national direct and indirect costs of caring for AD patients are estimated to be as much as $100 billion. This suggests that the economic burden will grow as the population ages and the number of AD patients increases.

For more information on AD research, as well as on biological, epidemiological, clinical, and social and behavioral research on AD, several publications are available from the NIA at NIA's AD-dedicated website www.alzheimers.org, the Institute's Alzheimer's Disease Education and Referral (ADEAR) Center, or by calling ADEAR at 800-438-4380.

Chapter 62

Brain Autopsy and Brain Tissue for Scientific Research

You are probably familiar with organ donations of the heart, kidneys, or eyes to save the health and even the lives of ill people.

The donation of brain tissue for research is also a precious and special gift. It will help scientists to understand the causes of brain disorders and also how normal brains work.

Future generations will benefit from this gift, which could lead to successful treatment and prevention of various brain disorders.

Why is brain tissue needed for scientific research?

Direct examination of the brain after death opens the door to many of its mysteries. New scientific techniques are now being used to compare the changes caused by brain diseases with the patient's symptoms during life. In this way, we can better understand the causes of memory loss and other mental or behavioral problems.

How will information obtained from brain examination benefit the family?

Examination of the brain after death is often the only way to confirm the diagnosis made during life. There are various causes of dementia

This chapter begins with "Brain Tissue for Scientific Research," © 2006 Consortium to Establish a Registry for Alzheimer's Disease, Duke University Medical Center. Reprinted with permission. "Brain Banks Across the United States," is from the National Institute of Neurological Disorders and Stroke. All contact information was verified and updated in August 2007.

in the elderly. Alzheimer disease is the most common; other frequent causes are stroke, Parkinson disease, and alcoholism. These conditions may occur alone or in combination, which makes clinical diagnosis even more difficult.

Learning the precise cause of the patient's illness can be a great relief to the family, helping them to close this chapter in their lives.

Will the brain examination cost the family anything?

No. There is now a nationwide study of brain diseases in elderly, and most if not all of the costs of brain examination for patients participating in this study are paid by the local researchers. (There is no cost to those participating through the University Memory and Aging Center.)

How does the family provide consent for brain examination?

The consent for a postmortem examination of the brain is usually given by the patient's next of kin. The family should discuss the issue together, so that the doctor can be sure that the close relatives agree. A legal consent form permitting this procedure will be given to the next of kin to be signed. Copies of the signed form should go to the patient's doctor, the hospital pathologist, the funeral home, and to the nursing home, if needed.

How will the family find out what the brain examination showed?

The physician or the pathologist who examines the brain will send a letter to the family, explaining the major findings.

When should plans be made for this procedure?

Although some elderly patients with brain disorders may live for many years families should start thinking about brain donation in the early stages of the illness. It is important to make the necessary arrangements well in advance, since family members need time to discuss this issue.

What effect will the examination have on funeral arrangements?

None. The removal of brain tissue, under the supervision of a pathologist, does not leave any visible marks. It is still possible to have an open-casket funeral. Funeral directors are usually very cooperative about transporting the body for the examination.

Is tissue from normal brains also needed for research?

Yes. It is also very important to study the brains of normal, healthy people after death.

As surprising as it seems, we still do not know how the brains of healthy persons change as they age. Scientist need to study normal brains to find out which changes in the brain are caused by disease and which are due to aging. It is especially valuable to study brain tissue from normal elderly persons who have had their memory tested as they age.

Brain Banks Across the United States

Brain banking is an important resource for the study of many diseases and disorders. There are currently several brain and tissue banks all over the world that focus specifically on Parkinson and/or Alzheimer research.

The following resources will provide you information on brain banks with websites, phone numbers, where they are available, and a short description of each. Note that some of these resources may be available to study participants only.

Alabama

Alzheimer's Disease Center
Department of Neurology
University of Alabama at Birmingham
640 Sparks Center
1720 7th Avenue South
Birmingham, AL 35294-0017
Phone: 205-934-1668
Fax: 205-975-7365
Website: http://main.uab.edu/neurology/Templates/Inner
.aspx?durki=11627&pid=11627
Information on Brain Donation: http://main.uab.edu/neurology/
Templates/Inner.aspx?pid=61773

Arizona

Sun Health Research Institute
10515 W. Santa Fe Drive
Sun City, AZ 85351
Phone: 623-876-5328

Website: http://www.shri.org/index.cfm
Info on Brain Donation: http://www.shri.org/brainbank

Scientists at Sun Health Research Institute have had a significant impact on how physicians diagnose and treat diseases such as Alzheimer disease, Parkinson disease, and arthritis. Founded in 1986, the Institute is one of just 29 national Alzheimer's Disease Core Centers in the nation. One key to the successes at the Institute has been its Brain Donation Program, which has provided researchers in Sun City and around the world with brain tissue to aid in their search for the cause and cure of those diseases.

California

Alzheimer Disease Research Center
Andrus Gerontology Center
University of Southern California
3715 McClintock Avenue, MC-0191
Los Angeles, CA 90089-0191
Phone: 213-740-7777
Website: http://www.usc.edu/dept/gero/ADRC

The focus of the USC ADRC is reducing the cognitive and behavioral impact of Alzheimer disease and cerebrovascular dementia among ethnically diverse populations. The objective of the ADRC is to provide a mechanism for integrating, coordinating, fostering, and developing interdisciplinary cooperation of a group of established investigators conducting programs of research on Alzheimer disease (AD), cardiovascular disease (CVD), and related disorders of older people. The ADRC provides financial, intellectual, patients, biological specimen resources to support cooperative interactions among scientists at USC, other Alzheimer centers, and the community at large. It also fosters an environment that will 1) strengthen research on AD, CVD, and related disorders, 2) increase productivity, and 3) generate new ideas, through formal interdisciplinary collaborations, both locally and nationally. The ADRC collaborates specifically with the National Alzheimer Coordinating Center (NACC) to contribute to a standardized clinical and neuropathological database and in the future anticipates working with the National Cell Repository for Alzheimer Disease (NCRAD) to share biological specimens.

Human Brain and Spinal and Spinal Fluid Resource Center
VA West Los Angeles Healthcare Center
11301 Wilshire Blvd.

Los Angeles, CA 90073
Phone: 310-268-3536
Fax: 310-268-4768
Website: http://www.loni.ucla.edu/uclabrainbank

The Human Brain and Spinal Fluid Resource Center was established in 1961 to provide a vital service to neuroscientists. The center collects, cryogenically stores, and distributes donated tissue to research scientists around the world. Collection occurs through their "Gift of Hope" anatomical donor program which accepts tissue donation from people with neurological/psychiatric disorders. These disorders include Alzheimer disease, Parkinson disease, multiple sclerosis, and many others as well as individuals without neurological/psychiatric disorders. The center is a consortium of two banks, the Neurological and Psychiatric Disorders Bank and the Multiple Sclerosis Human Neurospecimen Bank.

Stanford/VA Alzheimer's Disease Core Center
Aging Clinical Research Center
3801 Miranda Ave., 151 Y
Palo Alto, CA 94304
Phone: 650-852-3287
Fax: 650-852-3297
Website: http://alzheimer.stanford.edu
Information on donation: http://www.stanford.edu/~yesavage/neuropathology.shtml

The center is part of the Aging Clinical Research Center, supported by both Stanford and the VA and the National Institute on Aging. It currently has more than 1,000 samples from about 40 brains, available to researchers at any academic research center.

UC Davis Alzheimer's Disease Center
Lawrence J. Ellison Ambulatory Care Center
4860 Y Street, Suite 3900
Sacramento, CA 95817
Phone: 916-734-5496
Website: http://alzheimer.ucdavis.edu

Brain banking for this facility is open to patients of the clinical research being conducted at the center only. If you wish to discuss participation in the clinical research you can call the number listed above to speak to the facility representative. The center is located within the Department of Neurosciences in the Ambulatory Care Building at the UC Davis Medical Center. Under the direction of Professor and Chair W. Jagust, MD, the NIH-funded Alzheimer's Disease Center (ADC) provides a fully staffed site for the care and etiologic studies of up to 250 new dementia patients per year, 90% of whom carry the diagnosis of Alzheimer disease. An electronic base of clinical, cognitive, and imaging characteristics and of DNA samples is maintained on over 500 live patients with a complementary brain bank. Access to patients, the data base, DNA, and other tissue specimens is available to funded CNRU investigators with approved and relevant protocols though application to the ADC. Current examples of CNRU research interactions include ongoing and projected studies by former CNRU New Investigator J.W. Miller, PhD, on folate, vitamin B_{12}, and hyperhomocysteinemia in dementia syndromes, and of Program Director C.H. Halsted, MD, and Genetics Subcore Director C.H. Warden, PhD, on potential folate hydrolase polymorphisms in patients with Alzheimer disease.

UC San Francisco Memory and Aging Center
Alzheimer's Disease Research Center
350 Parnassus Avenue, Suite 706
San Francisco, CA 94143
Phone: 415-476-1820
Website: http://memory.ucsf.edu
Brain Donation Information: http://memory.ucsf.edu/Research/autopsy.html

The UCSF Memory and Aging Center provides a brain autopsy service for patients registered and seen at UCSF. Their autopsy program is associated primarily with various ongoing research projects.

Florida

Since 1987, Florida has conducted a Brain Bank program as part of the State Alzheimer's Disease Initiative (ADI). The Florida Brain Bank conducts analysis on postmortem brains clinically diagnosed with Alzheimer disease or other related dementia. Besides providing brain tissue for Alzheimer research that may lead to finding a cause and developing ways to treat or prevent Alzheimer disease, the Brain Bank provides families with a confirmation or correction of the clinical diagnosis. Services include accepting referrals from all respite and model day care service providers and conducting subsequent diagnostic workups for all referred consumers and for the general public. The Florida Brain Bank is located in Miami Beach, at the Mount Sinai

Medical Center, 305-674-2543. The Alzheimer's Resource Center in Orlando coordinates Brain Bank activities for Pasco, Pinellas, and nine other counties in west central Florida. For an application or information, call them toll-free at 800-330-1910. They also have a website, www.alzheimerorlando.com.

Alzheimer's Disease Initiative
Wien Center Memory Disorder Clinic
Mt. Sinai Medical Center
4300 Alton Road
Miami Beach, FL 33140
Phone: 305-674-2018
Website: http://citease.netspacetoday.com/msmc/door

The Wien Center is on the cutting edge of memory disorder diagnosis and treatment. Utilizing the combined resources of Mount Sinai Medical Center and the University of Miami's Department of Psychiatry, genetic and medical research is continuously conducted. Clinical drug trials allow the center to provide patients with the most current treatments available. Additionally, the Wien Center actively participates in and coordinates the State of Florida Brain Bank program.

The Alzheimer Resource Center
1506 Lake Highland Drive
Orlando, FL 32803
Toll-Free: 800-330-1910
Phone: 407-843-1910
Fax: 407-381-4155
Website: http://www.alzheimerresourcecenter.cc
Information on Donation: http://www.alzheimerresourcecenter.cc/Brain_Bank_Program.htm

The Alzheimer Resource Center coordinates the State of Florida Brain Bank Research Program for a 17 county area. The purpose of this program is to coordinate the donation of brain tissue for study and research and assists the medical community in finding the cause of Alzheimer disease so that it can become preventable and treatable.

Abigail Van Buren's Alzheimer's Disease Research Center
Mayo Clinic Jacksonville
Neuropathology Laboratory

4500 San Pablo Road
Jacksonville, FL 32224
Phone: 904-953-2000
Website: http://mayoresearch.mayo.edu/mayo/research/
alzheimers_center/index.cfm
E-mail: mayoadc@mayo.edu

The Mayo Alzheimer's Disease Research Center (ADRC) is one of 30 Alzheimer disease research centers across the country designated and funded by the National Institute on Aging of the National Institutes of Health. The Mayo ADRC is jointly based in Rochester, MN, and Jacksonville, FL. The Mayo ADRC is organized into five cores. The neuropathology core performs detailed neuropathologic examinations on patients with mild cognitive impairment and dementia such that a definite diagnosis of the cause of cognitive impairment/dementia can be determined. This Core also provides a mechanism for characterizing cognitively normal elderly individuals, as well as provides tissue to other investigators who are researching aging and dementia.

Brain Endowment Bank
Department of Neurology
University of Miami School of Medicine
1501 North West 9th Avenue
Miami, FL 33136
Phone: 800-862-7246
Fax: 305-243-3649
Website: http://neurology.med.miami.edu
Information on the Brain Endowment Bank: http://neurology.med
.miami.edu/research_div_basic_research.asp.

The Department of Neurology is home to the Brain Endowment Bank, which conducts clinical and basic research of the human brain including Parkinson disease and other movement disorders, drug addiction, and aging; the Sleep Disorders Center, which provides a wide range of services for individuals with sleep related disturbances; and the International Center for Epilepsy, to name a few. Headed by Deborah Mash, PhD, professor, director of research, and Levey Chair in Parkinson Disease Research, the bank's research team educates the public about the importance of brain donation as a permanent and invaluable research resource. The donor base includes normal and diseased brains from individuals with neurodegenerative and neuropsychiatric disorders.

Georgia

Alzheimer's Research Center
Medical College of Georgia
1120 15th Street
Augusta, GA 30912
Phone: 706-721-6356
Website: http://www.mcg.edu/centers/alz/bbank.html

The Alzheimer's Research Center was developed to support collaborative basic and clinical research in the area of Alzheimer disease and related neurodegenerative disorders, by 1) promoting interdisciplinary approaches to answering research questions, 2) providing a venue for regular meetings of its members for the purpose of sharing members' research findings, the latest published works in the field, and supporting visits to this campus by outside experts, 3) providing course materials and lectures related to Alzheimer disease for undergraduate, graduate, and postgraduate student instruction, and 4) supporting two core facilities, the Neurological Disorder Database Registry and the Animal Behavior Center.

Alzheimer's Disease Center
Emory University
Wesley Woods Health Center, 3rd Floor
1841 Clifton Road
Atlanta, GA 30329
Phone: 404-728-6950
Website: http://www.med.emory.edu/ADC/index.html

The Alzheimer's Disease Center at Emory University provides an Autopsy Program for patients who have and have not been seen by a physician at Emory. For information concerning autopsies you can contact the Alzheimer's Disease Center Autopsy Coordinator at 404-728-4881.

Illinois

Center for Alzheimer's Disease and Related Disorders
P.O. Box 19643
Southern Illinois School of Medicine
Springfield, IL 62794-9643
Phone: 217-545-8249
Fax: 217-545-7363
Website: http://www.siumed.edu/cadrd/cadrd.html

The SIU Center for Alzheimer Disease and Related Disorders (CADRD) was established in 1987 when the Illinois legislature mandated two regional Alzheimer disease assistance centers. Of the two centers established as a result, CADRD serves rural Illinois, a total of 93 counties. The second, Rush Medical Center, serves the greater Chicago area (Cook county and the eight collar counties). A third center, Northwestern Alzheimer's Disease Center was added through legislation in 1997 and also serves the greater Chicago area. Doctors working at CADRD study and treat patients suffering from Parkinson disease, and devote considerable time and effort to the study of other disorders affecting older people, including locomotor disorders (gait disturbances) and tremor.

- CADRD provides clinical services to patients and their families.

- CADRD supports research through a brain bank autopsy program.

- CADRD provides educational services to both medical professionals and lay persons.

Cognitive Neurology and Alzheimer's Disease Center
Northwestern University, Feinberg School of Medicine
320 E. Superior
Chicago, IL 60611
Phone: 312-908-9339
Fax: 312-908-8789
Website: http://www.brain.northwestern.edu/index.html
Information on Brain Endowment: http://www.brain.northwestern
.edu/mdad/brainendowment.html

Rush Alzheimer's Disease Center
Rush Presbyterian St. Luke's Medical Center
Armour Academic Center
600 S. Paulina Street, Suite 1038
Chicago, IL 60612
Phone: 312-942-8974
Website: http://www.rush.edu/rumc/page-R12388.html

The Rush Alzheimer's Disease Center Laboratory continues to serve the Northern Illinois community through the postmortem evaluation of brain tissue of persons from two sources:

- People clinically evaluated by RADC staff

- Participants in the Religious Orders Study and the Memory and Aging Project

Indiana

Indiana Alzheimer's Disease Center
Indiana University Medical Center
Department of Pathology and Lab Medicine
635 Barnhill Dr., MS A142
Indianapolis, IN 46202
Phone: 317-274-1590
Fax: 317-274-0504
Website: http://iadc.iupui.edu/index.htm

Kansas

Brain Tissue Bank and Research Laboratory
Kansas University Medical Center
3901 Rainbow Blvd.
Kansas City, KS 66160
Phone: 913-588-0103
Fax: 913-588-6414

Kentucky

Sanders-Brown Research Center on Aging
University of Kentucky
101 Sanders-Brown Bldg.
Lexington KY 40536
Phone: 859-323-6040
Fax: 859-323-2866
Website: http://web1.mccs.uky.edu/coa/ADRC/adrc.htm

The Neuropathology Core performs short postmortem interval autopsies on patients with AD and age-related dementing disorders and control subjects, and provides fresh and frozen specimens to AD investigators at UK and outside institutions. It maintains a tissue bank of brain specimens, cerebrospinal fluid, and synaptosome preparations from autopsied subjects.

Massachusetts

Harvard Brain Tissue Resource Center
McLean Hospital
115 Mill St.
Belmont, Ma 02178
Toll-Free: 800-272-4622 (information on donations)

Phone: 617-855-2400
Fax: 617-855-3199
Website: http://www.brainbank.mclean.org

The Harvard Brain Tissue Resource Center has been established at McLean Hospital as a centralized resource for the collection and distribution of human brain specimens for brain research.

Mass General Institute for Neurodegenerative Disease
Massachusetts General Hospital
Building 114 16th Street, 114-2001
Charlestown, MA 02129-4404
Phone: 617-726-1278
Fax: 617-724-1480
Website: http://www.mghmind.org

Mass General Institute for Neurodegenerative Disease was founded in 2001 with a mission to translate laboratory discoveries into prevention, treatment and cures for Alzheimer disease, ALS, Huntington disease, Parkinson disease, and other neurodegenerative diseases. Their infrastructure includes equipment and resources that are essential for translational research: high-tech microscopes, gene sequencing machines, a human brain bank, drug screening robotics, and a laboratory for testing new disease-fighting strategies in mice.

Massachusetts Alzheimer's Disease Research Center
Massachusetts General Hospital
WACC 830
Boston, MA 02114
Phone: 617-726-3987
Fax: 617-726-4101
Website: http://madrc.org

The Neuropathology Core was established as an integral part of the Massachusetts ADRC in 1985. The goals of the core are:

- to establish accurate neuropathological diagnoses on all brains donated to the ADRC Tissue Resource Center;

- to submit a standardized report with clinical-pathological correlation and interpretation of findings to investigators in the Clinical Core;

- to prepare brain tissues in a standardized manner for use by qualified investigators in the field of AD research;

- to maintain the ADRC Tissue Resource Center as a source of brain tissue for investigators studying AD;

- to facilitate correlative studies of pathology with clinical, behavioral, anatomic, genetic and neuroimaging aspects of AD;

- to serve as a resource for training and educating future investigators in the neuroanatomy and neuropathology of disorders of dementia.

Michigan

Michigan Alzheimer's Disease Research Center
University of Michigan
300 N. Ingalls, Room 3D05
Ann Arbor, MI 48109-0489
Phone: 734-936-8764
Fax: 734-936-8967
Website: http://sitemaker.med.umich.edu/madrc

The MADRC is one of 32 centers in the nation that are devoted to research, clinical care, neuropathologic studies, and educational activities in Alzheimer disease (AD) and related disorders. The Center was established in 1989 at the University of Michigan. The Neuropathology Core coordinates the collection, storage and postmortem analysis of brain tissue for research purposes.

Minnesota

Abigail Van Buren's Alzheimer's Disease Research Center
Mayo Clinic Rochester
Department of Laboratory Medicine and Pathology
200 First St., SW
Rochester, MN 55905
Phone: 507-284-6828
Website: http://mayoresearch.mayo.edu/mayo/research/
alzheimers_center/index.cfm

The purpose of the center is to provide care for dementia patients and promote research and education on Alzheimer disease and related dementias. The Mayo ADRC is organized into five cores. The neuropathology core performs detailed neuropathologic examinations on patients with mild cognitive impairment and dementia such that a definite diagnosis of the cause of cognitive impairment/dementia can be determined. This Core also provides a mechanism for characterizing cognitively normal elderly individuals, as well as provides tissue to other investigators who are researching aging and dementia.

Missouri

Alzheimer's Disease Research Center
Department of Neurology
Washington University
4488 Forest Park Avenue, Suite 130
St. Louis, MO 63108
Phone: 314-286-2881
Fax: 314-286-2763
Website: http://alzheimer.wustl.edu/adrc2/default.htm

The Neuropathology Core provides postmortem research assessments of brain changes in participants who died and have granted autopsy permission. Families gain a report from the neuropathologist of the final diagnosis. The information gained from autopsy is especially important for research purposes to aid in the search for clues in the brains of Alzheimer patients which may lead to a better understanding of the causes of this illness. Equally important to the analysis of Alzheimer brains is the study of brain tissue from healthy elderly persons. Without such efforts, our ability to discern meaningful changes in brain pathology would be impossible. In addition, the Neuropathology Core banks portions of these tissues, as well as blood and cerebrospinal fluid (CSF) for future studies.

New York

Alzheimer's Disease and Memory Research Center (ADRC)
Mount Sinai School of Medicine
Department of Psychiatry
One Gustave L. Levy Place, Box 1230
New York, NY 10029-6574
Phone: 212-241-1844
Website: http://www.mssm.edu/psychiatry/adrc
Tissue Donation Program: http://www.mssm.edu/psychiatry/adrc/brain_tissue_donation.shtml

The goals of the Brain Tissue Donation Program are to improve our ability to diagnose Alzheimer disease as early as possible, to improve existing treatments, to develop new treatments for Alzheimer disease, and to learn more about the disease process. The Brain and Biologic Studies of Aging, Dementia, and Alzheimer's Disease Research Program of Mount Sinai School of Medicine is dedicated to furthering the scientific understanding of both healthy aging and of brain disorders such as Alzheimer disease (AD), and to the development of new treatments. This research effort has been ongoing for more than 20 years and has been continuously funded by the National Institutes of Health.

Taub Institute for Research on Alzheimer's
Disease and the Aging Brain
630 West 168th Street, P.O. Box 16
New York, NY 10032
Phone 212-305-1818
Fax 212-342-2849
Website: http://www.cumc.columbia.edu/dept/taub/index.html

The Taub Institute's Alzheimer's Disease Research Center performs an essential research procedure to learn about memory disorders: brain autopsy or brain donation. True diagnosis of memory disorder is dependent upon studying both diseased and normal brain tissue at death. Our ability to understand how Alzheimer disease affects the brain and causes debilitating memory loss, confusion, and eventually death, is dependent upon studying brain tissue. Brain autopsy is also useful in clarifying risks to relatives of people with Alzheimer disease, which in some cases has been identified as a genetic disorder.

New York Brain Bank
Columbia University
3959 Broadway
New York, NY 10032
Telephone: 212-305-2299
Fax: 212-342-0083
Website: http://www.nybb.hs.columbia.edu

The New York Brain Bank (NYBB) at Columbia University was established to collect postmortem human brains to meet the needs of neuroscientists investigating specific psychiatric and neurological disorders.

Alzheimer's Disease Center
Department of Pathology
New York University Medical Center

560 First Ave, Room THN314
New York, NY 10016
Phone: 212-263-8088
Autopsy Information: 212-263-6262
Website: http://www.med.nyu.edu/adc

The NYU Alzheimer's Disease Center (ADC) is part of the Department of Psychiatry at New York University School of Medicine, located in midtown Manhattan, in New York City, New York. The Neuropathology Core is best known to research participants and their families for its brain donation program. Through the brain donation program and other efforts, this core conducts thorough postmortem examinations (autopsies) and maintains a brain bank for continued study by Alzheimer researchers.

New York University School of Medicine
Aging and Dementia Research Center
Brain Donation Program
560 First Avenue THN #314
New York, NY 10016
Phone: 212-263-6262
Fax: 212-263-6991

North Carolina

Kathleen Price Bryan Brain Bank
Joseph and Kathleen Bryan Alzheimer's Disease Research Center
Division of Neurology, Department of Medicine
Duke University Medical Center
2200 W. Main Street
Suite A200
Box 3503 DUMC
Durham, NC 27705
Toll-Free: 866-444-2372
Phone: 919-668-0820
Website: http://adrc.mc.duke.edu/BB.htm

The Kathleen Price Bryan Brain Bank is a repository of nearly 1200 human brains that contains approximately 750 brains from patients with Alzheimer disease and related dementing disorders and 250 brains with other neurological disorders such as Parkinson disease, amyotrophic lateral sclerosis, Huntington disease, and muscular dystrophy. Approximately 200 normal control brains are available.

Ohio

Human Tissue Procurement Facility
Institute of Pathology
Case Western Reserve University
11100 Euclid Avenue
Cleveland, OH 44106
Phone: 216-844-5335
Website: http://path-www.path.cwru.edu

The purpose of the Human Tissue Procurement Facility (HTPF) is to prospectively collect, prepare, and distribute high quality human tissue samples to researchers studying cancer and other diseases.

Human Tissue Resource Network
Department of Pathology
Ohio State University College of Medicine
Starling-Loving Hall
2001 Polaris Parkway
Polaris Innovative Center
Columbus, OH 43240
Phone: 614-293-8528
Fax: 614-293-7013
Website: http://www.pathology.osu.edu/htrn/default.asp

The Human Tissue Resource Network (HTRN) is funded through federal and corporate research programs for the collection, banking, and distribution of human tissue and fluid specimens. The HTRN is comprised of the Research Histology Core Facility (RHCF), Tissue Archive Service, Tissue Procurement Service, AIDS and Cancer Specimen Bank, the Cancer and Leukemia Group B (CALGB) Pathology Coordinating Office (PCO), and an Adenoma Polyp Specimen Bank. The HTRN unites tissue-based research resources within the OSU Department of Pathology and promotes collaborative research within the OSU Medical Center and related national human research projects.

University Memory and Aging Center
Alzheimer's Disease Research Center
University Hospitals of Cleveland
12200 Fairhill Road
Cleveland, OH 44120
Toll-Free: 800-252-5048
Phone: 216-844-6400

Website: http://www.ohioalzcenter.org
Tissue Donation: http://www.ohioalzcenter.org/autopsy.htm

Oregon

Oregon Brain Bank
Division of Pathology, L-113
Neuropath Section
Oregon Health and Science University
3181 S.W. Sam Jackson Park Rd.
Portland, OR 97239
Phone: 503-494-6923
Fax: 503-494-7499
Website: http://www.ohsu.edu/pathology/win/MainOBBIndex.htm

The Organ Brain Bank was established in 1990 with the assistance of the Alzheimer's Research Alliance of Oregon. The bank serves two main functions; first to provide a neuropathologic diagnosis of organic dementias in a cohort of NIH sponsored research subjects and second to harvest, bank and disperse postmortem tissue for use in neurodegenerative research. Although the focus is on Alzheimer disease, tissue from patients with Huntington disease, Parkinson disease, amyotrophic lateral sclerosis, multiple sclerosis, controls, and other disorders are also available.

Pennsylvania

Alzheimer's Disease and Dementia Center
Department of Neurology
Thomas Jefferson University
600 Chestnut Street, Suite 200
Philadelphia, PA 19107
Phone: 215-955-6692
Fax: 215-955-3745
Website: http://www.jeffersonhospital.org/neurology/article4318.html

Jefferson's Alzheimer's Disease and Dementia Center is a major referral center in the Delaware Valley. The Center provides comprehensive and individualized diagnostic services and therapeutic options to patients with various types of dementia. Patients evaluated at the center may suffer from Alzheimer disease, Parkinson disease, stroke, cancer, infections, head trauma, and other degenerative central nervous system conditions. In addition to its clinical programs, the center is involved in a number of basic science research projects that are advancing fundamental knowledge on these dementing disorders, while pursuing new treatment modalities. It also provides educational programs for patient's families and caregivers. The center includes a brain bank that receives brains for diagnostic and research purposes.

National Disease Research Interchange
1628 John F. Kennedy Blvd.
8 Penn Center, 8th Floor
Philadelphia PA 19103
Toll-Free: 800-222-NDRI (6374)
Phone: 215-557-7361
Fax: 215-557-7154
Website: http://www.ndriresource.org/index.html

Our mission is to serve scientists with customized biomaterials for use in studies to understand human disease. Human cells, tissues, and organs are required to investigate how human disease progresses and to develop new drugs and therapies for treatments and cures.

Center for Neurodegenerative Disease Research
University of Pennsylvania Health System
Department of Pathology and Laboratory Medicine
University of Pennsylvania School of Medicine
3rd Floor Maloney Building
3600 Spruce St.
Philadelphia, PA 19104
Phone: 215-662-4708
Fax: 215-349-5909
Website: http://www.uphs.upenn.edu/cndr/index.html

The mission of the Center for Neurodegenerative Disease Research (CNDR) is to conduct multidisciplinary clinical and basic research studies that increase understanding of the causes and mechanisms that increase understanding of the causes and mechanisms leading to brain dysfunction and degeneration in Alzheimer disease (AD), Parkinson disease (PD), motor neuron disease and other less common neurodegenerative disorders that also occur with more frequently with advancing age.

Brain Tissue Donation Program
University of Pittsburgh Medical Center
Translational Neuroscience Program

Department of Psychiatry
3811 O'Hara St.
Biomedical Science Tower W1650
Pittsburgh, PA 15213
Phone: 412-624-7802
Website: http://cortex.psychiatry.pitt.edu/research/cnmdframe_mb
.htm

The Department of Psychiatry at the University of Pittsburgh has
established a brain tissue bank to which brain tissue can be donated
at no expense.

Texas

The Alzheimer's Disease and Memory Disorder Center
Baylor College of Medicine
Department of Neurology
6550 Fannon St.
Smith Tower #1801
Houston, TX 77030
Phone: 713-798-6660
Fax: 713-798-5326
Website: http://www.bcm.edu/neurology/struct/admdc/admdc.html

The ADMDC at Baylor participates in basic science research on Alzheimer disease, in part, through the maintenance of a brain tissue
donation program. The Brain Donation Autopsy Program is limited
to those individuals who were diagnosed and followed as a patient or
control subject of the Baylor Alzheimer's Disease and Memory Disorders Center (ADMDC).

Alzheimer's Disease Center
Department of Neurology
Southwestern Medical Center
James W. Aston Ambulatory Care Center
5323 Harry Hines Blvd.
Dallas, TX 75390-9170
Phone: 214-648-9574
Website: http://www.utsouthwestern.edu/utsw/cda/dept23589/files/
46161.html

The Neuropathology Core, directed by Charles White III, MD, provides
a comprehensive brain bank for tissue to be utilized for research purposes.

Washington

Pacific Northwest Dementia and Aging Neuropathology Group (PANDA)
Harborview Medical Center
Neuropathology
325 Ninth Avenue, Box 359791
Seattle, WA 98104
Phone: 206-731-6315
Fax: 206-731-8240
Website: http://www.pathology.washington.edu/clinical/neuropath/
brainbank.php

PANDA is a collaborative effort between Oregon Health and Sciences University (OHSU) in Portland, OR, and the University of Washington (UW) Medical Center in Seattle, WA. The goals of PANDA are twofold. First, we apply the most current structural and molecular criteria to the classification of neurodegenerative diseases so as to provide families of the deceased with contemporary, accurate diagnoses. Second, we procure and maintain donated tissue in optimal states for dissemination to scientists throughout the world.

Part Six

Additional
Help and Information

Chapter 63

Glossary of Terms Related to Alzheimer Disease and Other Dementias

acetylcholine: A neurotransmitter that is important for the formation of memories. Studies have shown that levels of acetylcholine are reduced in the brains of people with Alzheimer disease.[1]

akinesia: Decreased body movements.[2]

Alzheimer disease: The most common cause of dementia in people aged 65 and older. Nearly all brain functions, including memory, movement, language, judgment, behavior, and abstract thinking, are eventually affected.[1]

amyloid plaques: Unusual clumps of material found in the tissue between nerve cells. Amyloid plaques, which consist of a protein called beta amyloid along with degenerating bits of neurons and other cells, are a hallmark of Alzheimer disease.[1]

amyloid precursor protein (APP): A normal brain protein that is a precursor for beta amyloid, the abnormal substance found in the characteristic amyloid plaques of Alzheimer disease patients.[1]

The terms in this glossary were excerpted from the following publications: 1. "Dementia: Hope through Research," National Institute of Neurological Disorders and Stroke (NINDS), 2007; 2. "Huntington's Disease: Hope Through Research," (NINDS), 2007; and 3. Alzheimer Disease: Unraveling the Mystery, National Institute on Aging, December 2003.

apolipoprotein E: A protein that carries cholesterol in blood and that appears to play some role in brain function. The gene that produces ApoE comes in several forms, or alleles—ε2, ε3, and ε4. The ApoE ε2 allele is relatively rare and may provide some protection against Alzheimer disease (AD). ApoE ε3 is the most common allele and it appears to play a neutral role in AD. ApoE ε4 occurs in about 40 percent of all AD patients who develop the disease in later life; it increases the risk of developing AD.[3]

ataxia: A loss of muscle control.[1]

atherosclerosis: A blood vessel disease characterized by the buildup of plaque, or deposits of fatty substances and other matter in the inner lining of an artery.[1]

at-risk: A description of a person whose mother or father has Huntington disease (HD) or has inherited the HD gene and who therefore has a 50-50 chance of inheriting the disorder.[2]

autosomal dominant disorder: A non-sex-linked disorder that can be inherited even if only one parent passes on the defective gene.[2]

axon: The long, tube-like part of a neuron that transmits outgoing signals to other cells.[3]

basal ganglia: A region located at the base of the brain composed of four clusters of neurons, or nerve cells. This area is responsible for body movement and coordination. The neuron groups most prominently and consistently affected by HD—the pallidum and striatum—are located here.[2]

beta amyloid: A protein found in the characteristic clumps of tissue (called plaques) that appear in the brains of Alzheimer patients.[1]

Binswanger disease: A rare form of dementia characterized by damage to small blood vessels in the white matter of the brain. This damage leads to brain lesions, loss of memory, disordered cognition, and mood changes.[1]

brain stem: The part of the brain that connects the brain to the spinal cord and that controls automatic body functions, such as breathing, heart rate, and blood pressure.[3]

CADASIL: A rare hereditary disorder which is linked to a type of vascular dementia. It stands for cerebral autosomal dominant arteriopathy with subcortical infarct and leukoencephalopathy.[1]

caudate nuclei: Part of the striatum in the basal ganglia.[2]

cerebellum: The part of the brain that is responsible for maintaining the body's balance and coordination.[3]

cerebral cortex: The outer layer of nerve cells surrounding the cerebral hemispheres.[3]

cerebral hemispheres: The largest portion of the brain, composed of billions of nerve cells in two structures connected by the corpus callosum; the cerebral hemispheres control conscious thought, language, decision-making, emotions, movement, and sensory functions.[3]

cholinesterase inhibitors: Drugs that slow the breakdown of the neurotransmitter acetylcholine.[1]

chorea: Uncontrolled body movements. Chorea is derived from the Greek word for dance.[2]

chromosome: A threadlike structure in the nucleus of a cell that contains DNA, sequences of which make up genes; most human cells contain 23 pairs of chromosomes.[3]

clinical trial: A research study involving humans that rigorously tests how well an intervention works.[3]

cognitive functions: All aspects of conscious thought and mental activity, including learning, perceiving, making decisions, and remembering.[3]

cognitive training: A type of training in which patients practice tasks designed to improve mental performance. Examples include memory aids, such as mnemonics, and computerized recall devices.[1]

computed tomography (CT): A technique used for diagnosing brain disorders. CT uses a computer to produce a high-quality image of brain structures. These images are called CT scans.[2]

corpus callosum: The thick bundle of nerves that connects the two hemispheres of the cerebral hemispheres.[3]

cortex: Part of the brain responsible for thought, perception, and memory. HD affects the basal ganglia and cortex.[2]

cortical atrophy: Degeneration of the brain's cortex (outer layer). Cortical atrophy is common in many forms of dementia and may be visible on a brain scan.[1]

cortical dementia: A type of dementia in which the damage primarily occurs in the brain's cortex, or outer layer.[1]

corticobasal degeneration: A progressive disorder characterized by nerve cell loss and atrophy in multiple areas of the brain.[1]

Creutzfeldt-Jakob disease: A rare, degenerative, fatal brain disorder believed to be linked to an abnormal form of a protein called a prion.[1]

dementia: A broad term referring to the symptoms associated with a decline in cognitive function to the extent that it interferes with daily life and activities.[3]

dementia pugilistica: A form of dementia caused by head trauma such as that experienced by boxers. It is also called chronic traumatic encephalopathy or Boxer's syndrome.[1]

dendrite: The branchlike extension of neurons that receive messages from other neurons.[3]

deoxyribonucleic acid (DNA): The substance of heredity containing the genetic information necessary for cells to divide and produce proteins. DNA carries the code for every inherited characteristic of an organism.[2]

dominant: A trait that is apparent even when the gene for that disorder is inherited from only one parent.[2]

early-onset Alzheimer disease: A rare form of AD that usually begins to affect people between ages 30 and 60; it is called familial AD (FAD) if it runs in the family.[3]

electroencephalogram (EEG): A medical procedure that records patterns of electrical activity in the brain.[1]

entorhinal cortex: An area deep within the brain where damage from AD first begins.[3]

enzyme: A substance that causes or speeds up a chemical reaction.[3]

fatal familial insomnia: An inherited disease that affects a brain region called the thalamus, which is partially responsible for controlling sleep. The disease causes dementia and a progressive insomnia that eventually leads to a complete lack of sleep.[1]

free radical: A highly reactive oxygen molecule that combines easily with other molecules, sometimes causing damage to cells.[3]

frontotemporal dementias: A group of dementias characterized by degeneration of nerve cells, especially those in the frontal and temporal lobes of the brain.[1]

FTDP-17: One of the frontotemporal dementias, linked to a mutation in the tau gene. It is much like other types of the frontotemporal dementias but often includes psychiatric symptoms such as delusions and hallucinations.[1]

gene: The biologic unit of heredity passed from parent to child; genes are segments of DNA and they contain instructions that tell a cell how to make specific proteins.[3]

genetic risk factor: A change in a cell's DNA that does not cause a disease but may increase the chance that a person will develop a disease.[3]

glial cell: A specialized cell that supports, protects, or nourishes nerve cells.[3]

Gerstmann-Straussler-Scheinker disease: A rare, fatal hereditary disease that causes ataxia and progressive dementia.[1]

hippocampus: A structure in the brain that plays a major role in learning and memory and is involved in converting short-term to long-term memory.[3]

HIV-associated dementia: A dementia that results from infection with the human immunodeficiency virus (HIV) that causes AIDS. It can cause widespread destruction of the brain's white matter.[1]

huntingtin: The protein encoded by the gene that carries the Huntington disease (HD) defect. The repeated CAG sequence in the gene causes an abnormal form of huntingtin to be formed. The function of the normal form of huntingtin is not yet known.[2]

Huntington disease: A degenerative hereditary disorder caused by a faulty gene for a protein called huntingtin. The disease causes degeneration in many regions of the brain and spinal cord and patients eventually develop severe dementia.[1]

hypothalamus: A structure in the brain under the thalamus that monitors activities such as body temperature and food intake.[3]

kindred: A group of related persons, such as a family or clan.[2]

late-onset Alzheimer disease: The most common form of AD; it occurs in people aged 65 and older.[3]

Lewy body dementia: One of the most common types of progressive dementia, characterized by the presence of abnormal structures called Lewy bodies in the brain. In many ways the symptoms of this disease overlap with those of Alzheimer disease.[1]

limbic system: A brain region that links the brain stem with the higher reasoning elements of the cerebral cortex; it controls emotions, instinctive behavior, and the sense of smell.[3]

magnetic resonance imaging (MRI): A diagnostic and research technique that uses magnetic fields to generate a computer image of internal structures in the body; MRIs are very clear and are particularly good for imaging the brain and soft tissues.[3]

marker: A piece of DNA that lies on the chromosome so close to a gene that the two are inherited together. Like a signpost, markers are used during genetic testing and research to locate the nearby presence of a gene.[2]

metabolism: All the chemical processes that take place inside the body. In some metabolic reactions, complex molecules are broken down to release energy; in others, the cells use energy to make complex compounds out of simpler ones (like making proteins from amino acids).[3]

microtubules: The internal support structure for neurons that guides nutrients and molecules from the body of the cell to the end of the axon and back.[3]

mild cognitive impairment: A condition associated with impairments in understanding and memory not severe enough to be diagnosed as dementia, but more pronounced than those associated with normal aging.[1]

Mini-Mental State Examination: A test used to assess cognitive skills in people with suspected dementia. The test examines orientation, memory, and attention, as well as the ability to name objects, follow verbal and written commands, write a sentence spontaneously, and copy a complex shape.[1]

mitochondria: Microscopic, energy-producing bodies within cells that are the cells' "power plants."[2]

multi-infarct dementia: A type of vascular dementia caused by numerous small strokes in the brain.[1]

mutation: A rare change in a cell's DNA that can cause a disease.[3]

myelin: A fatty substance that coats and insulates nerve cells.[1]

myoclonus: A condition in which muscles or portions of muscles contract involuntarily in a jerky fashion.[2]

nerve growth factor (NGF): A substance that maintains the health of nerve cells. NGF also promotes the growth of axons and dendrites, the parts of the nerve cell that are essential to its ability to communicate with other nerve cells.[3]

neurofibrillary tangles: Bundles of twisted filaments found within neurons, and a characteristic feature found in the brains of Alzheimer patients. These tangles are largely made up of a protein called tau.[1]

neuron: Greek word for a nerve cell, the basic impulse-conducting unit of the nervous system. Nerve cells communicate with other cells through an electrochemical process called neurotransmission.[2]

neurotransmitter: A chemical messenger between neurons; a substance that is released by the axon on one neuron and excites or inhibits activity in a neighboring neuron.[3]

nucleus: The organ within a cell that contains the chromosomes and controls many of its activities.[3]

organic brain syndrome: A term that refers to physical disorders (not psychiatric in origin) that impair mental functions.[1]

pallidum: Part of the basal ganglia of the brain. The pallidum is composed of the globus pallidus and the ventral pallidum.[2]

Parkinson dementia: A secondary dementia that sometimes occurs in people with advanced Parkinson disease, which is primarily a movement disorder. Many Parkinson patients have the characteristic amyloid plaques and neurofibrillary tangles found in Alzheimer disease, but it is not yet clear if the diseases are linked.[1]

Pick disease: A type of frontotemporal dementia where certain nerve cells become abnormal and swollen before they die. The brains of people with Pick disease have abnormal structures, called Pick bodies, inside the neurons. The symptoms are very similar to those of Alzheimer disease.[1]

541

plaques: Unusual clumps of material found between the tissues of the brain in Alzheimer disease.[1]

positron emission tomography (PET): A tool used to diagnose brain functions and disorders. PET produces three-dimensional, colored images of chemicals or substances functioning within the body. These images are called PET scans. PET shows brain function, in contrast to CT or MRI, which show brain structure.[2]

post-traumatic dementia: A dementia brought on by a single traumatic brain injury. It is much like dementia pugilistica, but usually also includes long-term memory problems.[1]

presenilin 1 and 2: Proteins produced by genes that influence susceptibility to early-onset Alzheimer disease.[1]

prevalence: The number of cases of a disease that are present in a particular population at a given time.[2]

primary dementia: A dementia, such as Alzheimer disease, that is not the result of another disease.[1]

primary progressive aphasia: A type of frontotemporal dementia resulting in deficits in language functions. Many, but not all, people with this type of aphasia eventually develop symptoms of dementia.[1]

progressive dementia: A dementia that gets worse over time, gradually interfering with more and more cognitive abilities.[1]

putamen: An area of the brain that decreases in size as a result of the damage produced by Huntington disease.[2]

receptor: Proteins that serve as recognition sites on cells and cause a response in the body when stimulated by chemicals called neurotransmitters. They act as on-and-off switches for the next nerve cell.[2]

recessive: A trait that is apparent only when the gene or genes for it are inherited from both parents.[2]

secondary dementia: A dementia that occurs as a consequence of another disease or an injury.[1]

senile chorea: A relatively mild and rare disorder found in elderly adults and characterized by choreic movements. It is believed by some scientists to be caused by a different gene mutation than that causing HD.[2]

senile dementia: An outdated term that reflects the formerly widespread belief that dementia was a normal part of aging. The word senile is derived from a Latin term that means, roughly, "old age."[1]

single photon emission computerized tomography (SPECT): An imaging technique that allows researchers to monitor blood flow to different parts of the brain.[3]

striatum: Part of the basal ganglia of the brain. The striatum is composed of the caudate nucleus, putamen, and ventral striatum.[2]

subcortical dementia: Dementia that affects parts of the brain below the outer brain layer, or cortex.[1]

substance-induced persisting dementia: Dementia caused by abuse of substances such as alcohol and recreational drugs that persists even after the substance abuse has ended.[1]

synapse: The tiny gap between nerve cells across which neurotransmitters pass.[3]

tau protein: A protein that helps the functioning of microtubules, which are part of the cell's structural support and help to deliver substances throughout the cell. In Alzheimer disease, tau is changed in a way that causes it to twist into pairs of helical filaments that collect into tangles.[1]

thalamus: A small organ in the front of the cerebral hemispheres that sends sensory information to the cerebral cortex and sends other information back to the body.[3]

trait: Any genetically determined characteristic.[2]

transgenic mice: Mice that receive injections of foreign genes during the embryonic stage of development. Their cells then follow the "instructions" of the foreign genes, resulting in the development of a certain trait or characteristic. Transgenic mice can serve as an animal model of a certain disease, telling researchers how genes work in specific cells.[2]

transmissible spongiform encephalopathies (TSEs): Part of a family of human and animal diseases in which brains become filled with holes resembling sponges when examined under a microscope. Creutzfeldt-Jakob disease (CJD) is the most common of the known transmissible spongiform encephalopathies.[1]

vascular dementia: A type of dementia caused by brain damage from cerebrovascular or cardiovascular problems: usually strokes. It accounts for up to 20 percent of all dementias.[1]

ventricle: Cavity within the brain that contains cerebrospinal fluid. During AD, brain tissue shrinks and the ventricles enlarge.[3]

Chapter 64

How to Enroll in The Safe Return® Program

How Safe Return Works

Alzheimer's Association Safe Return® is a nationwide identification, support, and enrollment program that provides assistance when a person with Alzheimer disease or a related dementia wanders and becomes lost locally or far from home.

Assistance is available 24 hours a day, 365 days a year. If an enrollee is missing, one call immediately activates a community support network to help reunite the lost person with his or her caregiver.

Safe Return faxes the enrolled person's information and photo (if provided) to local law enforcement. When the person is found, a citizen or law official calls the 800-number on the identification products and Safe Return notifies listed contacts. The nearest Alzheimer's Association office provides information and support during the search and rescue efforts.

Safe Return ID Products

With a $40 enrollment in Safe Return, you receive the following products:

- Engraved identification bracelet or necklace and iron-on clothing labels.

- "Five steps for a Safe Return" magnet card, key chain, wallet cards, Tips to Encourage the Use of Safe Return Identification Products, and About Wandering Behavior fact sheet.

- For an additional $15, you'll receive caregiver jewelry. In an emergency, it alerts others that you provide care for a person with dementia.

- There is a $20 annual program administrative fee.

Enroll in Safe Return

Enrolling a person with dementia in Safe Return is easy.

A caregiver fills out a simple form, supplies a photograph (if available), chooses the type of identification product that the enrollee will wear or carry, and pays a $40 enrollment fee.

After one year, you will receive an invoice for the $20 annual program administrative fee. This helps Safe Return respond to more than 6,000 calls for help each year.

Check with your local Alzheimer's Association to find out if scholarships are available in your area to cover the cost of enrollment.

There are three ways you can enroll:

1. Online. Enroll with our secure form. It's fast and easy.

2. Phone: Enroll by phone using a credit card. Call 888-572-8566 between 7 A.M.–1:30 P.M. (CST). Representatives are available Monday through Friday.

3. Mail: To enroll by mail, simply print out and complete the enrollment form and send payment and enrollee photo to: P.O. Box A3687, Chicago, IL 60690-3687. You may also phone 888-572-8566 to have an enrollment form mailed to you.

When enrolling online or by phone, you will be asked to provide the following information:

- Enrollee's name and contact information

- Enrollee's identifying characteristics (height, weight, eye color, distinguishing marks and characteristics)

- Enrollee's exact wrist measurement in inches (required when ordering a bracelet)

- At least two contact names, addresses, and phone numbers (more can be added, if needed)

- Local law enforcement phone number

- Credit card number and expiration date

Chapter 65

Alzheimer Disease Centers (ADCs) Program Directory

What do the ADCs do?

Researchers at NIA-funded Alzheimer's Disease Centers (ADC) are working to translate research advances into improved diagnosis and care for Alzheimer disease (AD) patients while, at the same time, focusing on the program's long-term goal—finding a way to cure and possibly prevent AD.

Areas of investigation range from the basic mechanisms of AD to managing the symptoms and helping families cope with the effects of the disease. Center staff conducts basic, clinical, and behavioral research and train scientists and health care providers who are new to AD research.

Although each center has its own unique area of emphasis, a common goal of the ADCs is to enhance research on AD by providing a network for sharing new ideas as well as research results. Collaborative studies draw upon the expertise of scientists from many different disciplines.

Some ADCs have satellite facilities, which offer diagnostic and treatment services and research opportunities in underserved, rural, and minority communities.

For patients and families affected by AD, the ADCs offer the following services:

"AD Research Centers," National Institute on Aging (http://www.nia.nih.gov), February 2007; all contact information was verified and updated in August 2007.

- Diagnosis and medical management (costs may vary—centers may accept Medicare, Medicaid, and private insurance)

- Information about the disease, services, and resources

- Opportunities for volunteers to participate in drug trials, support groups, clinical research projects, and other special programs for volunteers and their families

Two national AD resources are listed at the end of the directory. The National Alzheimer's Coordinating Center coordinates data collection and fosters collaborative research among the ADCs. The National Cell Repository for Alzheimer's Disease maintains a database of family histories and medical records and provides genetic researchers with cell lines or DNA samples.

For more information, contact any of the centers in the directory below.

ADC Directory

Alabama

Alzheimer's Disease Research Center
University of Alabama at Birmingham
Sparks Research Center
1720 7th Avenue South
Suite 650K
Birmingham, AL 35233-7340
Phone: 205-934-3847
Fax: 205-934-1569
Website: www.uab.edu/adc

Arizona

Arizona Alzheimer's Disease Center
Banner Alzheimer's Institute
901 E. Willeta Street
Phoenix, AZ 85006
Phone: 602-239-6999
Fax: 602-239-6253
Website: http://www.azalz.org

Arkansas

Alzheimer's Disease Center
Website: http://alzheimer.uams.edu

California

Stanford/VA Alzheimer's Disease Center
Department of Psychiatry, 5550
401 Quarry Road, C305
Stanford, CA 94305-5717
Phone: 650-852-3287
Fax: 650-852-3297
Website: http://alzheimer.stanford.edu

Alzheimer's Disease Center
University of California
Davis Medical Center
4860 Y Street
Suite 3900
Sacramento, CA 95817-4540
Phone: 916-734-5496
Fax: 916-703-5290
Website: http://alzheimer.ucdavis.edu

Alzheimer's Disease Research
Center
University of California, Irvine
Gillespie Neuroscience Research
Facility, Rm. 1113
Irvine, CA 92697-4540
Phone: 949-824-5847
Fax: 949-824-2071
Website: http://www.alz.uci.edu

Alzheimer's Disease Center
University of California
Los Angeles
10911 Weyburn Avenue
Suite 200
Los Angeles, CA 90095-1769
Phone: 310-206-6379
Fax: 310-794-3148
Website: http://www.adc.ucla.edu

Alzheimer's Disease Research
Center
University of California
San Diego
Department of Neurosciences
UCSD School of Medicine
8950 Villa La Jolla Dr.
Suite C129
La Jolla, CA 92037
Phone: 858-622-5800
Fax: 858-622-1012
Website: http://adrc.ucsd.edu
E-mail: adrc@ucsd.edu

Alzheimer's Disease Research
Center
University of California
San Francisco
Box 1207
350 Parnassus Avenue
Suite 706
San Francisco, CA 94143-1207
Phone: 415-476-6242
Fax: 415-476-4800
Website: http://memory.ucsf.edu
E-mail: adrc@memory.ucsf.edu

Alzheimer's Disease Research
Center
University of Southern California
Health Consultation Center
1510 San Pablo Street, HCC643
Los Angeles, CA 90033
Phone: 213-740-7777
Fax: 323-442-7689
Website: www.usc.edu/dept/gero/ADRC
E-mail: uscadrc@usc.edu

Florida

Florida Alzheimer's Disease
Research Center
Byrd Alzheimer's Institute
4001 East Fletcher Ave.
Tampa, FL 33613
Phone: 813-866-1600
Fax: 813-866-1601
Website: http://
www.floridaadrc.org

Georgia

Alzheimer's Disease Center
Emory University
Neurology Department
101 Woodruff Circle, #6000
Atlanta, GA 30322
Phone: 404-728-6950
Fax: 404-727-3999
Website: www.med.emory.edu/
ADC

Illinois

Cognitive Neurology and
Alzheimer's Disease Center
Feinberg School of Medicine
Northwestern University
320 East Superior
Searle Building
11th Floor, Rm. 453
Chicago, IL 60611
Phone: 312-908-9339
Fax: 312-908-8789
Website: http://
www.brain.northwestern.edu

Alzheimer's Disease Center
Rush University Medical Center
Armour Academic Center
600 South Paulina Street
Suite 1028
Chicago, IL 60612
Phone: 312-942-2362
Fax: 312-563-4605
Website: www.rush.edu/radc

Indiana

Indiana Alzheimer Disease
Center
Department of Pathology and
Lab Medicine
Indiana University School of
Medicine
635 Barnhill Drive, MS-A-138
Indianapolis, IN 46202-5120
Phone: 317-278-5500
Fax: 317-274-4882
Website: http://iadc.iupui.edu
E-mail: iadc@iupui.edu

Kentucky

University of Kentucky
Alzheimer's Disease Center
Sanders-Brown Center on Aging
Rm. 101
800 South Limestone St.
Lexington, KY 40536-0230
Phone: 859-323-6040
Fax: 859-323-2866
Website: www.mc.uky.edu/coa

Maryland

Alzheimer's Disease Research
Center
Division of Neuropathology
The Johns Hopkins University
Medical Institutions
558 Ross Research Building
720 Rutland Avenue
Baltimore, MD 21205-2196
Phone: 410-502-5169
Fax: 410-955-9777
Website: http://
www.alzresearch.org

Massachusetts

Alzheimer's Disease Center
Boston University
Bedford VA Medical Center
GRECC Program (182B)
715 Albany St.
Robinson Complex
Suite 7800
Boston, MA 02118
Phone: 617-638-5368
Fax: 781-687-3515
Website: www.bu.edu/alzresearch

Alzheimer's Disease Research
Center
Massachusetts General Hospital
114 16th Street
Room 2009
Charlestown, MA 02129
Phone: 617-726-3987
Fax: 617-724-1480
Website: http://madrc.org

Michigan

Alzheimer's Disease Research
Center
University of Michigan
Department of Neurology
300 North Ingalls, Room 3D15
Ann Arbor, MI 48109-0489
Phone: 734-764-2190
Fax: 734-963-1752
Website: www.med.umich.edu/
alzheimers
E-mail: neuro-ADresearch@med
.umich.edu

Minnesota

Mayo Clinic Alzheimer's Disease
Research Center
Department of Neurology
200 First Street, SW
Rochester, MN 55905
Phone: 507-284-1324
Fax: 507-538-0878
Website: http://mayoresearch
.mayo.edu/mayo/research/
alzheimers_center
E-mail: mayoADC@mayo.edu

Missouri

Alzheimer's Disease Research
Center
Washington University School of
Medicine
Department of Neurology
4488 Forest Park Avenue
Suite 130
St. Louis, MO 63108-2293
Phone: 314-286-2881
Fax: 314-286-2763
Website: http://
alzheimer.wustl.edu

New York

Columbia University
Alzheimer's Disease Center
630 West 168th Street
PH 19, Mailbox 16
New York, NY 10032
Phone: 212-305-1818
Fax: 212-305-5498
Website http://www.columbia
.edu [search for: Alzheimer]

Alzheimer's Disease Research
Center
Department of Psychiatry
Mount Sinai School of Medicine
One Gustave Levy Place
Box 1230
New York, NY 10029-6574
Phone: 212-241-8329
Fax: 718-562-9120
Website: www.mssm.edu/
psychiatry/adrc

Alzheimer's Disease Center
New York University
ADRC, Millhauser Labs
560 First Avenue
New York, NY 10016
Phone: 212-263-8088
Fax: 212-263-6991
Website: www.med.nyu.edu/adc

North Carolina

Joseph and Kathleen Bryan
Alzheimer's Disease Research
Center
Duke University Medical Center
2200 West Main Street
Suite A-200
Durham, NC 27705
Toll-free: 1-866-444-2372 (ADRC)
Fax: 919-668-0828
Website: http://adrc.mc.duke.edu

Oregon

Aging and Alzheimer's Disease
Center CR 131
Oregon Health and Science
University
3181 SW Sam Jackson Park Road
Portland, OR 97239-3098
Phone: 503-494-6976
Fax: 503-494-7499
Website: www.ohsu.edu/research/
alzheimers

Pennsylvania

Alzheimer's Disease Center
Department of Pathology and
Laboratory Medicine
University of Pennsylvania
School of Medicine
3615 Chestnut
Philadelphia, PA 19104-4283
Phone: 215-662-7810
Fax: 215-349-5909
Website: www.pennadc.org

Alzheimer's Disease Research
Center
University of Pittsburgh
Department of Neurology
4 West MH 200 Lothrop St.
Pittsburgh, PA 15213-2582
Phone: 412-692-2700
Fax: 412-692-2710
Website: http://www.adrc.pitt.edu

Texas

Alzheimer's Disease Research
Center
Department of Neurology
University of Texas SW Medical
Center
5323 Harry Hines Boulevard
Dallas, TX 75390-9036
Phone: 214-648-9376
Fax: 214-648-6824
Website:
www.utsouthwestern.edu/
alzheimers/research

Washington

Alzheimer's Disease Center
University of Washington
VA Puget Sound Health Care
System
Mental Health Services, S-116
1660 South Columbian Way
Seattle, WA 98108
Phone: 206-277-3281
Fax: 206-768-5456
Website: http://
depts.washington.edu/adrcweb

National Resources

National Alzheimer's Coordinat-
ing Center (NACC)
4311 11th Avenue NE, #300
Seattle, WA 98105
Phone: 206-543-8637
Fax: 206-616-5927
Website: http://
www.alz.washington.edu
E-mail: naccmail@u.washington
.edu

The NACC coordinates data collection and fosters collaborative
research among the ADCs.

National Cell Repository for
Alzheimer's Disease
Indiana University Medical
Center
Department of Medical and
Molecular Genetics
Hereditary Genomic Health
Information and Translational
Sciences Building
410 West 10th St., HS 4000
Indianapolis IN 46202-5251
Phone: 800-526-2839
Fax: 317-278-1100
Website: http://www.ncrad.org
E-mail: alzstudy@iupui.edu

Chapter 66

Directory of Resources for Additional Information about Alzheimer Disease and Other Dementias

Resources for Information about Alzheimer Disease

Administration on Aging (AoA)
Department of Health and Human Services
Washington, DC 20201
Phone: 202-619-0724
Fax: 202-357-3555
Website: http://www.aoa.gov
E-mail: AoAInfo@aoa.gov

Agency for Healthcare Research and Quality (AHRQ)
Publications Clearinghouse
P.O. Box 8547
Silver Spring, MD 20907-8547
Toll-Free: 800-358-9295
Website: http://www.ahrq.gov

Alliance for Aging Research
2021 K Street, NW, Suite 305
Washington, DC 20006
Phone: 202-293-2856
Fax: 202-785-8574
Website: http://www.agingresearch.org

Alzheimer's Association
225 North Michigan Avenue
Fl 17
Chicago, IL 60601-7633
Toll-Free: 800-272-3900
Phone: 312-335-8700
Fax: 312-335-1110
Website: http://www.alz.org
E-mail: info@alz.org

The resources listed in this chapter were compiled from many sources deemed accurate. They are listed alphabetically by topic under these three headings: Resources for Information about Alzheimer Disease; Resources for Information about Other Dementias; and Resources for Caregivers. Inclusion does not constitute endorsement and there is no implication associated with omission. All contact information was verified and updated in August 2007.

557

Alzheimer's Australia
Website: http://
www.alzheimers.org.au

Alzheimer's Disease Cooperative Study
University of California at San Diego (UCSD)-ADCS
8950 Villa La Jolla Dr.
Suite C129
La Jolla, CA 92037
Phone: 858-622-5880

Alzheimer's Disease Education and Referral (ADEAR) Center
P.O. Box 8250
Silver Spring, MD 20907-8250
Toll-Free: 800-438-4380
(English, Spanish)
Phone: 301-495-3311
Fax: 301-495-3334
Website: http://
www.alzheimers.org
E-mail: adear@alzheimers.org

Alzheimer's Disease International
64 Great Suffolk Street
London SE1 0BL UK
Phone: +44 20 79810880
Fax: +44 20 79282357
Website: http://www.alz.co.uk
E-mail: info@alz.co.uk

Alzheimer's Drug Discovery Foundation
(formerly, Institute for the Study of Aging)
1414 Avenue of the Americas, Suite 1502
New York, NY 10019
Phone: 212-935-2402
Fax: 212-935-2408
Website: http://
www.alzdiscovery.org

Alzheimer's Foundation of America
322 Eighth Avenue, 7th Floor
New York, NY 10001
Phone: 866-AFA-8484 (232-8484)
Fax: 646-638-1542
Website: http://www.alzfdn.org
E-mail: info@alzfdn.org

Alzheimer Society of Canada
20 Eglinton Avenue W.
Suite 1200
Toronto, ON M4R 1K8 Canada
Toll-Free: 800-616-8816 (Canada only)
Phone: 416-488-8772
Fax: 416-488-3778
Website: http://
www.alzheimer.ca
E-mail: info@alzheimer.ca

Alzheimer's Society (UK)
Gordon House
10 Greencoat Place
London, SW1P 1PH, UK
Website: http://
www.alzheimers.org.uk
E-mail:
enquiries@alzheimers.org.uk

American Academy of Neurology
1080 Montreal Avenue
St. Paul, MN 55116
Toll-Free: 800-879-1960
Phone: 651-695-2717
Fax: 651-695-2791
Website: http://www.aan.com

American Association for Geriatric Psychiatry
7910 Woodmont Avenue
Suite 1050
Bethesda, MD 20814-3004
Phone: 301-654-7850
Fax: 301-654-4137
Website: http://www.aagponline.org
E-mail: main@aagponline.org

American Association of Retired Persons (AARP)
601 E Street, NW
Washington, DC 20049
Toll-Free: 800-424-3410
(members only)
Phone: 202-434-2277
Website: http://www.aarp.org

American Federation for Aging Research
55 West 39th Street
New York, NY 10018
Toll-Free: 888-582-2327
Phone: 212-703-9977
Fax: 212-997-0030
Website: http://www.afar.org
E-mail: info@afar.org

American Geriatrics Society
350 Fifth Avenue
New York, NY 10118
Phone: 212-308-1414
Fax: 212-832-8646
Website: http://www.americangeriatrics.org
E-mail: info.amger@americangeriatrics.org

American Geriatrics Society Foundation for Health in Aging
Website: http://www.healthinaging.org

American Health Assistance Foundation
22512 Gateway Center Dr.
Clarksburg, MD 20871
Toll-Free: 800-437-AHAF (2423)
Phone: 301-948-3244
Fax: 301-258-9454
Website: http://www.ahaf.org

American Health Care Association
1201 L Street, NW
Washington, DC 20005
Phone: 202-842-4444
Fax: 202-842-3860
Website: http://www.ahca.org

American Medical Association (AMA)
515 North State Street
Chicago, IL 60610
Toll-Free: 800-621-8335
Phone: 312-464-5000
Fax: 312-464-5600
Website: http://www.ama-assn.org

American Psychiatric Association
1000 Wilson Blvd., Suite 1825
Arlington, VA 22209-3901
Toll-Free: 888-35-PSYCH
(888-357-7924)
Phone: 703-907-7300
Fax: 703-907-1085
Website: http://www.psych.org
E-mail: apa@psych.org

American Psychological Association
750 First Street, NE
Washington, DC 20002-4242
Toll-Free: 800-374-2721
Phone: 202-336-5500
Website: http://www.apa.org
E-mail: webmaster@apa.org

American Society on Aging
833 Market Street, Suite 511
San Francisco, CA 94103
Toll-Free: 800-537-9728
Phone: 415-974-9600
Fax: 415-974-0300
Website: http://www.asaging.org
E-mail: info@asaging.org

Brain Resources and Information Network (BRAIN)
P.O. Box 5801
Bethesda, MD 20824
Phone: 800-352-9424
Website: http://
www.ninds.nih.gov

Brookdale Center on Aging (BCOA) of Hunter College
425 East 25th Street
New York, NY 10010
Phone: 212-481-3780
Fax: 212-481-3791
Website: http://
www.brookdale.org
E-mail: info@brookdale.org

Center for Healthy Aging
Website: http://
www.helpguide.org

Center for Neurologic Study
9850 Genesee, Suite 320
La Jolla, CA 92037
Phone: 858-455-5463
Fax: 858-455-1713
Website: http://www.cnsonline.org
E-mail: cns@cts.com

Center for the Study of Aging and Human Development
P.O. Box 3003
Duke University Medical Center
Durham NC 27710
Phone: 919-660-7502
Fax: 919-684-8569
Website: http://
www.geri.duke.edu

Clearinghouse on Aging and Developmental Disabilities
University of Chicago
1640 West Roosevelt Rd.
Chicago, IL 60608-6904
Website: http://www.uic.edu/
orgs/rrtcamr/clearinghouse.htm

Cleveland Clinic Health Information Center

9500 Euclid Avenue
Cleveland, OH 44195
Phone: 216-444-3371
Website: http://
www.clevelandclinic.org/health

Cognitive Neurology and Alzheimer's Disease Center at Northwestern University

320 East Superior Street
Chicago, IL 60611-3008
Phone: 312-908-9339
Fax: 312-908-8789
Website: http://
www.brain.nwu.edu

Dana Alliance for Brain Initiatives

745 Fifth Avenue, Suite 900
New York, NY 10151
Phone: 212-223-4040
Fax: 212-317-8721
Website: http://www.dana.org
E-mail:
dabiinfo@danany.dana.org

Fisher Center for Alzheimer's Research

One Intrepid Square
West 46th Street & 12th Avenue
New York, NY 10036
Toll-Free: 800-259-4636
Phone: 212-245-5434
Website: http://www.alzinfo.org
E-mail: info@alzinfo.org

John Douglas French Alzheimer's Foundation

11620 Wilshire Boulevard
Suite 270
Los Angeles, CA 90025
Toll-Free: 800-477-2243
Phone: 310-445-4650
Fax: 310-479-0516
Website: http://www.jdfaf.org

Gerontological Society of America

1220 L Street NW, Suite 901
Washington, DC 20005
Phone: 202-842-1275
Fax: 202-842-1150
Website: http://www.geron.org
E-mail: geron@geron.org

Institute for Advanced Studies in Aging and Geriatric Medicine

1700 Wisconsin Ave., NW
1st Floor
Washington, DC 20007
Phone: 202-333-8845
Fax: 202-333-8898
Website: http://www.iasia.org
E-mail: iasia@iasia.org

International Center for the Disabled (ICD)

340 East 24th St.
New York, NY 10010
Phone: 212-585-6000
Fax: 212-585-6161
TTY: 212-585-6262
Website: http://www.icdnyc.org
E-mail: info@icdrehab.org

Mental Health America
2000 N. Beauregard Street
6th Floor
Alexandria, VA 22311
Toll-Free: 800-969-NMHA (6642)
(Mental Health Resource Center)
Phone: 703-684-7722
Fax: 703-684-5968
TTY: 800-433-5959
Website: http://www.nmha.org

**National Association of
Community Health Centers**
7200 Wisconsin Avenue
Suite 210
Bethesda, MD 20814
Phone: 301-347-0400
Fax: 301-347-0459
Website: http://www.nachc.com
E-mail: contact@nachc.com

**National Association of
Area Agencies on Aging
(N4A)**
1730 Rhode Island Ave., NW
Suite 1200
Washington, DC 20036
Phone: 202-872-0888
Website: http://www.n4a.org

**National Association of
Nutrition and Aging Service
Programs**
1612 K Street, NW, Suite 400
Washington, DC 20006
Phone: 202-682-6899
Fax: 202-223-2099
Website: http://www.nanasp.org

**National Association of
State Units on Aging**
1201 15th St., NW, Suite 350
Washington, DC 20005
Phone: 202-898-2578
Fax: 202-898-2583
Website: http://www.nasua.org
E-mail: info@nasua.org

**National Center for Health
Statistics**
3311 Toledo Road
Hyattsville, MD 20782-2003
Toll-Free: 866-441-NCHS
(441-6247)
Phone: 301-458-4000
Phone: 301-458-4636
Website: http://www.cdc.gov/nchs
E-mail: nchsquery@cdc.gov

**National Center on Women
and Aging**
Heller School for Social Policy
and Management
Mail Stop 035
Brandeis University
Waltham, MA 02454-9110
Phone: 781-736-3863
Fax: 781-736-3865
Website: http://www.brandeis
.edu/heller/national
E-mail: natwomctr@brandeis.edu

**National Council on Aging,
Inc.**
1901 L Street, NW, 4th Floor
Washington, DC 20036
Phone: 202-479-1200
TDD: 202-479-6674
Fax: 202-479-0735
Website: http://www.ncoa.org
E-mail: info@ncoa.org

National Council of Senior Citizens

8403 Colesville Rd., Suite 1200
Silver Spring, MD 20910
Phone: 301-578-8800
Website: http://www.ncscinc.org

National Gerontological Nursing Association

7794 Grow Drive
Pensacola, FL 32514
Toll-Free: 800-723-0560
Phone: 850-473-1174
Fax: 850-484-8762
Website: http://www.ngna.org
E-mail: ngna@puetzamc.com

National Health Information Center

P.O. Box 1133
Washington, DC 20013-1133
Toll-Free: 800-336-4797
Phone: 301-565-4167
Fax: 301-984-4256
Website: http://www.health.gov/
NHIC
E-mail: nhicinfo@health.org

National Hispanic Council on Aging

734 15th St., NW, Suite 1050
Washington, DC 20005
Phone: 202-347-9733
Fax: 202-347-9735
Website: http://www.nhcoa.org
E-mail: nhcoa@nhcoa.org

National Indian Council on Aging

10501 Montgomery Boulevard,
NE, Suite 210
Albuquerque, NM 87111-3846
Phone: 505-292-2001
Fax: 505-292-1922
Website: http://www.nicoa.org
E-mail: dave@nicoa.org

National Institute of Mental Health

6001 Executive Boulevard
Room 8184, MSC 9663
Bethesda, MD 20892-9663
Toll-Free: 800-421-4211
Phone: 301-443-4513
Fax: 301-443-4279
TTY: 866-415-8051
Website: http://www.nimh.nih.gov
E-mail: nimhinfo@nih.gov

National Institute of Neurological Disorders and Stroke

P.O. Box 5801
Bethesda, MD 20892-2540
Toll-Free: 800-352-9424
Phone: 301-496-5751
Fax: 301-402-2186
Website: http://www.ninds.nih.org

National Institute on Aging (NIA)

P.O. Box 8057
Gaithersburg, MD 20898-8057
Toll-Free: 800-222-2225
(NIA Information Center)
TTY: 800-222-4225
Phone: 301-496-1752
Website: http://www.nia.nih.gov

National Resource Center on Native American Aging
501 North Columbia Rd.
Grand Forks, ND 58202
Toll-Free: 800-896-7628
Phone: 701-777-6780
Fax: 701-777-6779
Website: http://www.med.und
.nodak.edu/depts/rural/nrcnaa

Northwestern University Medical School-Cognitive Neurology and Alzheimer's Disease Center
320 East Superior
Searle Building, 11th Floor
Rm. 453
Chicago, IL 60611
Phone: 312-908-9339
Fax: 312-908-8789
Website: http://
www.brain.northwestern.edu

Older Women's League (OWL)
3300 N. Fairfax Drive, Suite 218
Arlington, VA 22201
Toll-Free: 800-825-3695
Phone: 703-812-7990
Fax: 703-812-0687
Website: http://www.
owl-national.org
E-mail: owlinfo@owl-national.org

Society for Neuroscience
1121 14th St. NW
Suite 1010
Washington DC 20005
Phone: 202-462-6688
Fax: 202-462-9740
Website: http://www.sfn.org
E-mail: info@sfn.org

Taub Institute for Research on Alzheimer's Disease and the Aging Brain
College of Physicians and
Surgeons, Columbia University
630 West 168th St.
P.O. Box 16
New York, NY 10032
Phone: 212-305-1818
Fax: 212-342-2849
Website: http://
www.healthsciences.columbia.edu/
dept/taub/index.html

University of California San Francisco Memory and Aging Center
350 Parnassus Avenue
Suite 706
San Francisco CA 94143-1207
Phone: 415-476-6242
Fax: 415-476-4800
Website: http://memory.ucsf.edu
E-mail: adrc@memory.ucsf.edu

Resources for Information about Other Dementias

American Parkinson's Disease Association
135 Parkinson Avenue
Staten Island, NY 10305
Toll-Free: 800-223-2732
Phone: 718-981-8001
Fax: 718-981-4399
Website: http://www
.apdaparkinson.org/user/index
.asp
E-mail:
apda@apdaparkinson.org

Association for Frontotemporal Dementias (AFTD)
100 North 17th Street
Suite 600
Philadelphia, PA 19103
Toll-Free: 866-507-7222
Phone: 267-514-7221
Website: http://www.ftd-picks.org
E-mail: info@FTD-Picks.org

CJD Aware!
2527 South Carrollton Ave.
New Orleans, LA 70118-3013
Website: http://www.cjdaware.com
E-mail: cjdaware@iwon.com

Creutzfeldt-Jakob Disease (CJD) Foundation Inc.
P.O. Box 5312
Akron, OH 44334
Phone: 800-659-1991
Phone: 330-668-2474
Website: http://
www.cjdfoundation.org
E-mail: help@cjdfoundation.org

Huntington's Disease Society of America
158 West 29th Street, 7th Floor
New York, NY 10018
Toll-Free: 800-345-HDSA (4372)
Phone: 212-242-1968, ext. 10
Fax: 212-239-3430
Website: http://www.hdsa.org
E-mail: hdsainfo@hdsa.org

Lewy Body Dementia Association
P.O. Box 451429
Atlanta, GA 31145-9429
Toll-Free: 800-LEWYSOS
(539-9767)
Phone: 404-935-6444
Fax: 480-422-5434
Website: http://
www.lewybodydementia.org
E-mail: lbda@lbda.org

National Down Syndrome Society
666 Broadway
New York, NY 10012
Phone: 800-221-4602
Fax: 212-979-2873
Website: http://www.ndss.org
E-mail: info@ndss.org

National Institute on Alcohol Abuse and Alcoholism
5635 Fishers Lane, MSC 9304
Bethesda, MD 20892-9304
Phone: 301-443-3860
Website: http://pubs.niaaa.nih.gov
E-mail: niaaaweb-r@exchange
.nih.gov

National Organization for Rare Disorders (NORD)
55 Kenosia Avenue
P.O. Box 1968
Danbury, CT 06813-1968
Toll-Free: 800-999-NORD (6673)
Phone: 203-744-0100
Fax: 203-798-2291
Website: http://
www.rarediseases.org
E-mail: orphan@rarediseases.org

National Parkinson Foundation
1501 N.W. 9th Avenue
Miami, Florida 33136
Toll-Free: 800-327-4545
Phone: (305) 243-6666
Fax: (305) 243-5595
Website: http://
www.parkinson.org

Neurology Channel
Website: http://
www.neurologychannel.com

Parkinson's Association of the Rockies
1325 S. Colorado Blvd. #204-B
Denver, CO 80222
Phone: 303-830-1839
Fax : 303-830-2577
Toll-Free: 866-718-2996
Website: http://
www.parkinsonrockies.org
E-mail:info@parkinsonrockies.org

Parkinson's Disease Foundation
1359 Broadway, Suite 1509
New York, NY 10018
Toll-Free: 800-457-6676
Phone: 212-923-4700
Fax: 212-923-4778
Website: http://www.pdf.org
E-mail: info@pdf.org

The Pick's Disease Support Group
Website: http://www.pdsg.org.uk/
index.htm

Resources for Caregivers

Aging Network Services
4400 East-West Highway
Suite 907
Bethesda, MD 20814
Phone: 301-657-4329
Fax: 301-657-3250
Website: http://
www.agingnets.com
E-mail: ans@AgingNetS.com

Alzheimer's Disease Support Groups
Family Caregivers and Friends
Program
c/o Alzheimer's Association
225 North Michigan Avenue
Fl. 17
Chicago, IL 60601-7633
Toll-Free: 800-272-3900
Phone: 312-335-8700
Fax: 312-335-1110
TTY: 312-335-8882
Website: http://www.alz.org/
apps/findus.asp
E-mail: info@alz.org

American Association of Critical-Care Nurses
101 Columbia
Aliso Viejo, CA 92656-4109
Toll-Free: 800-899-AACN (2226)
Fax: 949-362-2020
Website: http://www.aacn.org
E-mail: info@aacn.org

American Association for Homecare
2011 Crystal Dr., Suite 725
Arlington, VA 22202
Phone: 703-836-6263
Website: http://
www.aahomecare.org

American Association of Homes and Services for the Aging
2519 Connecticut Avenue, NW
Washington, DC 20008-1520
Phone: 202-783-2242
Fax: 202-783-2255
Website: http://www.aahsa.org
E-mail: inform@aahsa.org

Assisted Living Federation of America
1650 King St., Suite 602
Alexandria, VA 22314-2747
Phone: 703-894-1805
Fax: 703-894-1831
Website: http://www.alfa.org

Caring Connections
Phone: 800-659-8898
Website: http://
www.caringinfo.org

Children of Aging Parents
1609 Woodbourne Road
Suite 302A
Levittown, PA 19057
Toll-Free: 800-227-7294
Fax: 215-945-8720
Website: http://
www.caps4caregivers.org

567

C-Mac Informational Services/Caregiver News
Website: http://
www.caregivernews.org
E-mail:
caregiver_cmi@hotmail.com

Eldercare Locator
Toll-Free: 800-677-1116
Website: http://www.eldercare.gov

Elderweb
1305 Chadwick Drive
Normal, IL 61761
Phone: 309-451-3319
Fax: 866-422-8995
Website: http://www.elderweb.com
E-mail: ksb@elderweb.com

Family Caregiver Alliance
180 Montgomery Street
Suite 1100
San Francisco, CA 94104
Toll-Free: 800-445-8106
Phone: 415-434-3388
Fax: 415-434-3508
Website: http://www.caregiver.org
E-mail: info @caregiver.org

Medicare Help Line
Toll-Free: 800-633-4227
Website: http://www.medicare.gov

MedSupport Friends Supporting Friends International
3132 Timberview Drive
Dunedin, FL 34698
Website: http://
www.medsupport.org

National Academy of Elder Law Attorneys, Inc.
1604 N. Country Club Rd.
Tucson, AZ 85716
Phone: 520-881-4005
Website: http://www.naela.org

National Association for Continence
P.O. Box 1019
Charleston, SC 29402
Toll-Free: 800-252-3337
Fax: 843-377-0905
Website: http://www.nafc.org
E-mail:
memberservices@nafc.org

National Association for Home Care
228 7th Street, SE
Washington, DC 20003
Phone: 202-547-7424
Fax: 202-547-3540
Website: http://www.nahc.org
E-mail: webmaster@nahc.org

National Caregiving Foundation
801 North Pitt St., Suite 116
Alexandria, VA 22314-1765
Toll-Free: 800-930-1357
Phone: 703-299 9300
Website: http://
www.caregivingfoundation.org
E-mail:
info@caregivingfoundation.org

National Center on Elder Abuse

1201 15th Street, NW, Suite 350
Washington, DC 20005
Phone: 202-898-2586
Fax: 202-898-2583
Website: http://www.elderabusecenter.org
E-mail: NCEA@nasua.org

National Family Caregivers Association

10400 Connecticut Avenue, #500
Kensington, MD 20895-3944
Toll-Free: 800-896-3650
Phone: 301-942-6430
Fax: 301-942-2302
Website: http://www.nfcacares.org
E-mail: info@nfcacares.org

National Hospice and Palliative Care Organization

1700 Diagonal Road, Suite 625
Alexandria, VA 22314
Toll-Free: 800-658-8898 (Hospice Helpline and Locator)
Toll-Free: 800-646-6460
Phone: 703-837-1500
Fax: 703-837-1233
Website: http://www.nhpco.org
E-mail: info@nhpco.org

National Respite Network and Resource Center

Website: http://www.archrespite.org

National Senior Citizens Law Center

1101 14th Street, NW
Suite 400
Washington, DC 20005
Phone: 202-289-6976
Fax: 202-289-7224
Website: http://www.nsclc.org
E-mail: nsclc@nsclc.org

Simon Foundation for Continence

P.O. Box 835
Wilmette, IL 60091
Toll-Free: 800-237-4666
Website: http://www.simonfoundation.org

United Seniors Health Cooperative

409 Third St., SW, Suite 200
Washington, DC 20024
Phone: 202-479-6973
Website: http://www.unitedseniorshealth.org

Visiting Nurse Associations of America

99 Summer Street, Suite 1700
Boston, MA 02110
Toll-Free: 888-866-8773
Phone: 617-737-3200
Fax: 617-737-1144
Website: http://www.vnaa.org
E-mail: vnaa@vnaa.org

Well Spouse Foundation

63 West Main Street, Suite H
Freehold, NJ 07728
Toll-Free: 800-838-0879
Phone: 732-577-8899
Fax: 732-577-8644
Website: http://
www.wellspouse.org

Chapter 67

Additional Reading about Alzheimer Disease and Other Dementias

Alzheimer's Early Stages: First Steps for Family, Friends and Caregivers, 2nd ed.
Published by Hunter House. 2003. 306 p. Available from Hunter House Publishers. P.O. Box 2914, Alameda, CA 94501-0914. 800-266-5592; 510-865-5282; FAX: 510-865-4295. Website: www.hunterhouse.com. PRICE: $15.95 paperback, $27.95 hardcover. ISBN: 0897933974 paperback; 0897933982 hardcover.

Alzheimer's Activities: Hundreds of Activities for Men and Women with Alzheimer's Disease and Related Disorders
By B. J. FitzRay. Published by Rayve Productions. 2001. 288 p. Available from Rayve Productions, P.O. Box 726, Windsor, CA 95492. 800-852-4890. PRICE $29.95. Website: http://www.rayveproductions.com.

Alzheimer's Research Review
A newsletter published by the American Health Assistance Foundation, 22512 Gateway Center Drive, Clarksburg, MD 20871. Available for free online at http://www.ahaf.org/pubs/ADRNewsLetters/ADRNewsletter.pdf or by calling 800-437-2423.

Resources listed in this chapter are listed alphabetically by title. They were compiled from suggestions by the National Institute on Aging, the Centers for Medicare and Medicaid Services, and other sources deemed reliable. Inclusion does not constitute endorsement and there is no implication associated with omission. Please verify current prices before ordering.

Alzheimer's: The Tangled Brain

An online feature produced by the University of Wisconsin at Madison. Available at http://www.whyfiles.org/117alzheimer

And Thou Shalt Honor: The Caregiver's Companion

Published by Rodale Books. 2002. 443 p. Available from Rodale Books. 400 South Tenth Street, Emmaus, PA 18098-0099. 800-848-4735; 610-967-8964; FAX: 610-967-8964. Website: www.rodalestore.com. PRICE: $15.95 and ISBN for paperback: 1579547745; ISBN for hardback: 1579545580.

Autopsy: A Lasting Gift for Your Family

Published by the Alzheimer's Association. 1996. 1 page (8 panels). Available from the Alzheimer's Association. 919 North Michigan Avenue, Suite 1000, Chicago, IL 60611-1676. 800-272-3900; 312-335-8700; TDD: 312-335-8882; FAX 312-335-1110. E-mail: info@alz.org. Website: www.alz.org. PRICE: Free print copy. Order Number: PF209Z.

Care Giving, Changing Needs

Produced by the American Association of Retired Persons (AARP). Available by calling 800-424-3410.

Caregiver's Handbook: A Guide to Caring for the Ill, Elderly, Disabled...and Yourself

Published by Harvard Medical School. 2004. 45 p. Available from Harvard Health Publications, P.O. Box 421073, Palm Coast, FL 32142-1073. Website: www.health.harvard.edu. PRICE: $16.00 for print or electronic versions.

Death in Slow Motion: A Memoir of a Daughter, Her Mother, and the Beast Called Alzheimer's

By Eleanor Cooney. Published by HarperCollins. 2004. 272 p. Available in bookstores and libraries. ISBN: 9780060937973

Family Guide to Alzheimer's Disease. Volume 5: Transitions

Produced by LifeView Resources, Inc. 2004. (videocassette, guidebook, 10 p.) Available from LifeView Resources, Inc., P.O. Box 290787, Nashville, TN 37229-0787. 800-395-5433. Website: www.lifeviewresources.com. PRICE: $24.95, or $99.95 for 5-volume set.

Getting Your Affairs in Order

An "Age Page" publication produced by the National Institute on Aging. June 2004. 1 p. (12 panels). Available from the National Institute on Aging Information Center (NIAIC). P.O. Box 8057, Gaithersburg, MD 20898-8057. 800-222-2225; TDD: 800-222-4225. Website: www .niapublications.org/agepages/affairs.asp . PRICE: Free print copies and free online access.

Honest Answers for the Recently Diagnosed Alzheimer Patient

Published by the American Health Assistance Foundation, 22512 Gateway Center Drive, Clarksburg, MD 20871. 43-page booklet. May be ordered online at http://www.ahaf.org or by calling 800-437-2426. PRICE: $2.00 (minimum order $5.00).

Hospice Care and the Medicare Hospice Benefit

Produced by the National Hospice Foundation. Available online at http://www.hospiceinfo.org

Hospice Care: A Consumer's Guide to Selecting a Hospice Program

Produced by the National Hospice Foundation. Available online at http://www.hospiceinfo.org

How to Care for Aging Parents, 2nd ed.

Published by Workman Publishing Company, Inc. 2004. 691 p. Available from the Workman Publishing Company, Inc. 708 Broadway, New York, NY 10003-9555. 212-254-5900; FAX: 212-254-8098. E-mail: info @workman.com. Website: www.workman.com. PRICE: $15.95 and ISBN: 1563054353 for paperback; $18.95 and ISBN: 0761134263 for book.

How To Select a Special Care Unit: A Consumer's Guide to Special Care Units For Persons With Dementia

Published by Kansas Department on Aging. 2002. 13 p. Available from Kansas Department on Aging, 503 South Kansas Avenue, Topeka, KS 66603-3404. 800-432-3535; 785-296-4986. Website: www.agingkansas .org/kdoa/publications/requestform.htm. PRICE: Single copy free.

Inside the Brain: An Interactive Tour

Produced by the Alzheimer's Association. Available online at http:// www.alz.org/alzheimers_disease_4719.asp

Learning to Speak Alzheimer's

By Joanne Koenig Coste and Robert N. Butler. Published by Houghton Mifflin. 2004. 256 p. Available in bookstores and libraries. ISBN: 9780618485178.

Living With Grief: Alzheimer's Disease

Published by Hospice Foundation of America. 2004. 290 p. Available from the Hospice Foundation of America, 1621 Connecticut Avenue, Suite 300, N.W., Washington, DC 20009. 202-638-5419; FAX: 202-638-5312. E-mail: info@hospicefoundation.org. Website: www.hospicefoundation .org. PRICE: $24.95 plus shipping fee. ISBN: 1893349055.

Losing my Mind: An Intimate Look at Life with Alzheimer's

By Thomas DeBaggio. Published by Simon and Schuster. 2003. 224 p. Available in bookstores and libraries. ISBN: 9780743205665.

Medicare Basics

Produced by Centers for Medicare and Medicaid Services; available on-line: http:// http://www.medicare.gov/publications/pubs/pdf/11034.pdf or by calling 800-MEDICARE (800-633-4227). TTY users should call 877-486-2048.

Medicare Coverage of Skilled Nursing Facility Care

CMS Pub. No. 10153
Produced by Centers for Medicare and Medicaid Services. Available on-line: http:// http://www.medicare.gov/publications/pubs/pdf/11034.pdf or by calling 800-MEDICARE (800-633-4227). TTY users should call 877-486-2048.

Medicare Hospice Benefits

CMS Pub. No. 02154
Produced by Centers for Medicare and Medicaid Services. Available on-line: http:// http://www.medicare.gov/publications/pubs/pdf/11034.pdf or by calling 800-MEDICARE (800-633-4227). TTY users should call 877-486-2048.

Palliative Care: Complete Care Everyone Deserves

Published by the National Alliance for Caregiving. 2003. 14 p. Available from the National Alliance for Caregiving. 4720 Montgomery Lane, Bethesda, MD 20814. 301-718-8444. E-mail: info@caregiving.org. Website: www.caregiving.org. PRICE: free online access and free print format for 1 to 10 copies; over 10 copies, pay postage.

Rush Manual for Caregivers, 6th ed.

Published by Rush Alzheimer's Disease Center. 2004. 116 p. Available from the Rush Alzheimer's Disease Center, Rush Presbyterian-St. Luke's Medical Center. 710 South Paulina Street, Suite 8 North, Chicago, IL 60612-3872. (312) 942-4463. E-mail: info@alz.org. Website: www.

rush.edu/rumc/page-R12399.html or www.rush.edu/Rush_Document/CaregiversManual.pdf. PRICE: $14.95 for printed version, and free online access.

Safety and the Older Driver
Published by the American Health Assistance Foundation, 22512 Gateway Center Drive, Clarksburg, MD 20871. Available for free online at http://www.ahaf.org/pubs/Safety_OlderDriver_ADR.pdf or by calling 800-437-2423.

Senior Legal Hotline Directory
Published by the Administration on Aging. Available online at http://www.aoa.gov/eldfam/Elder_Rights/Legal_Assistance/SRdirclient.pdf.

Shoppers Guide to Long-Term Care Insurance
Produced by the National Association of Insurance Commissioners. Available by calling 816-783-8500.

Steps to Caring for a Person with Late-Stage Alzheimer's Disease: Responding to the Individual's Increasing Needs
Published by the Alzheimer's Association. 2000. 15 p. Available from Alzheimer's Association. 225 North Michigan Avenue, Suite 1700, Chicago, IL 60601. 800-272-3900. FAX: 312-335-1110. PRICE: Single copy free, $10 for 50 copies. E-mail: info@alz.org. Website: www.alz.org. Item number: ED486Z.

Ten Legal and Financial Issues Everyone Should Consider
An article from *Reflections: Indiana Alzheimer Disease Center Newsletter.* 9(1): 7-9. Winter 2002-2003. Available from the Indiana Alzheimer Disease Center, Indiana University School of Medicine, 541 Clinical Drive, Suite CL 590, Indianapolis, IN 46202-5111. 317-274-4939. Website: http://iadc.iupui.edu/htm/newsletter.htm. PRICE: free.

There's Still a Person in There: The Complete Guide to Treating and Coping with Alzheimer's
By Michael Castleman, and others. Published by Penguin. 2000. 384 p. Available in bookstores and libraries. ISBN 9780399526350.

Understanding Alzheimer's Disease
Published by the American Health Assistance Foundation, 22512 Gateway Center Drive, Clarksburg, MD 20871. Available for free online at http://www.ahaf.org/pubs/UnderstandingAlzheimersNEW.pdf or by calling 800-437-2423.

Your Guide to Choosing a Nursing Home
CMS Pub. No. 02174
Produced by Centers for Medicare and Medicaid Services. Available online: http:// http://www.medicare.gov/publications/pubs/pdf/11034 .pdf or by calling 800-MEDICARE (800-633-4227). TTY users should call 877-486-2048.

Index

Index

Page numbers followed by 'n' indicate a footnote. Page numbers in *italics* indicate a table or illustration.

A

AAA *see* Area Agency on Aging
AAFP *see* American Academy of Family Physicians
AARP *see* American Association of Retired Persons
ABA *see* American Bar Association
Abeta-derived diffusible ligands (ADDL)
  described 30–31
  plaque formation 37
ACCORD *see* Action to Control Cardiovascular Risk in Diabetes
acetylcholine
  defined 535
  dementia treatment 117–18
Action to Control Cardiovascular Risk in Diabetes (ACCORD) 71
ACTIVE *see* Advanced Cognitive Training for Independent and Vital Elderly
"Activities at Home: Planning the Day for the Person with Dementia" (Alzheimer's Association) 369n

activities of daily living
  caregivers 309, 311–14
  coping strategies 388–91
  hospitalizations 422–23
  long-term care insurance 287
activity planning, overview 369–75
"Acute Hospitalization and Alzheimer's Disease: A Special Kind of Care" (North Carolina Department of Health and Human Services) 411n
ADAPT *see* Alzheimer's Disease Anti-Inflammatory Prevention Trial
ADC *see* AIDS dementia complex; Alzheimer Disease Centers
"AD Clinical Trials: Questions and Answers" (NIA) 447n
ADCS *see* Alzheimer's Disease Cooperative Study
ADDF *see* Alzheimer's Drug Discovery Foundation
ADDL *see* Abeta-derived diffusible ligands
ADEAR *see* Alzheimer's Disease Education and Referral Center
AD Genetics Study 6–7, 277

579

DeArmond, Stephen 175
dehydration, memory loss 238
Delaware
    Alzheimer disease death rates *18*
    Alzheimer disease statistics *13*
delirium
    causes 132
    versus dementia 129–36, *130*
    described 110
"Delirium (Sudden Confusion)"
    (American Geriatrics Society
    Foundation for Health in Aging)
    129n
delusions
    caregiving 315–16
    home safety 356–57
dementia
    Alzheimer disease 231
    caregivers 23–25
    causes 110–12
    coexisting medical conditions 16
    defined 538
    versus delirium 129–36, *130*
    described 3
    diagnosis 114–17
    overview 97–127
    patient care 121–23
    prevention 119–21
    research 44–45, 123–27, 483–84
    risk factors 112–14
    see also AIDS dementia complex;
        Alzheimer disease; Binswanger
        disease; frontotemporal
        dementia; Gerstmann-
        Straussler-Scheinker disease;
        HIV-associated dementia;
        Huntington disease; Lewy body
        dementia; mild cognitive
        impairment; multi-infarct
        dementia; Parkinson dementia;
        Pick disease; post-traumatic
        dementia; primary dementia;
        primary progressive aphasia;
        progressive dementia; secondary
        dementia; subcortical dementia;
        substance-induced persisting
        dementia; vascular dementia
"Dementia and Its Implications for
    Public Health" (Chapman) 141n

"Dementia: Hope through Research"
    (NINDS) 97n, 535n
dementia pugilistica, defined 538
dementia-related behaviors, coping
    strategies 381–92
dementia with Lewy bodies 149
dendrites
    defined 538
    described 27–28
dentate gyrus, described 33–34
deoxyribonucleic acid (DNA)
    defined 538
    described 27–28
depression
    aging process 228–29
    Alzheimer disease 365–67
    caregivers 338
    described 110
    memory loss 239
"Depression and Alzheimer's
    Disease" (AAFP) 365n
"Diabetes Linked to Increased
    Risk of Alzheimer's in Long-Term
    Study" (NIA) 489n
diabetes mellitus
    Alzheimer disease research
        56–58, 70–71, 486
    dementia risk factor 113
"Diagnosing Lewy Body
    Dementia" (Lewy Body
    Dementia Association) 149n
diazepam 167
diet and nutrition
    aging process 226–27
    Alzheimer disease 263–65
    Alzheimer disease research
        52–54
    cognitive function 92–93
    coping strategies 389–90
    memory loss 236
    Parkinson disease 199–200
diffuse Lewy body disease 149
directive to physicians, defined 302
District of Columbia (Washington,
    DC)
    Alzheimer disease death rates *18*
    Alzheimer disease statistics *13*
divalproex sodium, clinical trial 87
DNA *see* deoxyribonucleic acid

Health Reference Series
COMPLETE CATALOG
List price $87 per volume. **School and library price $78 per volume.**

Adolescent Health Sourcebook, 2nd Edition

Basic Consumer Health Information about the Physical, Mental, and Emotional Growth and Development of Adolescents, Including Medical Care, Nutritional and Physical Activity Requirements, Puberty, Sexual Activity, Acne, Tanning, Body Piercing, Common Physical Illnesses and Disorders, Eating Disorders, Attention Deficit Hyperactivity Disorder, Depression, Bullying, Hazing, and Adolescent Injuries Related to Sports, Driving, and Work

Along with Substance Abuse Information about Nicotine, Alcohol, and Drug Use, a Glossary, and Directory of Additional Resources

Edited by Joyce Brennfleck Shannon. 683 pages. 2006. 978-0-7808-0943-7.

"It is written in clear, nontechnical language aimed at general readers. . . . Recommended for public libraries, community colleges, and other agencies serving health care consumers."
— *American Reference Books Annual, 2003*

"Recommended for school and public libraries. Parents and professionals dealing with teens will appreciate the easy-to-follow format and the clearly written text. This could become a 'must have' for every high school teacher." — *E-Streams, Jan '03*

"A good starting point for information related to common medical, mental, and emotional concerns of adolescents." — *School Library Journal, Nov '02*

"This book provides accurate information in an easy to access format. It addresses topics that parents and caregivers might not be aware of and provides practical, useable information."
— *Doody's Health Sciences Book Review Journal, Sep-Oct '02*

"Recommended reference source."
— *Booklist, American Library Association, Sep '02*

AIDS Sourcebook, 3rd Edition

Basic Consumer Health Information about Acquired Immune Deficiency Syndrome (AIDS) and Human Immunodeficiency Virus (HIV) Infection, Including Facts about Transmission, Prevention, Diagnosis, Treatment, Opportunistic Infections, and Other Complications, with a Section for Women and Children, Including Details about Associated Gynecological Concerns, Pregnancy, and Pediatric Care

Along with Updated Statistical Information, Reports on Current Research Initiatives, a Glossary, and Directories of Internet, Hotline, and Other Resources

Edited by Dawn D. Matthews. 664 pages. 2003. 978-0-7808-0631-3.

"The 3rd edition of the *AIDS Sourcebook*, part of Omnigraphics' *Health Reference Series*, is a welcome update. . . . This resource is highly recommended for academic and public libraries."
— *American Reference Books Annual, 2004*

"Excellent sourcebook. This continues to be a highly recommended book. There is no other book that provides as much information as this book provides."
— *AIDS Book Review Journal, Dec-Jan '00*

"Recommended reference source."
— *Booklist, American Library Association, Dec '99*

Alcoholism Sourcebook, 2nd Edition

Basic Consumer Health Information about Alcohol Use, Abuse, and Dependence, Featuring Facts about the Physical, Mental, and Social Health Effects of Alcohol Addiction, Including Alcoholic Liver Disease, Pancreatic Disease, Cardiovascular Disease, Neurological Disorders, and the Effects of Drinking during Pregnancy

Along with Information about Alcohol Treatment, Medications, and Recovery Programs, in Addition to Tips for Reducing the Prevalence of Underage Drinking, Statistics about Alcohol Use, a Glossary of Related Terms, and Directories of Resources for More Help and Information

Edited by Amy L. Sutton. 653 pages. 2006. 978-0-7808-0942-0.

"This title is one of the few reference works on alcoholism for general readers. For some readers this will be a welcome complement to the many self-help books on the market. Recommended for collections serving general readers and consumer health collections."
— *E-Streams, Mar '01*

"This book is an excellent choice for public and academic libraries."
— *American Reference Books Annual, 2001*

"Recommended reference source."
— *Booklist, American Library Association, Dec '00*

"Presents a wealth of information on alcohol use and abuse and its effects on the body and mind, treatment, and prevention." — *SciTech Book News, Dec '00*

"Important new health guide which packs in the latest consumer information about the problems of alcoholism." — *Reviewer's Bookwatch, Nov '00*

SEE ALSO Drug Abuse Sourcebook

Allergies Sourcebook, 3rd Edition

Basic Consumer Health Information about Allergic Disorders, Such as Anaphylaxis, Hives, Eczema, Rhinitis, Sinusitis, and Conjunctivitis, and Their Triggers, Including Pollen, Mold, Dust Mites, Animal Dander, Insects, Chemicals, Food, Food Additives, and Medications;

Along with Advice about the Diagnosis and Treatment of Allergy Symptoms, a Glossary of Related Terms, a Directory of Resources for Help and Information, and Suggestions for Additional Reading

Edited by Amy L. Sutton. 598 pages. 2007. 978-0-7808-0950-5.

"This book brings a great deal of useful material together. . . . This is an excellent addition to public and consumer health library collections."
— *American Reference Books Annual, 2003*

"This second edition would be useful to laypersons with little or advanced knowledge of the subject matter. This book would also serve as a resource for nursing and other health care professions students. It would be useful in public, academic, and hospital libraries with consumer health collections."
— *E-Streams, Jul '02*

■

Alternative Medicine Sourcebook

SEE Complementary & Alternative Medicine Sourcebook

■

Alzheimer's Disease Sourcebook, 3rd Edition

Basic Consumer Health Information about Alzheimer's Disease, Other Dementias, and Related Disorders, Including Multi-Infarct Dementia, AIDS Dementia Complex, Dementia with Lewy Bodies, Huntington's Disease, Wernicke-Korsakoff Syndrome (Alcohol-Related Dementia), Delirium, and Confusional States

Along with Information for People Newly Diagnosed with Alzheimer's Disease and Caregivers, Reports Detailing Current Research Efforts in Prevention, Diagnosis, and Treatment, Facts about Long-Term Care Issues, and Listings of Sources for Additional Information

Edited by Karen Bellenir. 645 pages. 2003. 978-0-7808-0666-5.

"This very informative and valuable tool will be a great addition to any library serving consumers, students and health care workers."
— *American Reference Books Annual, 2004*

"This is a valuable resource for people affected by dementias such as Alzheimer's. It is easy to navigate and includes important information and resources."
— *Doody's Review Service, Feb '04*

"Recommended reference source."
— *Booklist, American Library Association, Oct '99*

***SEE ALSO** Brain Disorders Sourcebook*

Arthritis Sourcebook, 2nd Edition

Basic Consumer Health Information about Osteoarthritis, Rheumatoid Arthritis, Other Rheumatic Disorders, Infectious Forms of Arthritis, and Diseases with Symptoms Linked to Arthritis, Featuring Facts about Diagnosis, Pain Management, and Surgical Therapies

Along with Coping Strategies, Research Updates, a Glossary, and Resources for Additional Help and Information

Edited by Amy L. Sutton. 593 pages. 2004. 978-0-7808-0667-2.

"This easy-to-read volume is recommended for consumer health collections within public or academic libraries."
— *E-Streams, May '05*

"As expected, this updated edition continues the excellent reputation of this series in providing sound, usable health information. . . . Highly recommended."
— *American Reference Books Annual, 2005*

"Excellent reference." — *The Bookwatch, Jan '05*

■

Asthma Sourcebook, 2nd Edition

Basic Consumer Health Information about the Causes, Symptoms, Diagnosis, and Treatment of Asthma in Infants, Children, Teenagers, and Adults, Including Facts about Different Types of Asthma, Common Co-Occurring Conditions, Asthma Management Plans, Triggers, Medications, and Medication Delivery Devices

Along with Asthma Statistics, Research Updates, a Glossary, a Directory of Asthma-Related Resources, and More

Edited by Karen Bellenir. 609 pages. 2006. 978-0-7808-0866-9.

"A worthwhile reference acquisition for public libraries and academic medical libraries whose readers desire a quick introduction to the wide range of asthma information."
— *Choice, Association of College & Research Libraries, Jun '01*

"Recommended reference source."
— *Booklist, American Library Association, Feb '01*

"Highly recommended." — *The Bookwatch, Jan '01*

"There is much good information for patients and their families who deal with asthma daily."
— *American Medical Writers Association Journal, Winter '01*

"This informative text is recommended for consumer health collections in public, secondary school, and community college libraries and the libraries of universities with a large undergraduate population."
— *American Reference Books Annual, 2001*

■

Attention Deficit Disorder Sourcebook

Basic Consumer Health Information about Attention Deficit/Hyperactivity Disorder in Children and Adults,

Including Facts about Causes, Symptoms, Diagnostic Criteria, and Treatment Options Such as Medications, Behavior Therapy, Coaching, and Homeopathy

Along with Reports on Current Research Initiatives, Legal Issues, and Government Regulations, and Featuring a Glossary of Related Terms, Internet Resources, and a List of Additional Reading Material

Edited by Dawn D. Matthews. 470 pages. 2002. 978-0-7808-0624-5.

"Recommended reference source."
— Booklist, American Library Association, Jan '03

"This book is recommended for all school libraries and the reference or consumer health sections of public libraries." — American Reference Books Annual, 2003

■

Back & Neck Sourcebook, 2nd Edition

Basic Consumer Health Information about Spinal Pain, Spinal Cord Injuries, and Related Disorders, Such as Degenerative Disk Disease, Osteoarthritis, Scoliosis, Sciatica, Spina Bifida, and Spinal Stenosis, and Featuring Facts about Maintaining Spinal Health, Self-Care, Pain Management, Rehabilitative Care, Chiropractic Care, Spinal Surgeries, and Complementary Therapies

Along with Suggestions for Preventing Back and Neck Pain, a Glossary of Related Terms, and a Directory of Resources

Edited by Amy L. Sutton. 633 pages. 2004. 978-0-7808-0738-9.

"Recommended . . . an easy to use, comprehensive medical reference book." — E-Streams, Sep '05

"The strength of this work is its basic, easy-to-read format. Recommended." — Reference and User Services Quarterly, American Library Association, Winter '97

■

Blood & Circulatory Disorders Sourcebook, 2nd Edition

Basic Consumer Health Information about the Blood and Circulatory System and Related Disorders, Such as Anemia and Other Hemoglobin Diseases, Cancer of the Blood and Associated Bone Marrow Disorders, Clotting and Bleeding Problems, and Conditions That Affect the Veins, Blood Vessels, and Arteries, Including Facts about the Donation and Transplantation of Bone Marrow, Stem Cells, and Blood and Tips for Keeping the Blood and Circulatory System Healthy

Along with a Glossary of Related Terms and Resources for Additional Help and Information

Edited by Amy L. Sutton. 659 pages. 2005. 978-0-7808-0746-4.

"Highly recommended pick for basic consumer health reference holdings at all levels."
— The Bookwatch, Aug '05

"Recommended reference source."
— Booklist, American Library Association, Feb '99

"An important reference sourcebook written in simple language for everyday, non-technical users."
— Reviewer's Bookwatch, Jan '99

■

Brain Disorders Sourcebook, 2nd Edition

Basic Consumer Health Information about Acquired and Traumatic Brain Injuries, Infections of the Brain, Epilepsy and Seizure Disorders, Cerebral Palsy, and Degenerative Neurological Disorders, Including Amyotrophic Lateral Sclerosis (ALS), Dementias, Multiple Sclerosis, and More

Along with Information on the Brain's Structure and Function, Treatment and Rehabilitation Options, Reports on Current Research Initiatives, a Glossary of Terms Related to Brain Disorders and Injuries, and a Directory of Sources for Further Help and Information

Edited by Sandra J. Judd. 625 pages. 2005. 978-0-7808-0744-0.

"Highly recommended pick for basic consumer health reference holdings at all levels."
— The Bookwatch, Aug '05

"Belongs on the shelves of any library with a consumer health collection." — E-Streams, Mar '00

"Recommended reference source."
— Booklist, American Library Association, Oct '99

SEE ALSO Alzheimer's Disease Sourcebook

■

Breast Cancer Sourcebook, 2nd Edition

Basic Consumer Health Information about Breast Cancer, Including Facts about Risk Factors, Prevention, Screening and Diagnostic Methods, Treatment Options, Complementary and Alternative Therapies, Post-Treatment Concerns, Clinical Trials, Special Risk Populations, and New Developments in Breast Cancer Research

Along with Breast Cancer Statistics, a Glossary of Related Terms, and a Directory of Resources for Additional Help and Information

Edited by Sandra J. Judd. 595 pages. 2004. 978-0-7808-0668-9.

"This book will be an excellent addition to public, community college, medical, and academic libraries."
— American Reference Books Annual, 2006

"It would be a useful reference book in a library or on loan to women in a support group."
— Cancer Forum, Mar '03

"Recommended reference source."
— Booklist, American Library Association, Jan '02

"This reference source is highly recommended. It is quite informative, comprehensive and detailed in nature, and yet it offers practical advice in easy-to-read language. It could be thought of as the 'bible' of breast cancer for the consumer."   — *E-Streams, Jan '02*

"From the pros and cons of different screening methods and results to treatment options, *Breast Cancer Sourcebook* provides the latest information on the subject."
— *Library Bookwatch, Dec '01*

"This thoroughgoing, very readable reference covers all aspects of breast health and cancer. . . . Readers will find much to consider here. Recommended for all public and patient health collections."
— *Library Journal, Sep '01*

SEE ALSO *Cancer Sourcebook for Women, Women's Health Concerns Sourcebook*

▪

Breastfeeding Sourcebook

Basic Consumer Health Information about the Benefits of Breastmilk, Preparing to Breastfeed, Breastfeeding as a Baby Grows, Nutrition, and More, Including Information on Special Situations and Concerns Such as Mastitis, Illness, Medications, Allergies, Multiple Births, Prematurity, Special Needs, and Adoption

Along with a Glossary and Resources for Additional Help and Information

Edited by Jenni Lynn Colson. 388 pages. 2002. 978-0-7808-0332-9.

"Particularly useful is the information about professional lactation services and chapters on breastfeeding when returning to work. . . . *Breastfeeding Sourcebook* will be useful for public libraries, consumer health libraries, and technical schools offering nurse assistant training, especially in areas where Internet access is problematic."
— *American Reference Books Annual, 2003*

SEE ALSO *Pregnancy & Birth Sourcebook*

▪

Burns Sourcebook

Basic Consumer Health Information about Various Types of Burns and Scalds, Including Flame, Heat, Cold, Electrical, Chemical, and Sun Burns

Along with Information on Short-Term and Long-Term Treatments, Tissue Reconstruction, Plastic Surgery, Prevention Suggestions, and First Aid

Edited by Allan R. Cook. 604 pages. 1999. 978-0-7808-0204-9.

"This is an exceptional addition to the series and is highly recommended for all consumer health collections, hospital libraries, and academic medical centers."
— *E-Streams, Mar '00*

"This key reference guide is an invaluable addition to all health care and public libraries in confronting this ongoing health issue."
— *American Reference Books Annual, 2000*

"Recommended reference source."
— *Booklist, American Library Association, Dec '99*

SEE ALSO *Dermatological Disorders Sourcebook*

Cancer Sourcebook, 5th Edition

Basic Consumer Health Information about Major Forms and Stages of Cancer, Featuring Facts about Head and Neck Cancers, Lung Cancers, Gastrointestinal Cancers, Genitourinary Cancers, Lymphomas, Blood Cell Cancers, Endocrine Cancers, Skin Cancers, Bone Cancers, Metastatic Cancers, and More

Along with Facts about Cancer Treatments, Cancer Risks and Prevention, a Glossary of Related Terms, Statistical Data, and a Directory of Resources for Additional Information

Edited by Karen Bellenir. 1,133 pages. 2007. 978-0-7808-0947-5.

"With cancer being the second leading cause of death for Americans, a prodigious work such as this one, which locates centrally so much cancer-related information, is clearly an asset to this nation's citizens and others."
— *Journal of the National Medical Association, 2004*

"This title is recommended for health sciences and public libraries with consumer health collections."
— *E-Streams, Feb '01*

". . . can be effectively used by cancer patients and their families who are looking for answers in a language they can understand. Public and hospital libraries should have it on their shelves."
— *American Reference Books Annual, 2001*

"Recommended reference source."
— *Booklist, American Library Association, Dec '00*

SEE ALSO *Breast Cancer Sourcebook, Cancer Sourcebook for Women, Pediatric Cancer Sourcebook, Prostate Cancer Sourcebook*

▪

Cancer Sourcebook for Women, 3rd Edition

Basic Consumer Health Information about Leading Causes of Cancer in Women, Featuring Facts about Gynecologic Cancers and Related Concerns, Such as Breast Cancer, Cervical Cancer, Endometrial Cancer, Uterine Sarcoma, Vaginal Cancer, Vulvar Cancer, and Common Non-Cancerous Gynecologic Conditions, in Addition to Facts about Lung Cancer, Colorectal Cancer, and Thyroid Cancer in Women

Along with Information about Cancer Risk Factors, Screening and Prevention, Treatment Options, and Tips on Coping with Life after Cancer Treatment, a Glossary of Cancer Terms, and a Directory of Resources for Additional Help and Information

Edited by Amy L. Sutton. 715 pages. 2006. 978-0-7808-0867-6.

"An excellent addition to collections in public, consumer health, and women's health libraries."
— *American Reference Books Annual, 2003*

"Overall, the information is excellent, and complex topics are clearly explained. As a reference book for the consumer it is a valuable resource to assist them to make informed decisions about cancer and its treatments."
— *Cancer Forum, Nov '02*

"Highly recommended for academic and medical reference collections." — *Library Bookwatch, Sep '02*

"This is a highly recommended book for any public or consumer library, being reader friendly and containing accurate and helpful information."
— *E-Streams, Aug '02*

"Recommended reference source."
—*Booklist, American Library Association, Jul '02*

SEE ALSO *Breast Cancer Sourcebook, Women's Health Concerns Sourcebook*

Cancer Survivorship Sourcebook

Basic Consumer Health Information about the Physical, Educational, Emotional, Social, and Financial Needs of Cancer Patients from Diagnosis, through Cancer Treatment, and Beyond, Including Facts about Researching Specific Types of Cancer and Learning about Clinical Trials and Treatment Options, and Featuring Tips for Coping with the Side Effects of Cancer Treatments and Adjusting to Life after Cancer Treatment Concludes

Along with Suggestions for Caregivers, Friends, and Family Members of Cancer Patients, a Glossary of Cancer Care Terms, and Directories of Related Resources

Edited by Karen Bellenir. 6561 pages. 2007. 978-0-7808-0985-7.

Cardiovascular Diseases & Disorders Sourcebook, 3rd Edition

Basic Consumer Health Information about Heart and Vascular Diseases and Disorders, Such as Angina, Heart Attacks, Arrhythmias, Cardiomyopathy, Valve Disease, Atherosclerosis, and Aneurysms, with Information about Managing Cardiovascular Risk Factors and Maintaining Heart Health, Medications and Procedures Used to Treat Cardiovascular Disorders, and Concerns of Special Significance to Women

Along with Reports on Current Research Initiatives, a Glossary of Related Medical Terms, and a Directory of Sources for Further Help and Information

Edited by Sandra J. Judd. 713 pages. 2005. 978-0-7808-0739-6.

"This updated sourcebook is still the best first stop for comprehensive introductory information on cardiovascular diseases."
— *American Reference Books Annual, 2006*

"Recommended for public libraries and libraries supporting health care professionals."
— *E-Streams, Sep '05*

"This should be a standard health library reference."
—*The Bookwatch, Jun '05*

"Recommended reference source."
—*Booklist, American Library Association, Dec '00*

"... comprehensive format provides an extensive overview on this subject."
—*Choice, Association of College & Research Libraries*

Caregiving Sourcebook

Basic Consumer Health Information for Caregivers, Including a Profile of Caregivers, Caregiving Responsibilities and Concerns, Tips for Specific Conditions, Care Environments, and the Effects of Caregiving

Along with Facts about Legal Issues, Financial Information, and Future Planning, a Glossary, and a Listing of Additional Resources

Edited by Joyce Brennfleck Shannon. 600 pages. 2001. 978-0-7808-0331-2.

"Essential for most collections."
— *Library Journal, Apr 1, 2002*

"An ideal addition to the reference collection of any public library. Health sciences information professionals may also want to acquire the *Caregiving Sourcebook* for their hospital or academic library for use as a ready reference tool by health care workers interested in aging and caregiving." —*E-Streams, Jan '02*

"Recommended reference source."
—*Booklist, American Library Association, Oct '01*

Child Abuse Sourcebook

Basic Consumer Health Information about the Physical, Sexual, and Emotional Abuse of Children, with Additional Facts about Neglect, Munchausen Syndrome by Proxy (MSBP), Shaken Baby Syndrome, and Controversial Issues Related to Child Abuse, Such as Withholding Medical Care, Corporal Punishment, and Child Maltreatment in Youth Sports, and Featuring Facts about Child Protective Services, Foster Care, Adoption, Parenting Challenges, and Other Abuse Prevention Efforts

Along with a Glossary of Related Terms and Resources for Additional Help and Information

Edited by Dawn D. Matthews. 620 pages. 2004. 978-0-7808-0705-1.

"A valuable and highly recommended resource for school, academic and public libraries whether used on its own or as a starting point for more in-depth research."
— *E-Streams, Apr '05*

"Every week the news brings cases of child abuse or neglect, so it is useful to have a source that supplies so much helpful information. . . . Recommended. Public and academic libraries, and child welfare offices."
— *Choice, Association of College & Research Libraries, Mar '05*

"Packed with insights on all kinds of issues, from foster care and adoption to parenting and abuse prevention."
—*The Bookwatch, Nov '04*

SEE ALSO: *Domestic Violence Sourcebook*

Childhood Diseases & Disorders Sourcebook

Basic Consumer Health Information about Medical Problems Often Encountered in Pre-Adolescent Children, Including Respiratory Tract Ailments, Ear Infections, Sore Throats, Disorders of the Skin and Scalp, Digestive and Genitourinary Diseases, Infectious Diseases, Inflammatory Disorders, Chronic Physical and Developmental Disorders, Allergies, and More

Along with Information about Diagnostic Tests, Common Childhood Surgeries, and Frequently Used Medications, with a Glossary of Important Terms and Resource Directory

Edited by Chad T. Kimball. 662 pages. 2003. 978-0-7808-0458-6.

"This is an excellent book for new parents and should be included in all health care and public libraries."
—*American Reference Books Annual, 2004*

SEE ALSO: Healthy Children Sourcebook

Colds, Flu & Other Common Ailments Sourcebook

Basic Consumer Health Information about Common Ailments and Injuries, Including Colds, Coughs, the Flu, Sinus Problems, Headaches, Fever, Nausea and Vomiting, Menstrual Cramps, Diarrhea, Constipation, Hemorrhoids, Back Pain, Dandruff, Dry and Itchy Skin, Cuts, Scrapes, Sprains, Bruises, and More

Along with Information about Prevention, Self-Care, Choosing a Doctor, Over-the-Counter Medications, Folk Remedies, and Alternative Therapies, and Including a Glossary of Important Terms and a Directory of Resources for Further Help and Information

Edited by Chad T. Kimball. 638 pages. 2001. 978-0-7808-0435-7.

"A good starting point for research on common illnesses. It will be a useful addition to public and consumer health library collections."
—*American Reference Books Annual, 2002*

"Will prove valuable to any library seeking to maintain a current, comprehensive reference collection of health resources. . . . Excellent reference."
—*The Bookwatch, Aug '01*

"Recommended reference source."
—*Booklist, American Library Association, Jul '01*

Communication Disorders Sourcebook

Basic Information about Deafness and Hearing Loss, Speech and Language Disorders, Voice Disorders, Balance and Vestibular Disorders, and Disorders of Smell, Taste, and Touch

Edited by Linda M. Ross. 533 pages. 1996. 978-0-7808-0077-9.

"This is skillfully edited and is a welcome resource for the layperson. It should be found in every public and medical library." —*Booklist Health Sciences Supplement, American Library Association, Oct '97*

Complementary & Alternative Medicine Sourcebook, 3rd Edition

Basic Consumer Health Information about Complementary and Alternative Medical Therapies, Including Acupuncture, Ayurveda, Traditional Chinese Medicine, Herbal Medicine, Homeopathy, Naturopathy, Biofeedback, Hypnotherapy, Yoga, Art Therapy, Aromatherapy, Clinical Nutrition, Vitamin and Mineral Supplements, Chiropractic, Massage, Reflexology, Crystal Therapy, Therapeutic Touch, and More

Along with Facts about Alternative and Complementary Treatments for Specific Conditions Such as Cancer, Diabetes, Osteoarthritis, Chronic Pain, Menopause, Gastrointestinal Disorders, Headaches, and Mental Illness, a Glossary, and a Resource List for Additional Help and Information

Edited by Sandra J. Judd. 657 pages. 2006. 978-0-7808-0864-5.

"Recommended for public, high school, and academic libraries that have consumer health collections. Hospital libraries that also serve the public will find this to be a useful resource." —*E-Streams, Feb '03*

"Recommended reference source."
—*Booklist, American Library Association, Jan '03*

"An important alternate health reference."
—*MBR Bookwatch, Oct '02*

"A great addition to the reference collection of every type of library." —*American Reference Books Annual, 2000*

Congenital Disorders Sourcebook, 2nd Edition

Basic Consumer Health Information about Non-hereditary Birth Defects and Disorders Related to Prematurity, Gestational Injuries, Congenital Infections, and Birth Complications, Including Heart Defects, Hydrocephalus, Spina Bifida, Cleft Lip and Palate, Cerebral Palsy, and More

Along with Facts about the Prevention of Birth Defects, Fetal Surgery and Other Treatment Options, Research Initiatives, a Glossary of Related Terms, and Resources for Additional Information and Support

Edited by Sandra J. Judd. 647 pages. 2006. 978-0-7808-0945-1.

"Recommended reference source."
—*Booklist, American Library Association, Oct '97*

SEE ALSO Pregnancy & Birth Sourcebook

Contagious Diseases Sourcebook

Basic Consumer Health Information about Infectious Diseases Spread by Person-to-Person Contact through

Direct Touch, Airborne Transmission, Sexual Contact, or Contact with Blood or Other Body Fluids, Including Hepatitis, Herpes, Influenza, Lice, Measles, Mumps, Pinworm, Ringworm, Severe Acute Respiratory Syndrome (SARS), Streptococcal Infections, Tuberculosis, and Others

Along with Facts about Disease Transmission, Antimicrobial Resistance, and Vaccines, with a Glossary and Directories of Resources for More Information

Edited by Karen Bellenir. 643 pages. 2004. 978-0-7808-0736-5.

"This easy-to-read volume is recommended for consumer health collections within public or academic libraries." — E-Streams, May '05

"This informative book is highly recommended for public libraries, consumer health collections, and secondary schools and undergraduate libraries." — American Reference Books Annual, 2005

"Excellent reference." — The Bookwatch, Jan '05

Death & Dying Sourcebook, 2nd Edition

Basic Consumer Health Information about End-of-Life Care and Related Perspectives and Ethical Issues, Including End-of-Life Symptoms and Treatments, Pain Management, Quality-of-Life Concerns, the Use of Life Support, Patients' Rights and Privacy Issues, Advance Directives, Physician-Assisted Suicide, Caregiving, Organ and Tissue Donation, Autopsies, Funeral Arrangements, and Grief

Along with Statistical Data, Information about the Leading Causes of Death, a Glossary, and Directories of Support Groups and Other Resources

Edited by Joyce Brennfleck Shannon. 653 pages. 2006. 978-0-7808-0871-3.

"Public libraries, medical libraries, and academic libraries will all find this sourcebook a useful addition to their collections." — American Reference Books Annual, 2001

"An extremely useful resource for those concerned with death and dying in the United States." — Respiratory Care, Nov '00

"Recommended reference source." — Booklist, American Library Association, Aug '00

"This book is a definite must for all those involved in end-of-life care." — Doody's Review Service, 2000

Dental Care & Oral Health Sourcebook, 2nd Edition

Basic Consumer Health Information about Dental Care, Including Oral Hygiene, Dental Visits, Pain Management, Cavities, Crowns, Bridges, Dental Implants, and Fillings, and Other Oral Health Concerns, Such as Gum Disease, Bad Breath, Dry Mouth, Genetic and Developmental Abnormalities, Oral Cancers, Orthodontics, and Temporomandibular Disorders

Along with Updates on Current Research in Oral Health, a Glossary, a Directory of Dental and Oral Health Organizations, and Resources for People with Dental and Oral Health Disorders

Edited by Amy L. Sutton. 609 pages. 2003. 978-0-7808-0634-4.

"This book could serve as a turning point in the battle to educate consumers in issues concerning oral health." — American Reference Books Annual, 2004

"Unique source which will fill a gap in dental sources for patients and the lay public. A valuable reference tool even in a library with thousands of books on dentistry. Comprehensive, clear, inexpensive, and easy to read and use. It fills an enormous gap in the health care literature." — Reference & User Services Quarterly, American Library Association, Summer '98

"Recommended reference source." — Booklist, American Library Association, Dec '97

Depression Sourcebook

Basic Consumer Health Information about Unipolar Depression, Bipolar Disorder, Postpartum Depression, Seasonal Affective Disorder, and Other Types of Depression in Children, Adolescents, Women, Men, the Elderly, and Other Selected Populations

Along with Facts about Causes, Risk Factors, Diagnostic Criteria, Treatment Options, Coping Strategies, Suicide Prevention, a Glossary, and a Directory of Sources for Additional Help and Information

Edited by Karen Bellenir. 602 pages. 2002. 978-0-7808-0611-5.

"Depression Sourcebook is of a very high standard. Its purpose, which is to serve as a reference source to the lay reader, is very well served." — Journal of the National Medical Association, 2004

"Invaluable reference for public and school library collections alike." — Library Bookwatch, Apr '03

"Recommended for purchase." — American Reference Books Annual, 2003

Dermatological Disorders Sourcebook, 2nd Edition

Basic Consumer Health Information about Conditions and Disorders Affecting the Skin, Hair, and Nails, Such as Acne, Rosacea, Rashes, Dermatitis, Pigmentation Disorders, Birthmarks, Skin Cancer, Skin Injuries, Psoriasis, Scleroderma, and Hair Loss, Including Facts about Medications and Treatments for Dermatological Disorders and Tips for Maintaining Healthy Skin, Hair, and Nails

Along with Information about How Aging Affects the Skin, a Glossary of Related Terms, and a Directory of Resources for Additional Help and Information

Edited by Amy L. Sutton. 645 pages. 2005. 978-0-7808-0795-2.

"... comprehensive, easily read reference book."
—*Doody's Health Sciences Book Reviews, Oct '97*

SEE ALSO *Burns Sourcebook*

Diabetes Sourcebook, 3rd Edition

Basic Consumer Health Information about Type 1 Diabetes (Insulin-Dependent or Juvenile-Onset Diabetes), Type 2 Diabetes (Noninsulin-Dependent or Adult-Onset Diabetes), Gestational Diabetes, Impaired Glucose Tolerance (IGT), and Related Complications, Such as Amputation, Eye Disease, Gum Disease, Nerve Damage, and End-Stage Renal Disease, Including Facts about Insulin, Oral Diabetes Medications, Blood Sugar Testing, and the Role of Exercise and Nutrition in the Control of Diabetes

Along with a Glossary and Resources for Further Help and Information

Edited by Dawn D. Matthews. 622 pages. 2003. 978-0-7808-0629-0.

"This edition is even more helpful than earlier versions. . . . It is a truly valuable tool for anyone seeking readable and authoritative information on diabetes."
— *American Reference Books Annual, 2004*

"An invaluable reference." — *Library Journal, May '00*

Selected as one of the 250 "Best Health Sciences Books of 1999." — *Doody's Rating Service, Mar-Apr '00*

"Provides useful information for the general public."
— *Healthlines, University of Michigan Health Management Research Center, Sep/Oct '99*

". . . provides reliable mainstream medical information . . . belongs on the shelves of any library with a consumer health collection." — *E-Streams, Sep '99*

"Recommended reference source."
— *Booklist, American Library Association, Feb '99*

Diet & Nutrition Sourcebook, 3rd Edition

Basic Consumer Health Information about Dietary Guidelines and the Food Guidance System, Recommended Daily Nutrient Intakes, Serving Proportions, Weight Control, Vitamins and Supplements, Nutrition Issues for Different Life Stages and Lifestyles, and the Needs of People with Specific Medical Concerns, Including Cancer, Celiac Disease, Diabetes, Eating Disorders, Food Allergies, and Cardiovascular Disease

Along with Facts about Federal Nutrition Support Programs, a Glossary of Nutrition and Dietary Terms, and Directories of Additional Resources for More Information about Nutrition

Edited by Joyce Brennfleck Shannon. 633 pages. 2006. 978-0-7808-0800-3.

"This book is an excellent source of basic diet and nutrition information." — *Booklist Health Sciences Supplement, American Library Association, Dec '00*

"This reference document should be in any public library, but it would be a very good guide for beginning students in the health sciences. If the other books in this publisher's series are as good as this, they should all be in the health sciences collections."
— *American Reference Books Annual, 2000*

"This book is an excellent general nutrition reference for consumers who desire to take an active role in their health care for prevention. Consumers of all ages who select this book can feel confident they are receiving current and accurate information." — *Journal of Nutrition for the Elderly, Vol. 19, No. 4, 2000*

SEE ALSO *Digestive Diseases & Disorders Sourcebook, Eating Disorders Sourcebook, Gastrointestinal Diseases & Disorders Sourcebook, Vegetarian Sourcebook*

Digestive Diseases & Disorders Sourcebook

Basic Consumer Health Information about Diseases and Disorders that Impact the Upper and Lower Digestive System, Including Celiac Disease, Constipation, Crohn's Disease, Cyclic Vomiting Syndrome, Diarrhea, Diverticulosis and Diverticulitis, Gallstones, Heartburn, Hemorrhoids, Hernias, Indigestion (Dyspepsia), Irritable Bowel Syndrome, Lactose Intolerance, Ulcers, and More

Along with Information about Medications and Other Treatments, Tips for Maintaining a Healthy Digestive Tract, a Glossary, and Directory of Digestive Diseases Organizations

Edited by Karen Bellenir. 335 pages. 2000. 978-0-7808-0327-5.

"This title would be an excellent addition to all public or patient-research libraries."
— *American Reference Books Annual, 2001*

"This title is recommended for public, hospital, and health sciences libraries with consumer health collections." — *E-Streams, Jul-Aug '00*

"Recommended reference source."
— *Booklist, American Library Association, May '00*

SEE ALSO *Eating Disorders Sourcebook, Gastrointestinal Diseases & Disorders Sourcebook*

Disabilities Sourcebook

Basic Consumer Health Information about Physical and Psychiatric Disabilities, Including Descriptions of Major Causes of Disability, Assistive and Adaptive Aids, Workplace Issues, and Accessibility Concerns

Along with Information about the Americans with Disabilities Act, a Glossary, and Resources for Additional Help and Information

Edited by Dawn D. Matthews. 616 pages. 2000. 978-0-7808-0389-3.

"It is a must for libraries with a consumer health section." — *American Reference Books Annual, 2002*

"A much needed addition to the Omnigraphics *Health Reference Series*. A current reference work to provide people with disabilities, their families, caregivers or those who work with them, a broad range of information in one volume, has not been available until now. . . . It is recommended for all public and academic library reference collections."   — *E-Streams, May '01*

"An excellent source book in easy-to-read format covering many current topics; highly recommended for all libraries."   — *Choice, Association of College & Research Libraries, Jan '01*

"Recommended reference source."
    — *Booklist, American Library Association, Jul '00*

■

Domestic Violence Sourcebook, 2nd Edition

Basic Consumer Health Information about the Causes and Consequences of Abusive Relationships, Including Physical Violence, Sexual Assault, Battery, Stalking, and Emotional Abuse, and Facts about the Effects of Violence on Women, Men, Young Adults, and the Elderly, with Reports about Domestic Violence in Selected Populations, and Featuring Facts about Medical Care, Victim Assistance and Protection, Prevention Strategies, Mental Health Services, and Legal Issues

Along with a Glossary of Related Terms and Resources for Additional Help and Information

Edited by Dawn D. Matthews. 628 pages. 2004. 978-0-7808-0669-6.

"Educators, clergy, medical professionals, police, and victims and their families will benefit from this realistic and easy-to-understand resource."
    — *American Reference Books Annual, 2005*

"Recommended for all collections supporting consumer health information. It should also be considered for any collection needing general, readable information on domestic violence."   — *E-Streams, Jan '05*

"This sourcebook complements other books in its field, providing a one-stop resource . . . Recommended."
    — *Choice, Association of College & Research Libraries, Jan '05*

"Interested lay persons should find the book extremely beneficial. . . . A copy of *Domestic Violence and Child Abuse Sourcebook* should be in every public library in the United States."
    — *Social Science & Medicine, No. 56, 2003*

"This is important information. The Web has many resources but this sourcebook fills an important societal need. I am not aware of any other resources of this type."   — *Doody's Review Service, Sep '01*

"Recommended reference source."
    — *Booklist, American Library Association, Apr '01*

"Important pick for college-level health reference libraries."   — *The Bookwatch, Mar '01*

"Because this problem is so widespread and because this book includes a lot of issues within one volume, this work is recommended for all public libraries."
    — *American Reference Books Annual, 2001*

SEE ALSO *Child Abuse Sourcebook*

■

Drug Abuse Sourcebook, 2nd Edition

Basic Consumer Health Information about Illicit Substances of Abuse and the Misuse of Prescription and Over-the-Counter Medications, Including Depressants, Hallucinogens, Inhalants, Marijuana, Stimulants, and Anabolic Steroids

Along with Facts about Related Health Risks, Treatment Programs, Prevention Programs, a Glossary of Abuse and Addiction Terms, a Glossary of Drug-Related Street Terms, and a Directory of Resources for More Information

Edited by Catherine Ginther. 607 pages. 2004. 978-0-7808-0740-2.

"Commendable for organizing useful, normally scattered government and association-produced data into a logical sequence."
    — *American Reference Books Annual, 2006*

"This easy-to-read volume is recommended for consumer health collections within public or academic libraries."   — *E-Streams, Sep '05*

"An excellent library reference."
    — *The Bookwatch, May '05*

"Containing a wealth of information, this book will be useful to the college student just beginning to explore the topic of substance abuse. This resource belongs in libraries that serve a lower-division undergraduate or community college clientele as well as the general public."   — *Choice, Association of College & Research Libraries, Jun '01*

"Recommended reference source."
    — *Booklist, American Library Association, Feb '01*

SEE ALSO *Alcoholism Sourcebook*

■

Ear, Nose & Throat Disorders Sourcebook, 2nd Edition

Basic Consumer Health Information about Disorders of the Ears, Hearing Loss, Vestibular Disorders, Nasal and Sinus Problems, Throat and Vocal Cord Disorders, and Otolaryngologic Cancers, Including Facts about Ear Infections and Injuries, Genetic and Congenital Deafness, Sensorineural Hearing Disorders, Tinnitus, Vertigo, Ménière Disease, Rhinitis, Sinusitis, Snoring, Sore Throats, Hoarseness, and More

Along with Reports on Current Research Initiatives, a Glossary of Related Medical Terms, and a Directory of Sources for Further Help and Information

Edited by Sandra J. Judd. 659 pages. 2006. 978-0-7808-0872-0.

"Overall, this sourcebook is helpful for the consumer seeking information on ENT issues. It is recommended for public libraries."
—*American Reference Books Annual, 1999*

"Recommended reference source."
—*Booklist, American Library Association, Dec '98*

Eating Disorders Sourcebook, 2nd Edition

Basic Consumer Health Information about Anorexia Nervosa, Bulimia Nervosa, Binge Eating, Compulsive Exercise, Female Athlete Triad, and Other Eating Disorders, Including Facts about Body Image and Other Cultural and Age-Related Risk Factors, Prevention Efforts, Adverse Health Effects, Treatment Options, and the Recovery Process

Along with Guidelines for Healthy Weight Control, a Glossary, and Directories of Additional Resources

Edited by Joyce Brennfleck Shannon. 585 pages. 2007. 978-0-7808-0948-2.

"Recommended for health science libraries that are open to the public, as well as hospital libraries. This book is a good resource for the consumer who is concerned about eating disorders." —*E-Streams, Mar '02*

"This volume is another convenient collection of excerpted articles. Recommended for school and public library patrons; lower-division undergraduates; and two-year technical program students."
—*Choice, Association of College & Research Libraries, Jan '02*

"Recommended reference source."
—*Booklist, American Library Association, Oct '01*

SEE ALSO *Diet & Nutrition Sourcebook, Digestive Diseases & Disorders Sourcebook, Gastrointestinal Diseases & Disorders Sourcebook*

Emergency Medical Services Sourcebook

Basic Consumer Health Information about Preventing, Preparing for, and Managing Emergency Situations, When and Who to Call for Help, What to Expect in the Emergency Room, the Emergency Medical Team, Patient Issues, and Current Topics in Emergency Medicine

Along with Statistical Data, a Glossary, and Sources of Additional Help and Information

Edited by Jenni Lynn Colson. 494 pages. 2002. 978-0-7808-0420-3.

"Handy and convenient for home, public, school, and college libraries. Recommended."
—*Choice, Association of College & Research Libraries, Apr '03*

"This reference can provide the consumer with answers to most questions about emergency care in the United States, or it will direct them to a resource where the answer can be found."
—*American Reference Books Annual, 2003*

"Recommended reference source."
—*Booklist, American Library Association, Feb '03*

Endocrine & Metabolic Disorders Sourcebook

Basic Information for the Layperson about Pancreatic and Insulin-Related Disorders Such as Pancreatitis, Diabetes, and Hypoglycemia; Adrenal Gland Disorders Such as Cushing's Syndrome, Addison's Disease, and Congenital Adrenal Hyperplasia; Pituitary Gland Disorders Such as Growth Hormone Deficiency, Acromegaly, and Pituitary Tumors; Thyroid Disorders Such as Hypothyroidism, Graves' Disease, Hashimoto's Disease, and Goiter; Hyperparathyroidism; and Other Diseases and Syndromes of Hormone Imbalance or Metabolic Dysfunction

Along with Reports on Current Research Initiatives

Edited by Linda M. Shin. 574 pages. 1998. 978-0-7808-0207-0.

"Omnigraphics has produced another needed resource for health information consumers."
—*American Reference Books Annual, 2000*

"Recommended reference source."
—*Booklist, American Library Association, Dec '98*

Environmental Health Sourcebook, 2nd Edition

Basic Consumer Health Information about the Environment and Its Effect on Human Health, Including the Effects of Air Pollution, Water Pollution, Hazardous Chemicals, Food Hazards, Radiation Hazards, Biological Agents, Household Hazards, Such as Radon, Asbestos, Carbon Monoxide, and Mold, and Information about Associated Diseases and Disorders, Including Cancer, Allergies, Respiratory Problems, and Skin Disorders

Along with Information about Environmental Concerns for Specific Populations, a Glossary of Related Terms, and Resources for Further Help and Information

Edited by Dawn D. Matthews. 673 pages. 2003. 978-0-7808-0632-0.

"This recently updated edition continues the level of quality and the reputation of the numerous other volumes in Omnigraphics' *Health Reference Series.*"
—*American Reference Books Annual, 2004*

"An excellent updated edition."
—*The Bookwatch, Oct '03*

"Recommended reference source."
—*Booklist, American Library Association, Sep '98*

"This book will be a useful addition to anyone's library." —*Choice Health Sciences Supplement, Association of College & Research Libraries, May '98*

". . . a good survey of numerous environmentally induced physical disorders . . . a useful addition to anyone's library."
—*Doody's Health Sciences Book Reviews, Jan '98*

Ethnic Diseases Sourcebook

Basic Consumer Health Information for Ethnic and Racial Minority Groups in the United States, Including General Health Indicators and Behaviors, Ethnic Diseases, Genetic Testing, the Impact of Chronic Diseases, Women's Health, Mental Health Issues, and Preventive Health Care Services

Along with a Glossary and a Listing of Additional Resources

Edited by Joyce Brennfleck Shannon. 664 pages. 2001. 978-0-7808-0336-7.

"Recommended for health sciences libraries where public health programs are a priority."
— *E-Streams, Jan '02*

"Not many books have been written on this topic to date, and the *Ethnic Diseases Sourcebook* is a strong addition to the list. It will be an important introductory resource for health consumers, students, health care personnel, and social scientists. It is recommended for public, academic, and large hospital libraries."
— *American Reference Books Annual, 2002*

"Recommended reference source."
— *Booklist, American Library Association, Oct '01*

"Will prove valuable to any library seeking to maintain a current, comprehensive reference collection of health resources. . . . An excellent source of health information about genetic disorders which affect particular ethnic and racial minorities in the U.S."
— *The Bookwatch, Aug '01*

Eye Care Sourcebook, 2nd Edition

Basic Consumer Health Information about Eye Care and Eye Disorders, Including Facts about the Diagnosis, Prevention, and Treatment of Common Refractive Problems Such as Myopia, Hyperopia, Astigmatism, and Presbyopia, and Eye Diseases, Including Glaucoma, Cataract, Age-Related Macular Degeneration, and Diabetic Retinopathy

Along with a Section on Vision Correction and Refractive Surgeries, Including LASIK and LASEK, a Glossary, and Directories of Resources for Additional Help and Information

Edited by Amy L. Sutton. 543 pages. 2003. 978-0-7808-0635-1.

". . . a solid reference tool for eye care and a valuable addition to a collection."
— *American Reference Books Annual, 2004*

Family Planning Sourcebook

Basic Consumer Health Information about Planning for Pregnancy and Contraception, Including Traditional Methods, Barrier Methods, Hormonal Methods, Permanent Methods, Future Methods, Emergency Contraception, and Birth Control Choices for Women at Each Stage of Life

Along with Statistics, a Glossary, and Sources of Additional Information

Edited by Amy Marcaccio Keyzer. 520 pages. 2001. 978-0-7808-0379-4.

"Recommended for public, health, and undergraduate libraries as part of the circulating collection."
— *E-Streams, Mar '02*

"Information is presented in an unbiased, readable manner, and the sourcebook will certainly be a necessary addition to those public and high school libraries where Internet access is restricted or otherwise problematic." — *American Reference Books Annual, 2002*

"Recommended reference source."
— *Booklist, American Library Association, Oct '01*

"Will prove valuable to any library seeking to maintain a current, comprehensive reference collection of health resources. . . . Excellent reference."
— *The Bookwatch, Aug '01*

SEE ALSO Pregnancy & Birth Sourcebook

Fitness & Exercise Sourcebook, 3rd Edition

Basic Consumer Health Information about the Physical and Mental Benefits of Fitness, Including Cardiorespiratory Endurance, Muscular Strength, Muscular Endurance, and Flexibility, with Facts about Sports Nutrition and Exercise-Related Injuries and Tips about Physical Activity and Exercises for People of All Ages and for People with Health Concerns

Along with Advice on Selecting and Using Exercise Equipment, Maintaining Exercise Motivation, a Glossary of Related Terms, and a Directory of Resources for More Help and Information

Edited by Amy L. Sutton. 663 pages. 2007. 978-0-7808-0946-8.

"This work is recommended for all general reference collections."
— *American Reference Books Annual, 2002*

"Highly recommended for public, consumer, and school grades fourth through college." — *E-Streams, Nov '01*

"Recommended reference source."
— *Booklist, American Library Association, Oct '01*

"The information appears quite comprehensive and is considered reliable. . . . This second edition is a welcomed addition to the series."
— *Doody's Review Service, Sep '01*

Food Safety Sourcebook

Basic Consumer Health Information about the Safe Handling of Meat, Poultry, Seafood, Eggs, Fruit Juices, and Other Food Items, and Facts about Pesticides, Drinking Water, Food Safety Overseas, and the Onset, Duration, and Symptoms of Foodborne Illnesses, Including Types of Pathogenic Bacteria, Parasitic Protozoa, Worms, Viruses, and Natural Toxins

Along with the Role of the Consumer, the Food Handler, and the Government in Food Safety; a Glossary, and Resources for Additional Help and Information

Edited by Dawn D. Matthews. 339 pages. 1999. 978-0-7808-0326-8.

"This book is recommended for public libraries and universities with home economic and food science programs." — *E-Streams, Nov '00*

"Recommended reference source." — *Booklist, American Library Association, May '00*

"This book takes the complex issues of food safety and foodborne pathogens and presents them in an easily understood manner. [It does] an excellent job of covering a large and often confusing topic." — *American Reference Books Annual, 2000*

Forensic Medicine Sourcebook

Basic Consumer Information for the Layperson about Forensic Medicine, Including Crime Scene Investigation, Evidence Collection and Analysis, Expert Testimony, Computer-Aided Criminal Identification, Digital Imaging in the Courtroom, DNA Profiling, Accident Reconstruction, Autopsies, Ballistics, Drugs and Explosives Detection, Latent Fingerprints, Product Tampering, and Questioned Document Examination

Along with Statistical Data, a Glossary of Forensics Terminology, and Listings of Sources for Further Help and Information

Edited by Annemarie S. Muth. 574 pages. 1999. 978-0-7808-0232-2.

"Given the expected widespread interest in its content and its easy to read style, this book is recommended for most public and all college and university libraries." — *E-Streams, Feb '01*

"Recommended for public libraries." — *Reference & User Services Quarterly, American Library Association, Spring 2000*

"Recommended reference source." — *Booklist, American Library Association, Feb '00*

"A wealth of information, useful statistics, references are up-to-date and extremely complete. This wonderful collection of data will help students who are interested in a career in any type of forensic field. It is a great resource for attorneys who need information about types of expert witnesses needed in a particular case. It also offers useful information for fiction and nonfiction writers whose work involves a crime. A fascinating compilation. All levels." — *Choice, Association of College & Research Libraries, Jan '00*

"There are several items that make this book attractive to consumers who are seeking certain forensic data. . . . This is a useful current source for those seeking general forensic medical answers." — *American Reference Books Annual, 2000*

Gastrointestinal Diseases & Disorders Sourcebook, 2nd Edition

Basic Consumer Health Information about the Upper and Lower Gastrointestinal (GI) Tract, Including the Esophagus, Stomach, Intestines, Rectum, Liver, and Pancreas, with Facts about Gastroesophageal Reflux Disease, Gastritis, Hernias, Ulcers, Celiac Disease, Diverticulitis, Irritable Bowel Syndrome, Hemorrhoids, Gastrointestinal Cancers, and Other Diseases and Disorders Related to the Digestive Process

Along with Information about Commonly Used Diagnostic and Surgical Procedures, Statistics, Reports on Current Research Initiatives and Clinical Trials, a Glossary, and Resources for Additional Help and Information

Edited by Sandra J. Judd. 681 pages. 2006. 978-0-7808-0798-3.

". . . very readable form. The successful editorial work that brought this material together into a useful and understandable reference makes accessible to all readers information that can help them more effectively understand and obtain help for digestive tract problems." — *Choice, Association of College & Research Libraries, Feb '97*

SEE ALSO *Diet & Nutrition Sourcebook, Digestive Diseases & Disorders Sourcebook, Eating Disorders Sourcebook*

Genetic Disorders Sourcebook, 3rd Edition

Basic Consumer Health Information about Hereditary Diseases and Disorders, Including Facts about the Human Genome, Genetic Inheritance Patterns, Disorders Associated with Specific Genes, Such as Sickle Cell Disease, Hemophilia, and Cystic Fibrosis, Chromosome Disorders, Such as Down Syndrome, Fragile X Syndrome, and Turner Syndrome, and Complex Diseases and Disorders Resulting from the Interaction of Environmental and Genetic Factors, Such as Allergies, Cancer, and Obesity

Along with Facts about Genetic Testing, Suggestions for Parents of Children with Special Needs, Reports on Current Research Initiatives, a Glossary of Genetic Terminology, and Resources for Additional Help and Information

Edited by Karen Bellenir. 777 pages. 2004. 978-0-7808-0742-6.

"This text is recommended for any library with an interest in providing consumer health resources." — *E-Streams, Aug '05*

"This is a valuable resource for anyone wishing to have an understandable description of any of the topics or disorders included. The editor succeeds in making complex genetic issues understandable." — *Doody's Book Review Service, May '05*

"A good acquisition for public libraries." — *American Reference Books Annual, 2005*

Head Trauma Sourcebook

Basic Information for the Layperson about Open-Head and Closed-Head Injuries, Treatment Advances, Recovery, and Rehabilitation

Along with Reports on Current Research Initiatives

Edited by Karen Bellenir. 414 pages. 1997. 978-0-7808-0208-7.

Headache Sourcebook

Basic Consumer Health Information about Migraine, Tension, Cluster, Rebound and Other Types of Headaches, with Facts about the Cause and Prevention of Headaches, the Effects of Stress and the Environment, Headaches during Pregnancy and Menopause, and Childhood Headaches

Along with a Glossary and Other Resources for Additional Help and Information

Edited by Dawn D. Matthews. 362 pages. 2002. 978-0-7808-0337-4.

Healthy Aging Sourcebook

Basic Consumer Health Information about Maintaining Health through the Aging Process, Including Advice on Nutrition, Exercise, and Sleep, Help in Making Decisions about Midlife Issues and Retirement, and Guidance Concerning Practical and Informed Choices in Health Consumerism

Along with Data Concerning the Theories of Aging, Different Experiences in Aging by Minority Groups, and Facts about Aging Now and Aging in the Future; and Featuring a Glossary, a Guide to Consumer Help, Additional Suggested Reading, and Practical Resource Directory

Edited by Jenifer Swanson. 536 pages. 1999. 978-0-7808-0390-9.

SEE ALSO *Physical & Mental Issues in Aging Sourcebook*

Healthy Children Sourcebook

Basic Consumer Health Information about the Physical and Mental Development of Children between the Ages of 3 and 12, Including Routine Health Care, Preventative Health Services, Safety and First Aid,

Healthy Sleep, Dental Care, Nutrition, and Fitness, and Featuring Parenting Tips on Such Topics as Bedwetting, Choosing Day Care, Monitoring TV and Other Media, and Establishing a Foundation for Substance Abuse Prevention

Along with a Glossary of Commonly Used Pediatric Terms and Resources for Additional Help and Information

Edited by Chad T. Kimball. 647 pages. 2003. 978-0-7808-0247-6.

SEE ALSO *Childhood Diseases & Disorders Sourcebook*

Healthy Heart Sourcebook for Women

Basic Consumer Health Information about Cardiac Issues Specific to Women, Including Facts about Major Risk Factors and Prevention, Treatment and Control Strategies, and Important Dietary Issues

Along with a Special Section Regarding the Pros and Cons of Hormone Replacement Therapy and Its Impact on Heart Health, and Additional Help, Including Recipes, a Glossary, and a Directory of Resources

Edited by Dawn D. Matthews. 336 pages. 2000. 978-0-7808-0329-9.

SEE ALSO *Cardiovascular Diseases & Disorders Sourcebook, Women's Health Concerns Sourcebook*

Hepatitis Sourcebook

Basic Consumer Health Information about Hepatitis A, Hepatitis B, Hepatitis C, and Other Forms of Hepatitis, Including Autoimmune Hepatitis, Alcoholic Hepatitis, Nonalcoholic Steatohepatitis, and Toxic Hepatitis, with

Facts about Risk Factors, Screening Methods, Diagnostic Tests, and Treatment Options

Along with Information on Liver Health, Tips for People Living with Chronic Hepatitis, Reports on Current Research Initiatives, a Glossary of Terms Related to Hepatitis, and a Directory of Sources for Further Help and Information

Edited by Sandra J. Judd. 597 pages. 2005. 978-0-7808-0749-5.

"Highly recommended."
— American Reference Books Annual, 2006

∎

Household Safety Sourcebook

Basic Consumer Health Information about Household Safety, Including Information about Poisons, Chemicals, Fire, and Water Hazards in the Home

Along with Advice about the Safe Use of Home Maintenance Equipment, Choosing Toys and Nursery Furniture, Holiday and Recreation Safety, a Glossary, and Resources for Further Help and Information

Edited by Dawn D. Matthews. 606 pages. 2002. 978-0-7808-0338-1.

"This work will be useful in public libraries with large consumer health and wellness departments."
— American Reference Books Annual, 2003

"As a sourcebook on household safety this book meets its mark. It is encyclopedic in scope and covers a wide range of safety issues that are commonly seen in the home." — E-Streams, Jul '02

∎

Hypertension Sourcebook

Basic Consumer Health Information about the Causes, Diagnosis, and Treatment of High Blood Pressure, with Facts about Consequences, Complications, and Co-Occurring Disorders, Such as Coronary Heart Disease, Diabetes, Stroke, Kidney Disease, and Hypertensive Retinopathy, and Issues in Blood Pressure Control, Including Dietary Choices, Stress Management, and Medications

Along with Reports on Current Research Initiatives and Clinical Trials, a Glossary, and Resources for Additional Help and Information

Edited by Dawn D. Matthews and Karen Bellenir. 613 pages. 2004. 978-0-7808-0674-0.

"Academic, public, and medical libraries will want to add the Hypertension Sourcebook to their collections."
— E-Streams, Aug '05

"The strength of this source is the wide range of information given about hypertension."
— American Reference Books Annual, 2005

∎

Immune System Disorders Sourcebook, 2nd Edition

Basic Consumer Health Information about Disorders of the Immune System, Including Immune System Function and Response, Diagnosis of Immune Disorders, Information about Inherited Immune Disease, Acquired Immune Disease, and Autoimmune Diseases, Including Primary Immune Deficiency, Acquired Immunodeficiency Syndrome (AIDS), Lupus, Multiple Sclerosis, Type 1 Diabetes, Rheumatoid Arthritis, and Graves' Disease

Along with Treatments, Tips for Coping with Immune Disorders, a Glossary, and a Directory of Additional Resources.

Edited by Joyce Brennfleck Shannon. 671 pages. 2005. 978-0-7808-0748-8.

"Highly recommended for academic and public libraries." — American Reference Books Annual, 2006

"The updated second edition is a 'must' for any consumer health library seeking a solid resource covering the treatments, symptoms, and options for immune disorder sufferers. . . . An excellent guide."
— MBR Bookwatch, Jan '06

∎

Infant & Toddler Health Sourcebook

Basic Consumer Health Information about the Physical and Mental Development of Newborns, Infants, and Toddlers, Including Neonatal Concerns, Nutrition Recommendations, Immunization Schedules, Common Pediatric Disorders, Assessments and Milestones, Safety Tips, and Advice for Parents and Other Caregivers

Along with a Glossary of Terms and Resource Listings for Additional Help

Edited by Jenifer Swanson. 585 pages. 2000. 978-0-7808-0246-9.

"As a reference for the general public, this would be useful in any library." — E-Streams, May '01

"Recommended reference source."
— Booklist, American Library Association, Feb '01

"This is a good source for general use."
— American Reference Books Annual, 2001

∎

Infectious Diseases Sourcebook

Basic Consumer Health Information about Non-Contagious Bacterial, Viral, Prion, Fungal, and Parasitic Diseases Spread by Food and Water, Insects and Animals, or Environmental Contact, Including Botulism, E. Coli, Encephalitis, Legionnaires' Disease, Lyme Disease, Malaria, Plague, Rabies, Salmonella, Tetanus, and Others, and Facts about Newly Emerging Diseases, Such as Hantavirus, Mad Cow Disease, Monkeypox, and West Nile Virus

Along with Information about Preventing Disease Transmission, the Threat of Bioterrorism, and Current Research Initiatives, with a Glossary and Directory of Resources for More Information

Edited by Karen Bellenir. 634 pages. 2004. 978-0-7808-0675-7.

"This reference continues the excellent tradition of the *Health Reference Series* in consolidating a wealth of information on a selected topic into a format that is easy to use and accessible to the general public."
— *American Reference Books Annual, 2005*

"Recommended for public and academic libraries."
— *E-Streams, Jan '05*

Injury & Trauma Sourcebook

Basic Consumer Health Information about the Impact of Injury, the Diagnosis and Treatment of Common and Traumatic Injuries, Emergency Care, and Specific Injuries Related to Home, Community, Workplace, Transportation, and Recreation

Along with Guidelines for Injury Prevention, a Glossary, and a Directory of Additional Resources

Edited by Joyce Brennfleck Shannon. 696 pages. 2002. 978-0-7808-0421-0.

"This publication is the most comprehensive work of its kind about injury and trauma."
— *American Reference Books Annual, 2003*

"This sourcebook provides concise, easily readable, basic health information about injuries. . . . This book is well organized and an easy to use reference resource suitable for hospital, health sciences and public libraries with consumer health collections."
— *E-Streams, Nov '02*

"Practitioners should be aware of guides such as this in order to facilitate their use by patients and their families."
— *Doody's Health Sciences Book Review Journal, Sep-Oct '02*

"Recommended reference source."
— *Booklist, American Library Association, Sep '02*

"Highly recommended for academic and medical reference collections."
— *Library Bookwatch, Sep '02*

Kidney & Urinary Tract Diseases & Disorders Sourcebook

SEE *Urinary Tract & Kidney Diseases & Disorders Sourcebook*

Learning Disabilities Sourcebook, 2nd Edition

Basic Consumer Health Information about Learning Disabilities, Including Dyslexia, Developmental Speech and Language Disabilities, Non-Verbal Learning Disorders, Developmental Arithmetic Disorder, Developmental Writing Disorder, and Other Conditions That Impede Learning Such as Attention Deficit/Hyperactivity Disorder, Brain Injury, Hearing Impairment, Klinefelter Syndrome, Dyspraxia, and Tourette's Syndrome

Along with Facts about Educational Issues and Assistive Technology, Coping Strategies, a Glossary of Related Terms, and Resources for Further Help and Information

Edited by Dawn D. Matthews. 621 pages. 2003. 978-0-7808-0626-9.

"The second edition of Learning Disabilities Sourcebook far surpasses the earlier edition in that it is more focused on information that will be useful as a consumer health resource."
— *American Reference Books Annual, 2004*

"Teachers as well as consumers will find this an essential guide to understanding various syndromes and their latest treatments. [An] invaluable reference for public and school library collections alike."
— *Library Bookwatch, Apr '03*

Named "Outstanding Reference Book of 1999."
— *New York Public Library, Feb '00*

"An excellent candidate for inclusion in a public library reference section. It's a great source of information. Teachers will also find the book useful. Definitely worth reading."
— *Journal of Adolescent & Adult Literacy, Feb 2000*

"Readable . . . provides a solid base of information regarding successful techniques used with individuals who have learning disabilities, as well as practical suggestions for educators and family members. Clear language, concise descriptions, and pertinent information for contacting multiple resources add to the strength of this book as a useful tool."
— *Choice, Association of College & Research Libraries, Feb '99*

"Recommended reference source."
— *Booklist, American Library Association, Sep '98*

"A useful resource for libraries and for those who don't have the time to identify and locate the individual publications."
— *Disability Resources Monthly, Sep '98*

Leukemia Sourcebook

Basic Consumer Health Information about Adult and Childhood Leukemias, Including Acute Lymphocytic Leukemia (ALL), Chronic Lymphocytic Leukemia (CLL), Acute Myelogenous Leukemia (AML), Chronic Myelogenous Leukemia (CML), and Hairy Cell Leukemia, and Treatments Such as Chemotherapy, Radiation Therapy, Peripheral Blood Stem Cell and Marrow Transplantation, and Immunotherapy

Along with Tips for Life During and After Treatment, a Glossary, and Directories of Additional Resources

Edited by Joyce Brennfleck Shannon. 587 pages. 2003. 978-0-7808-0627-6.

"Unlike other medical books for the layperson, . . . the language does not talk down to the reader. . . . This volume is highly recommended for all libraries."
— *American Reference Books Annual, 2004*

". . . a fine title which ranges from diagnosis to alternative treatments, staging, and tips for life during and after diagnosis."
— *The Bookwatch, Dec '03*

Liver Disorders Sourcebook

Basic Consumer Health Information about the Liver and How It Works; Liver Diseases, Including Cancer, Cirrhosis, Hepatitis, and Toxic and Drug Related Diseases; Tips for Maintaining a Healthy Liver; Laboratory Tests, Radiology Tests, and Facts about Liver Transplantation

Along with a Section on Support Groups, a Glossary, and Resource Listings

Edited by Joyce Brennfleck Shannon. 591 pages. 2000. 978-0-7808-0383-1.

"A valuable resource."
—*American Reference Books Annual, 2001*

"This title is recommended for health sciences and public libraries with consumer health collections."
—*E-Streams, Oct '00*

"Recommended reference source."
—*Booklist, American Library Association, Jun '00*

■

Lung Disorders Sourcebook

Basic Consumer Health Information about Emphysema, Pneumonia, Tuberculosis, Asthma, Cystic Fibrosis, and Other Lung Disorders, Including Facts about Diagnostic Procedures, Treatment Strategies, Disease Prevention Efforts, and Such Risk Factors as Smoking, Air Pollution, and Exposure to Asbestos, Radon, and Other Agents

Along with a Glossary and Resources for Additional Help and Information

Edited by Dawn D. Matthews. 678 pages. 2002. 978-0-7808-0339-8.

"This title is a great addition for public and school libraries because it provides concise health information on the lungs."
—*American Reference Books Annual, 2003*

"Highly recommended for academic and medical reference collections." —*Library Bookwatch, Sep '02*

SEE ALSO *Respiratory Diseases & Disorders Sourcebook*

■

Medical Tests Sourcebook, 2nd Edition

Basic Consumer Health Information about Medical Tests, Including Age-Specific Health Tests, Important Health Screenings and Exams, Home-Use Tests, Blood and Specimen Tests, Electrical Tests, Scope Tests, Genetic Testing, and Imaging Tests, Such as X-Rays, Ultrasound, Computed Tomography, Magnetic Resonance Imaging, Angiography, and Nuclear Medicine

Along with a Glossary and Directory of Additional Resources

Edited by Joyce Brennfleck Shannon. 654 pages. 2004. 978-0-7808-0670-2.

"Recommended for hospital and health sciences libraries with consumer health collections."
—*E-Streams, Mar '00*

"This is an overall excellent reference with a wealth of general knowledge that may aid those who are reluctant to get vital tests performed."
—*Today's Librarian, Jan '00*

"A valuable reference guide."
—*American Reference Books Annual, 2000*

■

Men's Health Concerns Sourcebook, 2nd Edition

Basic Consumer Health Information about the Medical and Mental Concerns of Men, Including Theories about the Shorter Male Lifespan, the Leading Causes of Death and Disability, Physical Concerns of Special Significance to Men, Reproductive and Sexual Concerns, Sexually Transmitted Diseases, Men's Mental and Emotional Health, and Lifestyle Choices That Affect Wellness, Such as Nutrition, Fitness, and Substance Use

Along with a Glossary of Related Terms and a Directory of Organizational Resources in Men's Health

Edited by Robert Aquinas McNally. 644 pages. 2004. 978-0-7808-0671-9.

"A very accessible reference for non-specialist general readers and consumers." —*The Bookwatch, Jun '04*

"This comprehensive resource and the series are highly recommended."
—*American Reference Books Annual, 2000*

"Recommended reference source."
—*Booklist, American Library Association, Dec '98*

■

Mental Health Disorders Sourcebook, 3rd Edition

Basic Consumer Health Information about Mental and Emotional Health and Mental Illness, Including Facts about Depression, Bipolar Disorder, and Other Mood Disorders, Phobias, Post-Traumatic Stress Disorder (PTSD), Obsessive-Compulsive Disorder, and Other Anxiety Disorders, Impulse Control Disorders, Eating Disorders, Personality Disorders, and Psychotic Disorders, Including Schizophrenia and Dissociative Disorders

Along with Statistical Information, a Special Section Concerning Mental Health Issues in Children and Adolescents, a Glossary, and Directories of Resources for Additional Help and Information

Edited by Karen Bellenir. 661 pages. 2005. 978-0-7808-0747-1.

"Recommended for public libraries and academic libraries with an undergraduate program in psychology."
—*American Reference Books Annual, 2006*

"Recommended reference source."
—*Booklist, American Library Association, Jun '00*

Mental Retardation Sourcebook

Basic Consumer Health Information about Mental Retardation and Its Causes, Including Down Syndrome, Fetal Alcohol Syndrome, Fragile X Syndrome, Genetic Conditions, Injury, and Environmental Sources

Along with Preventive Strategies, Parenting Issues, Educational Implications, Health Care Needs, Employment and Economic Matters, Legal Issues, a Glossary, and a Resource Listing for Additional Help and Information

Edited by Joyce Brennfleck Shannon. 642 pages. 2000. 978-0-7808-0377-0.

"Public libraries will find the book useful for reference and as a beginning research point for students, parents, and caregivers."
— American Reference Books Annual, 2001

"The strength of this work is that it compiles many basic fact sheets and addresses for further information in one volume. It is intended and suitable for the general public. This sourcebook is relevant to any collection providing health information to the general public."
— E-Streams, Nov '00

"From preventing retardation to parenting and family challenges, this covers health, social and legal issues and will prove an invaluable overview."
— Reviewer's Bookwatch, Jul '00

■

Movement Disorders Sourcebook

Basic Consumer Health Information about Neurological Movement Disorders, Including Essential Tremor, Parkinson's Disease, Dystonia, Cerebral Palsy, Huntington's Disease, Myasthenia Gravis, Multiple Sclerosis, and Other Early-Onset and Adult-Onset Movement Disorders, Their Symptoms and Causes, Diagnostic Tests, and Treatments

Along with Mobility and Assistive Technology Information, a Glossary, and a Directory of Additional Resources

Edited by Joyce Brennfleck Shannon. 655 pages. 2003. 978-0-7808-0628-3.

". . . a good resource for consumers and recommended for public, community college and undergraduate libraries." *— American Reference Books Annual, 2004*

■

Muscular Dystrophy Sourcebook

Basic Consumer Health Information about Congenital, Childhood-Onset, and Adult-Onset Forms of Muscular Dystrophy, Such as Duchenne, Becker, Emery-Dreifuss, Distal, Limb-Girdle, Facioscapulohumeral (FSHD), Myotonic, and Ophthalmoplegic Muscular Dystrophies, Including Facts about Diagnostic Tests, Medical and Physical Therapies, Management of Co-Occurring Conditions, and Parenting Guidelines

Along with Practical Tips for Home Care, a Glossary, and Directories of Additional Resources

Edited by Joyce Brennfleck Shannon. 577 pages. 2004. 978-0-7808-0676-4.

"This book is highly recommended for public and academic libraries as well as health care offices that support the information needs of patients and their families."
— E-Streams, Apr '05

"Excellent reference." *— The Bookwatch, Jan '05*

■

Obesity Sourcebook

Basic Consumer Health Information about Diseases and Other Problems Associated with Obesity, and Including Facts about Risk Factors, Prevention Issues, and Management Approaches

Along with Statistical and Demographic Data, Information about Special Populations, Research Updates, a Glossary, and Source Listings for Further Help and Information

Edited by Wilma Caldwell and Chad T. Kimball. 376 pages. 2001. 978-0-7808-0333-6.

"The book synthesizes the reliable medical literature on obesity into one easy-to-read and useful resource for the general public."
— American Reference Books Annual, 2002

"This is a very useful resource book for the lay public."
— Doody's Review Service, Nov '01

"Well suited for the health reference collection of a public library or an academic health science library that serves the general population." *— E-Streams, Sep '01*

"Recommended reference source."
— Booklist, American Library Association, Apr '01

"Recommended pick both for specialty health library collections and any general consumer health reference collection." *— The Bookwatch, Apr '01*

■

Oral Health Sourcebook

SEE *Dental Care & Oral Health Sourcebook*

■

Osteoporosis Sourcebook

Basic Consumer Health Information about Primary and Secondary Osteoporosis and Juvenile Osteoporosis and Related Conditions, Including Fibrous Dysplasia, Gaucher Disease, Hyperthyroidism, Hypophosphatasia, Myeloma, Osteopetrosis, Osteogenesis Imperfecta, and Paget's Disease

Along with Information about Risk Factors, Treatments, Traditional and Non-Traditional Pain Management, a Glossary of Related Terms, and a Directory of Resources

Edited by Allan R. Cook. 584 pages. 2001. 978-0-7808-0239-1.

"This would be a book to be kept in a staff or patient library. The targeted audience is the layperson, but the therapist who needs a quick bit of information on a particular topic will also find the book useful."
— Physical Therapy, Jan '02

"This resource is recommended as a great reference source for public, health, and academic libraries, and is another triumph for the editors of Omnigraphics."
— *American Reference Books Annual, 2002*

"Recommended for all public libraries and general health collections, especially those supporting patient education or consumer health programs."
— *E-Streams, Nov '01*

"Will prove valuable to any library seeking to maintain a current, comprehensive reference collection of health resources. . . . From prevention to treatment and associated conditions, this provides an excellent survey."
— *The Bookwatch, Aug '01*

"Recommended reference source."
— *Booklist, American Library Association, Jul '01*

SEE ALSO *Healthy Aging Sourcebook, Physical & Mental Issues in Aging Sourcebook, Women's Health Concerns Sourcebook*

■

Pain Sourcebook, 2nd Edition

Basic Consumer Health Information about Specific Forms of Acute and Chronic Pain, Including Muscle and Skeletal Pain, Nerve Pain, Cancer Pain, and Disorders Characterized by Pain, Such as Fibromyalgia, Shingles, Angina, Arthritis, and Headaches

Along with Information about Pain Medications and Management Techniques, Complementary and Alternative Pain Relief Options, Tips for People Living with Chronic Pain, a Glossary, and a Directory of Sources for Further Information

Edited by Karen Bellenir. 670 pages. 2002. 978-0-7808-0612-2.

"A source of valuable information. . . . This book offers help to nonmedical people who need information about pain and pain management. It is also an excellent reference for those who participate in patient education."
— *Doody's Review Service, Sep '02*

"Highly recommended for academic and medical reference collections." — *Library Bookwatch, Sep '02*

"The text is readable, easily understood, and well indexed. This excellent volume belongs in all patient education libraries, consumer health sections of public libraries, and many personal collections."
— *American Reference Books Annual, 1999*

"The information is basic in terms of scholarship and is appropriate for general readers. Written in journalistic style . . . intended for non-professionals. Quite thorough in its coverage of different pain conditions and summarizes the latest clinical information regarding pain treatment." — *Choice, Association of College and Research Libraries, Jun '98*

"Recommended reference source."
— *Booklist, American Library Association, Mar '98*

■

Pediatric Cancer Sourcebook

Basic Consumer Health Information about Leukemias, Brain Tumors, Sarcomas, Lymphomas, and Other Cancers in Infants, Children, and Adolescents, Including Descriptions of Cancers, Treatments, and Coping Strategies

Along with Suggestions for Parents, Caregivers, and Concerned Relatives, a Glossary of Cancer Terms, and Resource Listings

Edited by Edward J. Prucha. 587 pages. 1999. 978-0-7808-0245-2.

"An excellent source of information. Recommended for public, hospital, and health science libraries with consumer health collections." — *E-Streams, Jun '00*

"Recommended reference source."
— *Booklist, American Library Association, Feb '00*

"A valuable addition to all libraries specializing in health services and many public libraries."
— *American Reference Books Annual, 2000*

SEE ALSO *Childhood Diseases & Disorders Sourcebook, Healthy Children Sourcebook*

■

Physical & Mental Issues in Aging Sourcebook

Basic Consumer Health Information on Physical and Mental Disorders Associated with the Aging Process, Including Concerns about Cardiovascular Disease, Pulmonary Disease, Oral Health, Digestive Disorders, Musculoskeletal and Skin Disorders, Metabolic Changes, Sexual and Reproductive Issues, and Changes in Vision, Hearing, and Other Senses

Along with Data about Longevity and Causes of Death, Information on Acute and Chronic Pain, Descriptions of Mental Concerns, a Glossary of Terms, and Resource Listings for Additional Help

Edited by Jenifer Swanson. 660 pages. 1999. 978-0-7808-0233-9.

"This is a treasure of health information for the layperson." — *Choice Health Sciences Supplement, Association of College & Research Libraries, May '00*

"Recommended for public libraries."
— *American Reference Books Annual, 2000*

"Recommended reference source."
— *Booklist, American Library Association, Oct '99*

SEE ALSO *Healthy Aging Sourcebook*

■

Podiatry Sourcebook, 2nd Edition

Basic Consumer Health Information about Disorders, Diseases, Deformities, and Injuries that Affect the Foot and Ankle, Including Sprains, Corns, Calluses, Bunions, Plantar Warts, Plantar Fasciitis, Neuromas, Clubfoot, Flat Feet, Achilles Tendonitis, and Much More

Along with Information about Selecting a Foot Care Specialist, Foot Fitness, Shoes and Socks, Diagnostic Tests and Corrective Procedures, Financial Assistance for Corrective Devices, a Glossary of Related Terms, and a Directory of Resources for Additional Help and Information

Edited by Ivy L. Alexander. 543 pages. 2007. 978-0-7808-0944-4.

"**Recommended reference source.**"
— *Booklist, American Library Association, Feb '02*

"**There is a lot of information presented here on a topic that is usually only covered sparingly in most larger comprehensive medical encyclopedias.**"
— *American Reference Books Annual, 2002*

■

Pregnancy & Birth Sourcebook, 2nd Edition

Basic Consumer Health Information about Conception and Pregnancy, Including Facts about Fertility, Infertility, Pregnancy Symptoms and Complications, Fetal Growth and Development, Labor, Delivery, and the Postpartum Period, as Well as Information about Maintaining Health and Wellness during Pregnancy and Caring for a Newborn

Along with Information about Public Health Assistance for Low-Income Pregnant Women, a Glossary, and Directories of Agencies and Organizations Providing Help and Support

Edited by Amy L. Sutton. 626 pages. 2004. 978-0-7808-0672-6.

"**Will appeal to public and school reference collections strong in medicine and women's health. . . . Deserves a spot on any medical reference shelf.**"
— *The Bookwatch, Jul '04*

"**A well-organized handbook. Recommended.**"
— *Choice, Association of College & Research Libraries, Apr '98*

"**Recommended reference source.**"
— *Booklist, American Library Association, Mar '98*

"**Recommended for public libraries.**"
— *American Reference Books Annual, 1998*

SEE ALSO Breastfeeding Sourcebook, Congenital Disorders Sourcebook, Family Planning Sourcebook

■

Prostate & Urological Disorders Sourcebook

Basic Consumer Health Information about Urogenital and Sexual Disorders in Men, Including Prostate and Other Andrological Cancers, Prostatitis, Benign Prostatic Hyperplasia, Testicular and Penile Trauma, Cryptorchidism, Peyronie Disease, Erectile Dysfunction, and Male Factor Infertility, and Facts about Commonly Used Tests and Procedures, Such as Prostatectomy, Vasectomy, Vasectomy Reversal, Penile Implants, and Semen Analysis

Along with a Glossary of Andrological Terms and a Directory of Resources for Additional Information

Edited by Karen Bellenir. 631 pages. 2005. 978-0-7808-0797-6.

Prostate Cancer Sourcebook

Basic Consumer Health Information about Prostate Cancer, Including Information about the Associated Risk Factors, Detection, Diagnosis, and Treatment of Prostate Cancer

Along with Information on Non-Malignant Prostate Conditions, and Featuring a Section Listing Support and Treatment Centers and a Glossary of Related Terms

Edited by Dawn D. Matthews. 358 pages. 2001. 978-0-7808-0324-4.

"**Recommended reference source.**"
— *Booklist, American Library Association, Jan '02*

"**A valuable resource for health care consumers seeking information on the subject. . . . All text is written in a clear, easy-to-understand language that avoids technical jargon. Any library that collects consumer health resources would strengthen their collection with the addition of the *Prostate Cancer Sourcebook*.**"
— *American Reference Books Annual, 2002*

SEE ALSO Men's Health Concerns Sourcebook

■

Reconstructive & Cosmetic Surgery Sourcebook

Basic Consumer Health Information on Cosmetic and Reconstructive Plastic Surgery, Including Statistical Information about Different Surgical Procedures, Things to Consider Prior to Surgery, Plastic Surgery Techniques and Tools, Emotional and Psychological Considerations, and Procedure-Specific Information

Along with a Glossary of Terms and a Listing of Resources for Additional Help and Information

Edited by M. Lisa Weatherford. 374 pages. 2001. 978-0-7808-0214-8.

"**An excellent reference that addresses cosmetic and medically necessary reconstructive surgeries. . . . The style of the prose is calm and reassuring, discussing the many positive outcomes now available due to advances in surgical techniques.**"
— *American Reference Books Annual, 2002*

"**Recommended for health science libraries that are open to the public, as well as hospital libraries that are open to the patients. This book is a good resource for the consumer interested in plastic surgery.**"
— *E-Streams, Dec '01*

"**Recommended reference source.**"
— *Booklist, American Library Association, Jul '01*

■

Rehabilitation Sourcebook

Basic Consumer Health Information about Rehabilitation for People Recovering from Heart Surgery, Spinal Cord Injury, Stroke, Orthopedic Impairments, Amputation, Pulmonary Impairments, Traumatic Injury, and More, Including Physical Therapy, Occupational Therapy, Speech/Language Therapy, Massage Therapy, Dance Therapy, Art Therapy, and Recreational Therapy

Along with Information on Assistive and Adaptive Devices, a Glossary, and Resources for Additional Help and Information

Edited by Dawn D. Matthews. 531 pages. 1999. 978-0-7808-0236-0.

"This is an excellent resource for public library reference and health collections."
— American Reference Books Annual, 2001

"Recommended reference source."
— Booklist, American Library Association, May '00

■

Respiratory Diseases & Disorders Sourcebook

Basic Information about Respiratory Diseases and Disorders, Including Asthma, Cystic Fibrosis, Pneumonia, the Common Cold, Influenza, and Others, Featuring Facts about the Respiratory System, Statistical and Demographic Data, Treatments, Self-Help Management Suggestions, and Current Research Initiatives

Edited by Allan R. Cook and Peter D. Dresser. 771 pages. 1995. 978-0-7808-0037-3.

"Designed for the layperson and for patients and their families coping with respiratory illness. . . . an extensive array of information on diagnosis, treatment, management, and prevention of respiratory illnesses for the general reader." — Choice, Association of College & Research Libraries, Jun '96

"A highly recommended text for all collections. It is a comforting reminder of the power of knowledge that good books carry between their covers."
— Academic Library Book Review, Spring '96

"A comprehensive collection of authoritative information presented in a nontechnical, humanitarian style for patients, families, and caregivers."
—Association of Operating Room Nurses, Sep/Oct '95

SEE ALSO Lung Disorders Sourcebook

■

Sexually Transmitted Diseases Sourcebook, 3rd Edition

Basic Consumer Health Information about Chlamydial Infections, Gonorrhea, Hepatitis, Herpes, HIV/AIDS, Human Papillomavirus, Pubic Lice, Scabies, Syphilis, Trichomoniasis, Vaginal Infections, and Other Sexually Transmitted Diseases, Including Facts about Risk Factors, Symptoms, Diagnosis, Treatment, and the Prevention of Sexually Transmitted Infections

Along with Updates on Current Research Initiatives, a Glossary of Related Terms, and Resources for Additional Help and Information

Edited by Amy L. Sutton. 629 pages. 2006. 978-0-7808-0824-9.

"Recommended for consumer health collections in public libraries, and secondary school and community college libraries."
— American Reference Books Annual, 2002

"Every school and public library should have a copy of this comprehensive and user-friendly reference book."
— Choice, Association of College & Research Libraries, Sep '01

"This is a highly recommended book. This is an especially important book for all school and public libraries."
— AIDS Book Review Journal, Jul-Aug '01

"Recommended reference source."
— Booklist, American Library Association, Apr '01

■

Sleep Disorders Sourcebook, 2nd Edition

Basic Consumer Health Information about Sleep and Sleep Disorders, Including Insomnia, Sleep Apnea, Restless Legs Syndrome, Narcolepsy, Parasomnias, and Other Health Problems That Affect Sleep, Plus Facts about Diagnostic Procedures, Treatment Strategies, Sleep Medications, and Tips for Improving Sleep Quality

Along with a Glossary of Related Terms and Resources for Additional Help and Information

Edited by Amy L. Sutton. 567 pages. 2005. 978-0-7808-0743-3.

"This book will be useful for just about everybody, especially the 40 million Americans with sleep disorders."
— American Reference Books Annual, 2006

"Recommended for public libraries and libraries supporting health care professionals." — E-Streams, Sep '05

". . . key medical library acquisition."
— The Bookwatch, Jun '05

■

Smoking Concerns Sourcebook

Basic Consumer Health Information about Nicotine Addiction and Smoking Cessation, Featuring Facts about the Health Effects of Tobacco Use, Including Lung and Other Cancers, Heart Disease, Stroke, and Respiratory Disorders, Such as Emphysema and Chronic Bronchitis

Along with Information about Smoking Prevention Programs, Suggestions for Achieving and Maintaining a Smoke-Free Lifestyle, Statistics about Tobacco Use, Reports on Current Research Initiatives, a Glossary of Related Terms, and Directories of Resources for Additional Help and Information

Edited by Karen Bellenir. 621 pages. 2004. 978-0-7808-0323-7.

"Provides everything needed for the student or general reader seeking practical details on the effects of tobacco use." — The Bookwatch, Mar '05

"Public libraries and consumer health care libraries will find this work useful."
— American Reference Books Annual, 2005

Sports Injuries Sourcebook, 3rd Edition

Basic Consumer Health Information about Sprains and Strains, Fractures, Growth Plate Injuries, Overtraining Injuries, and Injuries to the Head, Face, Shoulders, Elbows, Hands, Spinal Column, Knees, Ankles, and Feet, and with Facts about Heat-Related Illness, Steroids and Sport Supplements, Protective Equipment, Diagnostic Procedures, Treatment Options, and Rehabilitation

Along with a Glossary of Related Terms and a Directory of Resources for Additional Help and Information

Edited by Sandra J. Judd. 651 pages. 2007. 978-0-7808-0949-9.

"This is an excellent reference for consumers and it is recommended for public, community college, and undergraduate libraries."
— American Reference Books Annual, 2003

"Recommended reference source."
— Booklist, American Library Association, Feb '03

■

Stress-Related Disorders Sourcebook

Basic Consumer Health Information about Stress and Stress-Related Disorders, Including Stress Origins and Signals, Environmental Stress at Work and Home, Mental and Emotional Stress Associated with Depression, Post-Traumatic Stress Disorder, Panic Disorder, Suicide, and the Physical Effects of Stress on the Cardiovascular, Immune, and Nervous Systems

Along with Stress Management Techniques, a Glossary, and a Listing of Additional Resources

Edited by Joyce Brennfleck Shannon. 610 pages. 2002. 978-0-7808-0560-6.

"Well written for a general readership, the *Stress-Related Disorders Sourcebook* is a useful addition to the health reference literature."
— American Reference Books Annual, 2003

"I am impressed by the amount of information. It offers a thorough overview of the causes and consequences of stress for the layperson. . . . A well-done and thorough reference guide for professionals and nonprofessionals alike." *— Doody's Review Service, Dec '02*

■

Stroke Sourcebook

Basic Consumer Health Information about Stroke, Including Ischemic, Hemorrhagic, Transient Ischemic Attack (TIA), and Pediatric Stroke, Stroke Triggers and Risks, Diagnostic Tests, Treatments, and Rehabilitation Information

Along with Stroke Prevention Guidelines, Legal and Financial Information, a Glossary, and a Directory of Additional Resources

Edited by Joyce Brennfleck Shannon. 606 pages. 2003. 978-0-7808-0630-6.

"This volume is highly recommended and should be in every medical, hospital, and public library."
— American Reference Books Annual, 2004

"Highly recommended for the amount and variety of topics and information covered." *— Choice, Nov '03*

■

Surgery Sourcebook

Basic Consumer Health Information about Inpatient and Outpatient Surgeries, Including Cardiac, Vascular, Orthopedic, Ocular, Reconstructive, Cosmetic, Gynecologic, and Ear, Nose, and Throat Procedures and More

Along with Information about Operating Room Policies and Instruments, Laser Surgery Techniques, Hospital Errors, Statistical Data, a Glossary, and Listings of Sources for Further Help and Information

Edited by Annemarie S. Muth and Karen Bellenir. 596 pages. 2002. 978-0-7808-0380-0.

"Large public libraries and medical libraries would benefit from this material in their reference collections."
— American Reference Books Annual, 2004

"Invaluable reference for public and school library collections alike." *— Library Bookwatch, Apr '03*

■

Thyroid Disorders Sourcebook

Basic Consumer Health Information about Disorders of the Thyroid and Parathyroid Glands, Including Hypothyroidism, Hyperthyroidism, Graves Disease, Hashimoto Thyroiditis, Thyroid Cancer, and Parathyroid Disorders, Featuring Facts about Symptoms, Risk Factors, Tests, and Treatments

Along with Information about the Effects of Thyroid Imbalance on Other Body Systems, Environmental Factors That Affect the Thyroid Gland, a Glossary, and a Directory of Additional Resources

Edited by Joyce Brennfleck Shannon. 599 pages. 2005. 978-0-7808-0745-7.

"Recommended for consumer health collections."
— American Reference Books Annual, 2006

"Highly recommended pick for basic consumer health reference holdings at all levels."
— The Bookwatch, Aug '05

■

Transplantation Sourcebook

Basic Consumer Health Information about Organ and Tissue Transplantation, Including Physical and Financial Preparations, Procedures and Issues Relating to Specific Solid Organ and Tissue Transplants, Rehabilitation, Pediatric Transplant Information, the Future of Transplantation, and Organ and Tissue Donation

Along with a Glossary and Listings of Additional Resources

Edited by Joyce Brennfleck Shannon. 628 pages. 2002. 978-0-7808-0322-0.

"Along with these advances [in transplantation technology] have come a number of daunting questions for potential transplant patients, their families, and their health care providers. This reference text is the best single tool to address many of these questions. . . . It will be a much-needed addition to the reference collections in health care, academic, and large public libraries."
— *American Reference Books Annual, 2003*

"Recommended for libraries with an interest in offering consumer health information." — *E-Streams, Jul '02*

"This is a unique and valuable resource for patients facing transplantation and their families."
— *Doody's Review Service, Jun '02*

■

Traveler's Health Sourcebook

Basic Consumer Health Information for Travelers, Including Physical and Medical Preparations, Transportation Health and Safety, Essential Information about Food and Water, Sun Exposure, Insect and Snake Bites, Camping and Wilderness Medicine, and Travel with Physical or Medical Disabilities

Along with International Travel Tips, Vaccination Recommendations, Geographical Health Issues, Disease Risks, a Glossary, and a Listing of Additional Resources

Edited by Joyce Brennfleck Shannon. 613 pages. 2000. 978-0-7808-0384-8.

"Recommended reference source."
— *Booklist, American Library Association, Feb '01*

"This book is recommended for any public library, any travel collection, and especially any collection for the physically disabled."
— *American Reference Books Annual, 2001*

SEE ALSO Worldwide Health Sourcebook

■

Urinary Tract & Kidney Diseases & Disorders Sourcebook, 2nd Edition

Basic Consumer Health Information about the Urinary System, Including the Bladder, Urethra, Ureters, and Kidneys, with Facts about Urinary Tract Infections, Incontinence, Congenital Disorders, Kidney Stones, Cancers of the Urinary Tract and Kidneys, Kidney Failure, Dialysis, and Kidney Transplantation

Along with Statistical and Demographic Information, Reports on Current Research in Kidney and Urologic Health, a Summary of Commonly Used Diagnostic Tests, a Glossary of Related Terms, and a Directory of Resources for Additional Help and Information

Edited by Ivy L. Alexander. 649 pages. 2005. 978-0-7808-0750-1.

"A good choice for a consumer health information library or for a medical library needing information to refer to their patients."
— *American Reference Books Annual, 2006*

Vegetarian Sourcebook

Basic Consumer Health Information about Vegetarian Diets, Lifestyle, and Philosophy, Including Definitions of Vegetarianism and Veganism, Tips about Adopting Vegetarianism, Creating a Vegetarian Pantry, and Meeting Nutritional Needs of Vegetarians, with Facts Regarding Vegetarianism's Effect on Pregnant and Lactating Women, Children, Athletes, and Senior Citizens

Along with a Glossary of Commonly Used Vegetarian Terms and Resources for Additional Help and Information

Edited by Chad T. Kimball. 360 pages. 2002. 978-0-7808-0439-5.

"Organizes into one concise volume the answers to the most common questions concerning vegetarian diets and lifestyles. This title is recommended for public and secondary school libraries." — *E-Streams, Apr '03*

"Invaluable reference for public and school library collections alike." — *Library Bookwatch, Apr '03*

"The articles in this volume are easy to read and come from authoritative sources. The book does not necessarily support the vegetarian diet but instead provides the pros and cons of this important decision. The Vegetarian Sourcebook is recommended for public libraries and consumer health libraries."
— *American Reference Books Annual, 2003*

SEE ALSO Diet & Nutrition Sourcebook

■

Women's Health Concerns Sourcebook, 2nd Edition

Basic Consumer Health Information about the Medical and Mental Concerns of Women, Including Maintaining Health and Wellness, Gynecological Concerns, Breast Health, Sexuality and Reproductive Issues, Menopause, Cancer in Women, Leading Causes of Death and Disability among Women, Physical Concerns of Special Significance to Women, and Women's Mental and Emotional Health

Along with a Glossary of Related Terms and Directories of Resources for Additional Help and Information

Edited by Amy L. Sutton. 746 pages. 2004. 978-0-7808-0673-3.

"This is a useful reference book, which makes the reader knowledgeable about several issues that concern women's health. It is recommended for public libraries and home library collections." — *E-Streams, May '05*

"A useful addition to public and consumer health library collections."
— *American Reference Books Annual, 2005*

"A highly recommended title."
— *The Bookwatch, May '04*

"Handy compilation. There is an impressive range of diseases, devices, disorders, procedures, and other physical and emotional issues covered . . . well organized, illustrated, and indexed." — *Choice, Association of College & Research Libraries, Jan '98*

SEE ALSO *Breast Cancer Sourcebook, Cancer Sourcebook for Women, Healthy Heart Sourcebook for Women, Osteoporosis Sourcebook*

Workplace Health & Safety Sourcebook

Basic Consumer Health Information about Workplace Health and Safety, Including the Effect of Workplace Hazards on the Lungs, Skin, Heart, Ears, Eyes, Brain, Reproductive Organs, Musculoskeletal System, and Other Organs and Body Parts

Along with Information about Occupational Cancer, Personal Protective Equipment, Toxic and Hazardous Chemicals, Child Labor, Stress, and Workplace Violence

Edited by Chad T. Kimball. 626 pages. 2000. 978-0-7808-0231-5.

"As a reference for the general public, this would be useful in any library." — *E-Streams, Jun '01*

"Provides helpful information for primary care physicians and other caregivers interested in occupational medicine. . . . General readers; professionals."
— *Choice, Association of College & Research Libraries, May '01*

"Recommended reference source."
— *Booklist, American Library Association, Feb '01*

"Highly recommended." — *The Bookwatch, Jan '01*

Worldwide Health Sourcebook

Basic Information about Global Health Issues, Including Malnutrition, Reproductive Health, Disease Dispersion and Prevention, Emerging Diseases, Risky Health Behaviors, and the Leading Causes of Death

Along with Global Health Concerns for Children, Women, and the Elderly, Mental Health Issues, Research and Technology Advancements, and Economic, Environmental, and Political Health Implications, a Glossary, and a Resource Listing for Additional Help and Information

Edited by Joyce Brennfleck Shannon. 614 pages. 2001. 978-0-7808-0330-5.

"Named an Outstanding Academic Title."
— *Choice, Association of College & Research Libraries, Jan '02*

"Yet another handy but also unique compilation in the extensive *Health Reference Series*, this is a useful work because many of the international publications reprinted or excerpted are not readily available. Highly recommended." — *Choice, Association of College & Research Libraries, Nov '01*

"Recommended reference source."
— *Booklist, American Library Association, Oct '01*

SEE ALSO *Traveler's Health Sourcebook*

627

Teen Health Series
Helping Young Adults Understand, Manage, and Avoid Serious Illness

List price $65 per volume. **School and library price $58 per volume.**

Alcohol Information for Teens
Health Tips about Alcohol and Alcoholism

Including Facts about Underage Drinking, Preventing Teen Alcohol Use, Alcohol's Effects on the Brain and the Body, Alcohol Abuse Treatment, Help for Children of Alcoholics, and More

Edited by Joyce Brennfleck Shannon. 370 pages. 2005. 978-0-7808-0741-9.

"Boxed facts and tips add visual interest to the well-researched and clearly written text."
— *Curriculum Connection, Apr '06*

Allergy Information for Teens
Health Tips about Allergic Reactions Such as Anaphylaxis, Respiratory Problems, and Rashes

Including Facts about Identifying and Managing Allergies to Food, Pollen, Mold, Animals, Chemicals, Drugs, and Other Substances

Edited by Karen Bellenir. 410 pages. 2006. 978-0-7808-0799-0.

Asthma Information for Teens
Health Tips about Managing Asthma and Related Concerns

Including Facts about Asthma Causes, Triggers, Symptoms, Diagnosis, and Treatment

Edited by Karen Bellenir. 386 pages. 2005. 978-0-7808-0770-9.

"Highly recommended for medical libraries, public school libraries, and public libraries."
— *American Reference Books Annual, 2006*

"It is so clearly written and well organized that even hesitant readers will be able to find the facts they need, whether for reports or personal information. . . . A succinct but complete resource."
— *School Library Journal, Sep '05*

Body Information for Teens
Health Tips about Maintaining Well-Being for a Lifetime

Including Facts about the Development and Functioning of the Body's Systems, Organs, and Structures and the Health Impact of Lifestyle Choices

Edited by Sandra Augustyn Lawton. 458 pages. 2007. 978-0-7808-0443-2.

Cancer Information for Teens
Health Tips about Cancer Awareness, Prevention, Diagnosis, and Treatment

Including Facts about Frequently Occurring Cancers, Cancer Risk Factors, and Coping Strategies for Teens Fighting Cancer or Dealing with Cancer in Friends or Family Members

Edited by Wilma R. Caldwell. 428 pages. 2004. 978-0-7808-0678-8.

"Recommended for school libraries, or consumer libraries that see a lot of use by teens."
— *E-Streams, May '05*

"A valuable educational tool."
— *American Reference Books Annual, 2005*

"Young adults and their parents alike will find this new addition to the *Teen Health Series* an important reference to cancer in teens."
— *Children's Bookwatch, Feb '05*

Complementary and Alternative Medicine Information for Teens
Health Tips about Non-Traditional and Non-Western Medical Practices

Including Information about Acupuncture, Chiropractic Medicine, Dietary and Herbal Supplements, Hypnosis, Massage Therapy, Prayer and Spirituality, Reflexology, Yoga, and More

Edited by Sandra Augustyn Lawton. 405 pages. 2006. 978-0-7808-0966-6.

Diabetes Information for Teens
Health Tips about Managing Diabetes and Preventing Related Complications

Including Information about Insulin, Glucose Control, Healthy Eating, Physical Activity, and Learning to Live with Diabetes

Edited by Sandra Augustyn Lawton. 410 pages. 2006. 978-0-7808-0811-9.

Diet Information for Teens, 2nd Edition

Health Tips about Diet and Nutrition

Including Facts about Dietary Guidelines, Food Groups, Nutrients, Healthy Meals, Snacks, Weight Control, Medical Concerns Related to Diet, and More

Edited by Karen Bellenir. 432 pages. 2006. 978-0-7808-0820-1.

"Full of helpful insights and facts throughout the book. . . . An excellent resource to be placed in public libraries or even in personal collections."
— *American Reference Books Annual, 2002*

"Recommended for middle and high school libraries and media centers as well as academic libraries that educate future teachers of teenagers. It is also a suitable addition to health science libraries that serve patrons who are interested in teen health promotion and education."
— *E-Streams, Oct '01*

"This comprehensive book would be beneficial to collections that need information about nutrition, dietary guidelines, meal planning, and weight control. . . . This reference is so easy to use that its purchase is recommended."
— *The Book Report, Sep-Oct '01*

"This book is written in an easy to understand format describing issues that many teens face every day, and then provides thoughtful explanations so that teens can make informed decisions. This is an interesting book that provides important facts and information for today's teens."
— *Doody's Health Sciences Book Review Journal, Jul-Aug '01*

"A comprehensive compendium of diet and nutrition. The information is presented in a straightforward, plain-spoken manner. This title will be useful to those working on reports on a variety of topics, as well as to general readers concerned about their dietary health."
— *School Library Journal, Jun '01*

Drug Information for Teens, 2nd Edition

Health Tips about the Physical and Mental Effects of Substance Abuse

Including Information about Marijuana, Inhalants, Club Drugs, Stimulants, Hallucinogens, Opiates, Prescription and Over-the-Counter Drugs, Herbal Products, Tobacco, Alcohol, and More

Edited by Sandra Augustyn Lawton. 468 pages. 2006. 978-0-7808-0862-1.

"A clearly written resource for general readers and researchers alike."
— *School Library Journal*

"This book is well-balanced. . . . a must for public and school libraries."
— *VOYA: Voice of Youth Advocates, Dec '03*

"The chapters are quick to make a connection to their teenage reading audience. The prose is straightforward and the book lends itself to spot reading. It should be useful both for practical information and for research, and it is suitable for public and school libraries."
— *American Reference Books Annual, 2003*

"Recommended reference source."
— *Booklist, American Library Association, Feb '03*

"This is an excellent resource for teens and their parents. Education about drugs and substances is key to discouraging teen drug abuse and this book provides this much needed information in a way that is interesting and factual."
— *Doody's Review Service, Dec '02*

Eating Disorders Information for Teens

Health Tips about Anorexia, Bulimia, Binge Eating, and Other Eating Disorders

Including Information on the Causes, Prevention, and Treatment of Eating Disorders, and Such Other Issues as Maintaining Healthy Eating and Exercise Habits

Edited by Sandra Augustyn Lawton. 337 pages. 2005. 978-0-7808-0783-9.

"An excellent resource for teens and those who work with them."
— *VOYA: Voice of Youth Advocates, Apr '06*

"A welcome addition to high school and undergraduate libraries." — *American Reference Books Annual, 2006*

"This book covers the topic in a lucid manner but delves deeper into every aspect of an eating disorder. A solid addition for any nonfiction or reference collection."
— *School Library Journal, Dec '05*

Fitness Information for Teens

Health Tips about Exercise, Physical Well-Being, and Health Maintenance

Including Facts about Aerobic and Anaerobic Conditioning, Stretching, Body Shape and Body Image, Sports Training, Nutrition, and Activities for Non-Athletes

Edited by Karen Bellenir. 425 pages. 2004. 978-0-7808-0679-5.

"Another excellent offering from Omnigraphics in their *Teen Health Series*. . . . This book will be a great addition to any public, junior high, senior high, or secondary school library."
— *American Reference Books Annual, 2005*

Learning Disabilities Information for Teens

Health Tips about Academic Skills Disorders and Other Disabilities That Affect Learning

Including Information about Common Signs of Learning Disabilities, School Issues, Learning to Live with a Learning Disability, and Other Related Issues

Edited by Sandra Augustyn Lawton. 337 pages. 2005. 978-0-7808-0796-9.

"This book provides a wealth of information for any reader interested in the signs, causes, and consequences of learning disabilities, as well as related legal rights and educational interventions. . . . Public and academic libraries should want this title for both students and general readers."

— American Reference Books Annual, 2006

■

Mental Health Information for Teens, 2nd Edition
Health Tips about Mental Wellness and Mental Illness

Including Facts about Mental and Emotional Health, Depression and Other Mood Disorders, Anxiety Disorders, Behavior Disorders, Self-Injury, Psychosis, Schizophrenia, and More

Edited by Karen Bellenir. 400 pages. 2006. 978-0-7808-0863-8.

"In both language and approach, this user-friendly entry in the *Teen Health Series* is on target for teens needing information on mental health concerns."
— Booklist, American Library Association, Jan '02

"Readers will find the material accessible and informative, with the shaded notes, facts, and embedded glossary insets adding appropriately to the already interesting and succinct presentation."
— School Library Journal, Jan '02

"This title is highly recommended for any library that serves adolescents and parents/caregivers of adolescents." — E-Streams, Jan '02

"Recommended for high school libraries and young adult collections in public libraries. Both health professionals and teenagers will find this book useful."
— American Reference Books Annual, 2002

"This is a nice book written to enlighten the society, primarily teenagers, about common teen mental health issues. It is highly recommended to teachers and parents as well as adolescents."
— Doody's Review Service, Dec '01

■

Sexual Health Information for Teens
Health Tips about Sexual Development, Human Reproduction, and Sexually Transmitted Diseases

Including Facts about Puberty, Reproductive Health, Chlamydia, Human Papillomavirus, Pelvic Inflammatory Disease, Herpes, AIDS, Contraception, Pregnancy, and More

Edited by Deborah A. Stanley. 391 pages. 2003. 978-0-7808-0445-6.

"This work should be included in all high school libraries and many larger public libraries. . . . highly recommended."
— American Reference Books Annual, 2004

"*Sexual Health* approaches its subject with appropriate seriousness and offers easily accessible advice and information." — School Library Journal, Feb '04

Skin Health Information for Teens
Health Tips about Dermatological Concerns and Skin Cancer Risks

Including Facts about Acne, Warts, Hives, and Other Conditions and Lifestyle Choices, Such as Tanning, Tattooing, and Piercing, That Affect the Skin, Nails, Scalp, and Hair

Edited by Robert Aquinas McNally. 429 pages. 2003. 978-0-7808-0446-3.

"This volume, as with others in the series, will be a useful addition to school and public library collections." — American Reference Books Annual, 2004

"There is no doubt that this reference tool is valuable."
— VOYA: Voice of Youth Advocates, Feb '04

"This volume serves as a one-stop source and should be a necessity for any health collection."
— Library Media Connection

■

Sports Injuries Information for Teens
Health Tips about Sports Injuries and Injury Protection

Including Facts about Specific Injuries, Emergency Treatment, Rehabilitation, Sports Safety, Competition Stress, Fitness, Sports Nutrition, Steroid Risks, and More

Edited by Joyce Brennfleck Shannon. 405 pages. 2003. 978-0-7808-0447-0.

"This work will be useful in the young adult collections of public libraries as well as high school libraries."
— American Reference Books Annual, 2004

■

Suicide Information for Teens
Health Tips about Suicide Causes and Prevention

Including Facts about Depression, Risk Factors, Getting Help, Survivor Support, and More

Edited by Joyce Brennfleck Shannon. 368 pages. 2005. 978-0-7808-0737-2.

■

Tobacco Information for Teens
Health Tips about the Hazards of Using Cigarettes, Smokeless Tobacco, and Other Nicotine Products

Including Facts about Nicotine Addiction, Immediate and Long-Term Health Effects of Tobacco Use, Related Cancers, Smoking Cessation, Tobacco Use Prevention, and Tobacco Use Statistics

Edited by Karen Bellenir. 440 pages. 2007. 978-0-7808-0976-5.

Health Reference Series

Adolescent Health Sourcebook,
2nd Edition

AIDS Sourcebook, 3rd Edition

Alcoholism Sourcebook, 2nd Edition

Allergies Sourcebook, 3rd Edition

Alzheimer's Disease Sourcebook,
3rd Edition

Arthritis Sourcebook, 2nd Edition

Asthma Sourcebook, 2nd Edition

Attention Deficit Disorder Sourcebook

Back & Neck Sourcebook, 2nd Edition

Blood & Circulatory Disorders
Sourcebook, 2nd Edition

Brain Disorders Sourcebook, 2nd Edition

Breast Cancer Sourcebook, 2nd Edition

Breastfeeding Sourcebook

Burns Sourcebook

Cancer Sourcebook, 5th Edition

Cancer Sourcebook for Women,
3rd Edition

Cancer Survivorship Sourcebook

Cardiovascular Diseases & Disorders
Sourcebook, 3rd Edition

Caregiving Sourcebook

Child Abuse Sourcebook

Childhood Diseases & Disorders
Sourcebook

Colds, Flu & Other Common Ailments
Sourcebook

Communication Disorders Sourcebook

Complementary & Alternative Medicine
Sourcebook, 3rd Edition

Congenital Disorders Sourcebook,
2nd Edition

Contagious Diseases Sourcebook

Cosmetic & Reconstructive Surgery
Sourcebook, 2nd

Death & Dying Sourcebook, 2nd Edition

Dental Care & Oral Health Sourcebook,
2nd Edition

Depression Sourcebook

Dermatological Disorders Sourcebook,
2nd Edition

Diabetes Sourcebook, 3rd Edition

Diet & Nutrition Sourcebook,
3rd Edition

Digestive Diseases & Disorder
Sourcebook

Disabilities Sourcebook

Domestic Violence Sourcebook,
2nd Edition

Drug Abuse Sourcebook, 2nd Edition

Ear, Nose & Throat Disorders
Sourcebook, 2nd Edition

Eating Disorders Sourcebook, 2nd Edition

Emergency Medical Services Sourcebook

Endocrine & Metabolic Disorders
Sourcebook, 2nd Edition

EnvironmentalHealth Sourcebook,
2nd Edition

Ethnic Diseases Sourcebook

Eye Care Sourcebook, 2nd Edition

Family Planning Sourcebook

Fitness & Exercise Sourcebook,
3rd Edition

Food Safety Sourcebook

Forensic Medicine Sourcebook

Gastrointestinal Diseases & Disorders
Sourcebook, 2nd Edition

Genetic Disorders Sourcebook,
3rd Edition

Head Trauma Sourcebook

Headache Sourcebook

Health Insurance Sourcebook

Healthy Aging Sourcebook

Healthy Children Sourcebook

Healthy Heart Sourcebook for Women

Hepatitis Sourcebook

Household Safety Sourcebook

Hypertension Sourcebook

Immune System Disorders Sourcebook,
2nd Edition

Infant & Toddler Health Sourcebook

Infectious Diseases Sourcebook